LIVING
WITH
CANCER

Prior Books by **Dr. Rosenbaum**

LIVING WITH CANCER, New York, 1975, Praeger Publishers

MIND AND BODY, San Francisco, 1977, Life Mind & Body

HEALTH THROUGH NUTRITION, San Francisco, 1978, Alchemy Books

UP AND AROUND REHABILITATION EXERCISES FOR CANCER
PATIENTS, San Francisco, 1978, Life Mind & Body

COMPREHENSIVE GUIDE FOR CANCER PATIENTS, Palo Alto, Calif.,
1980, Bull Publishing Co.

DECISION FOR LIFE, Palo Alto, Calif., 1980, Bull Publishing Co.

NUTRITION FOR THE CANCER PATIENT, Palo Alto, Calif., 1980,
Bull Publishing Co.

REHABILITATION FOR CANCER PATIENTS, Palo Alto, Calif., 1980,
Bull Publishing Co.

SEXUALITY AND CANCER, Palo Alto, Calif., 1980, Bull Publishing Co.

About the Author
Dr. Rosenbaum, a hematologist and oncologist, is in private practice in San
Francisco. At the Mount Zion Hospital and Medical Center, he is Associate
Chief of Medicine and Codirector of the Immunology Research Laboratory.
He is also associated with the Claire Zellerbach Saroni Tumor Institute of the
Mount Zion Hospital and Medical Center, and the University of California
Medical School.

LIVING
WITH
CANCER

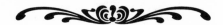

Ernest H. Rosenbaum, M.D.

with a contribution by
Patricia T. Kelly, Ph.D.
Director of Stanton and Corrine Genetic Counseling Service,
Mt. Zion Hospital and Medical Center, San Francisco;
Associate Research Geneticist, University of California, San Francisco

A PLUME BOOK

NEW AMERICAN LIBRARY

MOSBY

TIMES MIRROR
NEW YORK AND SCARBOROUGH, ONTARIO

Publisher: Thomas A. Manning
Assistant editor: Nancy L. Mullins
Manuscript editor: Judy Jamison
Production: Barbara Merritt

MOSBY MEDICAL LIBRARY

Library of Congress Cataloging in Publication Data

Rosenbaum, Ernest H.
Living with cancer.

Originally published: New York: Praeger, 1975
"A Plume book."
Bibliography: p.
1. Cancer. 2. Cancer—Psychological aspects.
I. Kelly, Patricia T., 1942— . II. Title.
RC263.R638 1982   362.1'96994   82-2125
ISBN 0-452-25340-3

ST/D/D 1 2 3 4 5 6 7 8 9 02/B/263

Printed in the United States of America

This book is dedicated to my wife

Isadora

my companion in life and assistant in medicine,

a woman whose daily efforts have enhanced the quality of my life

and given comfort to both my patients and me, and

to our patients

who have taught us so much about the meaning of life

Foreword

A diagnosis of cancer used to be thought of as a virtual death sentence. However, of the 815,000 Americans who will be diagnosed with the serious forms of cancer this year, 45 percent are expected to be cured of their disease. As greater numbers of those diagnosed live longer, new concerns arise. These are related to living with the disease—adjustment in daily living patterns, changing relationships with family and friends, changing employment status, and planning for the future.

In recognition of the above, the National Cancer Institute has developed a program designated "Coping with Cancer." Its goal is to provide those who have cancer and their family members the opportunity to control and improve the quality of their lives by giving them information on the disease, its treatment, and its psychosocial aspects.

Living with Cancer discusses, with candor and sensitivity, how average people from many walks of life and diverse ethnic backgrounds deal with cancer—its impact on their lives and on the lives of those who are close to them. An update of the 1975 edition of the same title, Dr. Rosenbaum's new book emphasizes how patients who have learned to cope successfully with cancer have added new depth to their lives. A number of very different, although exemplary, personal accounts are related by patients of the author.

Recognizing the changes that have occurred in public attitudes toward cancer since 1975, Dr. Rosenbaum has included new information on the sections entitled "Understanding Cancer" and "Supportive Services." Three patients whose stories were told in the first edition of the book—Elisabeth Lee, Darrell Ansbacher, and Anthony Verdi—update their cancer experiences from the perspective of time and cure.

Dr. Rosenbaum's messages are realistic: although cancer has a potentially devastating impact on many aspects of life, the disease is one that should not completely disrupt one's lifestyle. Establishment of a constructive and substantive relationship with physicians and others from whom the patient seeks information and support is the key to living well with cancer. Acknowledging the void that often exists between the patient and the health professional, Dr. Rosenbaum wisely advises members of the latter group to read the book as well.

Living with Cancer puts forth a challenge to the patient, the family, friends, and the health professional community with whom the patient interacts to live a satisfying life with a chronic and often debilitating disease. It advises seeking information, questioning, communicating, and sharing. Written from the viewpoint of a hematologist-oncologist of national repute, *Living with Cancer* belongs on the shelf of *all* those who *live* with cancer—patient, family, and health professional.

Vincent T. DeVita, Jr., M.D.

Director, National Cancer Institute,
National Cancer Program

Acknowledgment

I wish to thank Tina Anderson, my editor, who worked with me to capture an accurate pulse of what it means to live with cancer.

I wish to thank the following persons whose contributions appear in these pages: Patricia Kelly, Ph.D., Patricia Tobain, M.S.W., Irene Harrison, M.S.W., John Caton, M.S.W., Laura Williams, Shirley Shelby, Rhoda Gredman, Mary Lawton, R.N., Eileen Shepley, R.N., Fleur Frederick Stanley, S.R.N., Becky Moore, R.N., Liz Light, R.N., and Kim Drucker.

I received invaluable medical reviews from Eugene Monita, M.D., Kenneth McCormack, M.D., David Suffa, M.D., Jack Noyes, M.D., T. Stanley Meyer, M.D., Richard Miner, B.A., Erica Goode, M.D., Alan Glassberg, M.D., Phillip Purser, M.S.C., and Barbara Blumberg, Sc.M.

I also wish to thank Alexandra Renskoff, Eleanor Tida, Virginia Mapa, Grace Drummond, David Bull, and Liza O'Mallon for their help and encouragement.

Ernest H. Rosenbaum

Contents

Introduction:
The curability of cancer

Cancer is one of the most curable
chronic diseases in this country today.

VINCENT DeVITA
DIRECTOR, NATIONAL CANCER INSTITUTE
1981

The Dark Ages are over. It is no longer a sin to have cancer. It is no longer mentioned in hushed tones. People are more knowledgeable about the disease and more accepting of those who have it. Feature articles in newspapers and magazines report the latest medical progress or controversy over a new treatment. Television programs and books describe the problems of living with cancer. Cancer has become, as Dr. DeVita claims, the most curable chronic disease.

If cancer is so controllable and curable, why do we seem to hear more about it today than we did in the past? Why do statistics show a higher incidence and higher mortality rate? Moreover, if you have cancer, how do you begin to cope with it? This book attempts to answer some of these questions and offer suggestions on the prevention, treatment, and potential for living with cancer.

First, the statistics belie the facts. Forty-three percent of the people with cancer in the United States today will survive 5 years or more, which in most cases is the same as saying they are cured. This represents a 12% increase in the survival rate in the past 10 years. These figures result from sophisticated diagnostic techniques that reveal more cancers in the early curable stages and from improved methods of treating cancer, particularly with radiotherapy and chemotherapy. The survival rate would be even higher if people would heed the warning signals published by the American Cancer Society and seek earlier diagnosis, and if they would avoid some of the known carcinogens such as nicotine and sunlight.

Today's statistics must be viewed in the perspective of progress in other areas of medicine. The average age of the population has increased because people are living longer and the birth rate is low. In 1900 the average life span was 50 years of age; in 1982 it is 73 years. Today people rarely die of infectious diseases such as tuberculosis, scarlet fever, or diphtheria, or from infections such as one might develop from acute appendicitis or childbirth; they survive into old age, which is a time of higher risk for developing cancer. Even among older people, however, cancer is the number two killer, responsible for only 20% of deaths in the United States. Heart and arterial diseases are the number one killer, responsible for 50% of deaths in older people.

It is also important to appreciate that significant advances in diagnosis and therapy are not instantly reflected in cancer statistics. It takes years for new techniques to be applied and accepted all over the country before the statistical changes in prolongation of life or cure are registered.

For example, some of these new therapeutic techniques include a combined program of radiation therapy and multidrug chemotherapy. Although the majority of people who benefited from these new therapeutic approaches were diagnosed early, a small percentage were diagnosed when they had more extensive (or metastatic) disease. Early diagnosis is currently the best means of effecting a cure, although successful methods of treatment have been developed for all stages of cancer. An excellent example of this progress is Hodgkin's disease, for which the cure rate rose from 10% in 1960 to 85 to 90% in 1980. Currently, 13 other cancers, many in the advanced state, have a possibility of cure, a statement that could not have been made 10 years ago. These potentially curable cancers are acute lymphocytic leukemia, adult myelogenous leukemia, histiocytic lymphoma, Burkitt's lymphoma, nodular mixed lymphoma, Ewing's sarcoma, Wilms' tumor, rhabdomyosarcoma, choriocarcinoma, testicular carcinoma, ovarian cancer, breast cancer, and osteogenic sarcoma. The list will grow in time. For many other cancers, the disease-free interval before recurrence has also increased.

A recent study conducted by the American College of Surgeons analyzed the treatment and results on 468,288 cancer patients; this study indicates that the 5-year survival rate for forms of cancer has increased as much as 11%. The report further indicates an improved survival rate (up about 18%) for less common cancers such as leukemia and Hodgkin's disease. One member of the College's Commission on Cancer stated, "Survival rates are more sensitive than mortality rates in gauging improvements . . . I think that what we are seeing is that better treatment means better survival." Table 1 lists types of cancer and the 5-year relative survival rates.

About 58 million Americans now living will eventually have cancer. This represents one in four people—you or someone else you know. We are all affected by cancer. Over 3 million Americans alive today have a history of the disease. Of these 3 million, 2 million were diagnosed 5 or more years ago and can therefore be considered cured, whereas others still have evidence of cancer. The term cured means that a patient is free of disease and has the same life expectancy as a person who never had cancer. The decision as to when a patient may be considered cured is one that must be made by the physician after examining the individual patient. For most forms of cancer, 5 years without symptoms following treatment is the accepted time. However, some patients can be considered cured after 1 year, others after 3 years. Some people must be followed much longer than 5 years.

Practically all cancers are treatable. People not cured of their disease may

TABLE 1

Commission on Cancer of the American College of Surgeons
5-year relative survival rates (%)

Type	NCI study* 1965-1969	COC study† 1973-1979	Degree of change
Ten most frequent cancers			
Lung	9	11	22
Breast (female)	65	73	12
Colon	46	50	9
Prostate	57	68	19
Corpus uteri	75	84	12
Bladder	62	70	13
Rectal	42	49	17
Stomach	13	15	15
Cervix (invasive)	57	65	14
Pancreatic	2	3	50
Other types			
Multiple myeloma	16	22	38
Acute leukemia	3	18	500
Chronic leukemia	32	40	25
Bone	32	49	53
Soft-tissue sarcoma	42	54	29
Hodgkin's disease	54	72	33
Testicular embryonal cancer	50	63	26
Testicular malignant teratoma	60	77	28

*Cancer Patient Survival, Report No. 5, 1976, U.S. DHEW. These rates are for the white population, which gives slightly higher rates than if blacks were included. The rates also exclude in situ carcinomas.
†These rates include all races and in situ carcinomas, except in cervix.

live months, years, or their entire lives without a recurrence. Even when cancer invades certain organs, the disease may not be serious unless it causes functional impairment. The essential problem is not that one has cancer and that it has spread; more important is whether the disease will respond to treatment. The answer to that question may not be evident for weeks or months. Each person is unique as is the course of that person's disease. Unfortunately, time must pass before the effects of a particular treatment can be assessed.

In the next few years more people will go to their doctor for earlier diagnosis; we will continue to improve treatments and get longer remissions; and we will learn how to cure more types of cancer. Most important, we must be more successful in preventing cancer. The potential is there.

In the meantime, we all live with the risk of cancer. We live with the knowledge that if we don't get it, someone we love probably will. We have close friends with cancer who are anxious about the outcome of therapy. We have a parent or child who is dying from the disease. We all face cancer in one way or another.

How well we face cancer when it touches our lives will depend on many factors: our willingness to be informed about cancer, to have yearly check-ups, and to undergo conventional therapy as soon as possible if cancer is diagnosed; our disease and our body's response to treatment; and our psychological makeup.

In spite of today's progress and the hope it brings, being told you have cancer is still a terrible blow. It is like being hit by a truck. Your life is altered in a few seconds. You can't help being tormented by questions of whether you will suffer or die. It is hard to imagine feeling more isolated than you do at that moment. Undergoing diagnostic procedures reinforces a growing feeling that you have lost control of your life. There is an unpleasant awareness of a new dependence on others. Treatment and cure are to a large extent in the hands of others.

The depression, anxiety, and fear that usually accompany a diagnosis of cancer can be blinding. They can render a person unable to function in any area of life. It is a new experience for which one needs guidelines. It is the reason for this book, to promote the knowledge and understanding needed to cope with every aspect of living with cancer.

Early chapters give information as to what cancer is, on some of the contributing causes, and the importance of early detection. The most common diagnostic techniques are explained, along with my own approach to diagnosis.

My approach is to ask each patient to enter into an unwritten contract for candor and mutual trust. I give my assurance that I will do my best to cure or control the cancer, reduce any pain, and cope with any other problems that arise. I also let a patient know that I am interested in anything that concerns him or her—work, play, philosophy, family, sex life—because I know that if I can free people from worry, they may respond better to therapy as well as have more desire and energy to do the things they enjoy.

Also included in this book are descriptions of both conventional and experimental methods of treatment, as well as an assessment of some of the more unorthodox theories, such as the cure potential of megadoses of vitamins.

When you are ill, you have one overriding goal: to regain your health and return to an active, fulfilling life. An integrated program of overall care contributes to this goal. There are many things a person can do to combat the debilitating effects of therapy—namely, to keep one's body in as good shape as possible. It is important not to let muscles atrophy if confined to bed following surgery or prolonged bed rest; special nutritional supplements are also needed when the body is fighting disease. Moreover, cancer, like other chronic diseases, has important psychological and social dimensions. A patient's needs go far beyond medical treatment.

Exercise, diet, psychological support—these are all reasons cancer patients need a health care team to help them through the steps to recovery. The contributions of a team of professionals—dieticians, physical therapists, occupational therapists, nurses, psychologists, members of the clergy, and others—are described throughout these pages. Transcriptions of interviews with some of these people are also included. A well-organized program coordinated by the health care team can make the difference between chronic debility, disease control, and recovery.

However, the health care team is a resource to be used or not used by the patient. Throughout the book emphasis is also laid on the importance of patient responsibility. Patients who are active participants in their medical care and rehabilitation are better able to maintain a feeling of independence and faith in their ability to cope. Their rationality, courage, and decision-making ability are best mobilized when they know what they're fighting and how to fight it.

When facing a new experience, particularly a traumatic one such as a diagnosis of cancer and the fight to get well, we often want to hear what someone else who has been through the experience has to say. Twelve cancer patients share their emotions and thoughts in these pages. Only their names are changed. They often speak of resetting their priorities when they discovered their lives were threatened. They became more outspoken and developed a renewed appreciation of friends, nature, music, and art. They also speak of fear, depression, anger, and self-pity.

Yet in spite of these similar reactions, each person also has problems unique to his or her personality and life situation. One person has devoted parents, a wife, husband, or children; another lives alone. One person finds that her self-image has changed radically by having cancer; another is untouched in this respect. Several patients address the issues of maintaining self-esteem in a world of healthy people and of the emotional and practical support that family and friends can provide. Ellen Abbott speaks eloquently of the relationship between patient and physician and of the responsibility of anyone who is ill for setting the ground rules for the way in which he or she wishes to be treated by family and friends. Anthony Verdi and Alexander Jones exemplify what all these patients have—the will to live.

In short, this book is a compilation of my beliefs and my practices. I know that the more knowledge that is disseminated about cancer, the sooner people will have less fear and come for earlier diagnosis. I believe in the approach of a team of health care professionals who are resources a patient can draw on in every area of life. By combining knowledge and problem solving with action, a person can greatly increase his or her chances of recovery from cancer—if not recovery, then of prolonged survival. I hope this book provides a touchstone for those persons who have cancer, to help them help themselves to the best possible care.

PART ONE

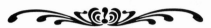

Understanding cancer

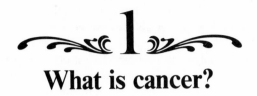

What is cancer?

Cancer has been found in prehistoric skeletons
1 million years old as well as in Egyptian
mummies who lived 5000 years ago.

Perhaps the least understood fact about cancer is that it is only a name for more than 200 diseases that have in common the production of abnormal cells capable of irregular, independent growth and the invasion of healthy tissue. Some of these diseases can be cured; others become chronic but are not necessarily fatal; and still others are eventually fatal as a result of their local or distant destructive activities. Unless a specific cancer is designated, the word cancer in this book will apply generally to the approximately 200 diseases represented by the word.

Our knowledge of cancer remains incomplete but there is common agreement among experts on some points. Most cancers develop from a normal cell or cells that receive multiple injuries, over many years, to the chromosomes in the cell. These injuries are caused by external factors such as sunlight, radiation, drugs, hormones, chemicals, food additives, industrial pollutants, water, and smoking. It is probable that environmental carcinogens initiate approximately 75 to 80% of cancers today, causing these changes in DNA—chromosomes and genes. (Some of these carcinogens are discussed in Chapter 3, Role of Early Detection in Preventing Cancer.) At the same time, it is also apparent that genetic predisposition, which accounts for the remaining 20% of cancers, may in part determine one's susceptibility to cancer. This predisposition may also include defects in the host immunologic defense system or an immunologic imbalance. A separate chapter on genetic counseling is included.

Animal experiments suggest that viruses may also play a role in causing cancer, but thus far only one virus (the Ebstein-Barr virus) has been shown to have a causal relationship to cancer in humans. The Ebstein-Barr virus has been implicated as the cause of infectious mononucleosis, Burkitt's lymphoma, nasopharyngeal cancer, and herpes. Of note is that a positive serum test for the Ebstein-Barr virus antibody (confirming past exposure) has been found in healthy children and adults. Thus other factors are required to develop cancer, such as a specific susceptibility. Age, sex, race, occupation, diet, and geographic location can also be factors in the development of cancer.

In recent years there has been much discussion of the role of the mind and stress in causing cancer. There is no scientific evidence that the mind is a major contributing factor in the development of cancer, although it may play a minor role in determining susceptibility to or acceleration of cancer growth.

It is known that during the first year of grief there is a small increase in mortality in the bereaved when compared to a control group. There is no doubt that during stress or an emotional crisis, changes occur in body chemistry with the release of cortisone, epinephrine, hormones, and other substances and a depression of the immune system. These substances may alter metabolic functions and accelerate disease or affect the growth of a cancer that is *already* present in an inactive or slowly growing rate.

Because there are so many types of cancer, it is highly improbable that research will unearth a single cause or a single cure. Until we have specific knowledge, it will be open season for speculation about the causes and cures of cancer, and it will be impossible to refute some of the wilder speculations that frighten and confuse people, such as the belief that cancer is contagious or that you can get it from using aluminum cookware. Those factors that we know contribute to the development of cancer are discussed in Chapter 3.

All growths, masses, or tumors are not malignant or cancerous. A tumor can be benign (noncancerous) or malignant (cancerous). Benign tumors remain localized and are not invasive or destructive. Malignant tumors are invasive and differ from normal cells in the chromosome (composed of deoxyribonucleic acid, DNA) number and structure. Cancer cells vary from low-grade malignancies to high-grade, more aggressive cancers. The grade of a tumor is classified by tissue examination under a microscope by a pathologist.

Each form of cancer has its own growth rate and pattern of spread. Some cancers remain localized; some invade adjacent structures; and others spread into the blood or lymphatic vessels where they are carried through the body to a distant site.

With both malignant and nonmalignant tumors, there is usually a long latency period of from 1 to 30 years before the tumor is clinically demonstrable (can be felt on physical examination or detected by x-ray examination, isotopic scan, or chemical or immunologic test). It is believed that a normal cell requires multiple chromosomal "hits" or injuries over months or years by a potential carcinogen (any cancer-causing substance) before cell mutation can occur, transforming a normal cell into a cancer cell.

Approximately 30 cell divisions must occur in order for cancer cells to reach a mass that is detectable on physical examination or chest x-ray examination (usually greater than 1 cubic centimeter or one-third square inch). When a cell becomes cancerous, it divides (reproduces) into two cells. After 1 to 2 years, it has doubled 20 times until it contains about 1 million cells. At this point, it weighs only 0.01 gram (0.00035 ounce) and is the size of a pinpoint—or 0.0004 inch. In the meantime, cells are being sloughed off or are falling from the tumor's surface, and hundreds or thousands may metastasize. Fortunately, most of these metastasized cells die. Because they do not implant (like a seed that does not grow), they do not become cancer growths when they reach another part of the body. By the time a cell has divided 30 times, the tumor has 1 billion cells, measuring approximately 1 cm in diameter (a pea-sized lump). This is the smallest size lesion that can be seen on an x-ray film, such as a chest roentgenogram. (The cure rate for lung cancer is 10% because the tumor has usually metastasized before it is diagnosed. If it is diagnosed before clinical metastasis, the cure rate is 33%.)

Cancers in the abdomen or chest cavity are detected late because they have to grow to a size where they will cause symptoms. For example, if a woman did not miss her period or have morning sickness, she would not know she was pregnant for many months. Improved diagnostic techniques capable of detecting early cell changes will dramatically increase the cure rate for most diseases, as it has for cervical cancer, which can be detected in its early stages by means of a Pap smear. Among those diseases for which earlier detection will be important are breast cancer, melanoma, certain lung cancers, and leukemias. New diagnostic tests are becoming available, but until these tests are perfected, most cancers will grow for months or years before causing symptoms that will lead to their discovery by physical examination, radiography, isotopic scan, or biopsy.

2

Genetics

PATRICIA T. KELLY

We differ from one another in many ways, including hair and eye color and body shape. We pass these genetic traits on to our offspring because our cells have chromosomes with DNA that determine these traits. They also determine genetic defects or abnormalities such as diabetes, birth defects, or cancer. The genetic susceptibility of cancer is not common and varies in strength from one person to another.

If you are concerned about your own genetic predisposition for cancer, a genetic counselor may be of help in determining your susceptibility and risks. For example, genetic counseling is useful where there is a family history of colon polyps (benign growths) because these frequently become colon cancer. Breast cancer and a small percentage of melanomas can also have a hereditary predisposition.

In the last few years, important advances have been made in our understanding of the genetics of cancer. These advances have made it possible, and will continue to make it more possible, for us to determine the risk of cancer to the relatives of cancer patients.

When one member of the family has cancer, the relatives often assume that their own risk of that cancer is increased. Sometimes this concern is justified. Often, however, a relative's cancer risk is no greater than that of a neighbor who has no relative with cancer.

It is the job of the genetic counselor to analyze who is and who is not at increased cancer risk due to family history, and—when a person is found to be at increased risk—to determine the extent of that risk. Once individuals know what their risk of a given cancer is, they can work out an appropriate health plan with their doctor. Such a plan may include an increase in periodic screening tests and changes in diet.

There are some families in which the genetic predisposition to a given cancer is very strong. There are even some families where there is a genetic predisposition not only to one, but to several different types of cancer.

Research for material in this chapter was supported by Grant CA 09348, from the National Institutes of Health, and Research Support Program of Mt. Zion Hospital and Medical Center, San Francisco, California.

Fortunately, these families are rare. In most families, if a genetic predisposition is present, it is *not* strong. The relatives of the cancer patient are at little if any increased risk.

The new studies on breast cancer risk in families show that a woman's risk is influenced by the ages at which her relatives were affected (pre- or postmenopausal) and by whether the affected relatives had breast cancer in one or both breasts. Usually women whose relatives had premenopausal breast cancer in both breasts are at higher risk than are women whose relatives had breast cancer after menopause and in only one breast. As mentioned earlier, some women with a family history are at no increased risk of breast cancer.

Currently genetic counselors can give information about cancer risk only in terms of probability or likelihood. Often the risk information is obtained from a group of families, each of which has several members with cancer. The risk of cancer to various relatives in this group is calculated and then used when similar types of families ask about their risk. Such information is rough and provides only an approximation of an individual's risk. The approximation is often useful, but not as useful as a test that would provide information about a specific individual's genetic susceptibility.

One such test has been developed and is currently being tested on an experimental basis. Dr. Mary Claire King of the University of California, Berkeley, analyzed 11 families that had a very high incidence of breast cancer. She found that in these families individuals who had breast cancer were more likely to carry a given enzyme in their blood (glutamate-pyruvate transaminase, or GPT) than were their relatives who did not have breast cancer. In these families, the gene that makes GPT is thought to be close to a gene that increases an individual's breast cancer susceptibility.

Dr. King's test is still in the experimental stage, so it cannot be used to test for breast cancer susceptibility in other families at this time. However, she has shown the usefulness of an approach that will probably be frequently used in the future to determine which individuals in a family are at high cancer risk. Those who are found to be at high risk will receive close medical attention. Those whose risk is not found to be increased will be spared much anxiety.

In my genetic counseling practice, I often see husbands and wives, mothers and daughters, and even whole families together. I have found that when a family gathers together to ask questions about risk and to face squarely whether some of them are at increased risk, a great feeling of peace can develop, regardless of the risk information they acquire.

During genetic counseling sessions, family members have an opportunity to ask questions about the possible causes of cancer in their family. Many experience a sense of relief when they realize they have received the very latest scientific and medical information. The risk figures obtained through genetic counseling, even when rough, give many people a sense of predictability that helps to reduce their fear of the unknown. As one woman said, "I can take hearing information, no matter how bad. It's worrying about the unknown that I can't take."

Many individuals use the counseling time to think about the type of health program they need to follow in order to avoid excessive worry. The information they receive and the health planning that results helps to keep them from feeling powerless and victimized.

As important as the risk information is, many individuals seem to gain even more relief from the process of exploring the causes and risks together. This process helps relieve guilt and blame and enables family members to realize that by loving, supporting, and helping each other they can all lead richer, fuller lives.

PART TWO

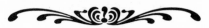

Early detection
and prevention of cancer

3

Role of early detection in preventing cancer

I am often asked, "What kind of vitamins can I take to avoid getting cancer?" or "Will I get cancer from a dental x-ray?" This chapter tries to answer some of these questions and stresses the importance of being aware of your body—of what you put into it and of the environmental hazards you can avoid.

Unfortunately, avoiding the known contributing causes of cancer discussed in these pages may not prevent you from developing the disease. Many patients who develop cancer believe they have caused it by something they did wrong in their lives. They should not feel guilty, because there still are many things over which people have no control that influence their likelihood of getting cancer. Examples include heredity, a defective immune system, and hundreds of environmental causes. However, there still are some things you can do to lower your risk of developing the disease or at least to help guarantee that it can be caught early at a curable stage.

EARLY DETECTION OF CANCER
Yearly medical examination

A yearly medical evaluation may save your life because early detection of cancer increases your chances of a cure. Being practical, this means 30 physician visits between the ages of 40 and 70, a minor inconvenience when you consider the value of your health in contrast to overlooking a cancer that might be cured. Fewer visits are needed for the adult under 40 years of age. The likelihood of finding a problem is much less in this age group.

A yearly physical examination will include many standard screening tests for cancer, such as a Pap smear for cancer of the cervix or a chest x-ray film for cancer of the lung. The cervical Pap smear is about 97% successful in detecting cancer at an early stage. It is the main reason for the significant reduction in the death rate from cervical cancer since the test was introduced 50 years ago. A yearly chest x-ray examination is also a good idea after the age of 50, especially for smokers.

Cancer costs can be measured not only with regard to their effects on our health but also, more broadly, in their effects on our families and all those whom our lives touch. Not surprisingly, even industry is affected. It has been estimated that U.S. industry could save $800 million yearly if workers would follow five cancer prevention and detection measures. An American Cancer Society (ACS) report analyzed about two-thirds of the U.S. work force in private industry. The findings indicated that preventive measures could save $2.8 billion in earnings lost by workers who develop the four cancers that are most preventable by early detection: lung, cervix, breast, and colon.

The five recommended prevention and detection activities could eliminate 15,000 cancer cases and nearly 17,000 deaths yearly. The activities are as follows:

1. Monthly breast self-examination by all female employees
2. Yearly breast physical examination for women employees between ages 20 and 65
3. After two initial negative Pap smears at least a year apart, a smear at least every 3 years for women employees between the ages of 20 and 65
4. A stool guaiac slide test yearly for all male and female employees between the ages of 50 and 65
5. Antismoking activities aimed at getting all employees to give up cigarettes. This activity alone would have enormous effect, because more men are in the industrial work force, more of them smoke, and the incidence of lung cancer is higher among men than among women.

Screening techniques to detect cancer are constantly being reassessed as to their effectiveness and as to how often and on whom they should be performed. For example, the screening test to detect lung cancer in heavy smokers can be done by a Pap smear of a sample of sputum or by a chest x-ray film. A special screening program is now in progress to evaluate whether one or the other, or a combination of the two tests, is more effective in the early detection of lung cancer. Such screening programs for lung and other cancers are becoming more prevalent throughout the United States. They are beginning to be used more routinely by physicians and requested more often by members of the public.

Self-examination

Breast self-examination. Women themselves find 90% of breast cancers, but unfortunately most women do not examine their own breasts and thus have a more advanced breast mass when they report for a physical examination.

Breast cancer is the number one cancer killer of women in the United States, although lung cancer is quickly gaining with the increased number of women who are heavy smokers for over 20 years. In 1973 the American Cancer Society conducted a survey to find out how many women who were informed as to the risks of breast cancer and the hope that might lie in self-examination, actually performed self-examinations. The survey found that 77% of women were educated with regard to the risks, but that only 18% examined their breasts on a regular basis. The ACS then launched a campaign to encourage self-examination, and the figure rose to 24%. It should be stressed that most breast lumps are benign—*not* malignant. It is critical that a woman follow up early on any new changes in a lump or report a new change to her physician.

The steps involved in self-examination are easy and require only a few minutes each month.

1. Examine each breast during your shower or bath when your skin is wet and reexamine when soapy. Gently glide your fingers over the breast. The right hand examines the left breast and the left hand, the right breast. You may find it easier if your hands are soapy or are moistened with lotion or oil.

2. The second step is carried out in front of a mirror when your hands are above your head and then on your hips. Examine your breasts for any lumps or changes in contour, swelling, or dimpling.

3. For the third step, lie down with a pillow under one shoulder and put the arm on the same side as the shoulder behind your head. Examine the breast with the other hand in a slow circular, clockwise pattern, starting at the outer rim. Rotate around the breast slowly, moving toward the nipple. Examine the nipple with the thumb and index finger for changes or abnormalities. Then squeeze the nipple to examine for discharge.

If you find any lumps, changes, or thickening with any of these maneuvers, consult your physician.

This examination should be done monthly, usually a week after the menstrual cycle or, if postmenopausal, on the first day of each month. (For a more complete description of breast self-examination, ask your local chapter of the ACS or your doctor for the ACS brochure on the subject.)

Testicular self-examination. Testicular cancer accounts for 1% of cancer in males and usually occurs in men between the ages of 20 and 35. The first sign of testicular cancer is a swelling, occasionally associated with pain, in or around the testicles. Pain usually means a benign infection or inflammation but, in more advanced testicular cancer, pain may be present. Fortunately, most testicular or scrotal swellings are benign. However, when a swelling or change is noted, one should check it out with a physician.

Testicular cancer, diagnosed early, has the best chance for cure if treated with surgery and/or radiation therapy. During the past 10 years, new chemotherapeutic programs have achieved cures in certain types of advanced testicular cancer in 90% of the patients treated.

For self-examination, examine each testicle gently with both hands after a bath or hot shower. Place the index and middle fingers underneath the scrotum and the thumb on top; gently roll the testicle as you would a golf ball in a small sock. Compare one testicle with the other. There usually is a difference in testicle size, but if lumps or masses are present, report to your physician immediately. A small fullness called the epididymis is normally present on the top of each testicle.

RECOMMENDATIONS OF THE AMERICAN CANCER SOCIETY

The ACS publishes guidelines on cancer-related checkups and periodically revises these guidelines according to the latest research results. For example, research may reveal that a given screening procedure is not as effective as was once believed or that a once-a-year test is preferable to a test every 2 years.

The ACS also urges every adult to "Talk with your doctor and ask how these guidelines relate to you." The guidelines are intended to help individual physicians and patients select the early-detection procedures that best meet the patient's needs and correlate with the beliefs of the individual doctor. For example, the ACS recommends a Pap smear at least every 3 years for women between the ages of 20 and 65 who are not a high risk. I do not agree with this recommendation. I still believe that a yearly Pap smear for all women is the best means of preventing death from cervical cancer.

Thus the following guidelines will be tailored to individual patients by their doctors, based on a case history and the results of a yearly physical examination.

- Women 20 and over, and those under 20 who are sexually active, should have a Pap test at least every 3 years, after two initial negative tests a year apart.
- Women 20 to 40 years of age should have a pelvic examination as part of a general physical examination every 3 years, and women over 40 should have a pelvic examination every year.
- Every woman should have a pelvic examination and Pap test at menopause. Those at high risk of endometrial cancer should also have an endometrial tissue sample examined. High risk is defined as having a history of infertility, obesity, failure of ovulation, abnormal uterine bleeding, or estrogen therapy.
- Women over 50 years old should have a mammogram every year. Women under 50 should consult their personal physicians about the need for mammography in their individual cases. All women should have a baseline mammogram between the ages of 35 and 40.
- Women 20 to 40 years old should have a breast physical examination every 3 years, and women over 40 should have a breast physical examination every year.
- All women over 20 years old should perform a breast self-examination monthly.
- Men and women over 50 years of age should have a stool occult blood slide every year.
- Men and women over 50 years old should have a sigmoidoscopic examination every 3 to 5 years after two initial negative examinations 1 year apart.
- Men and women over 40 years old should have a digital rectal examination every year.

Because of these schedules, a "cancer-related health checkup" is recommended for all persons over 20 years of age every 3 years, and for all persons older than 40 every year. In addition to including special tests and procedures at the designated frequencies during these checkups, patients should obtain health counseling (including consultation about smoking and other personal cancer-risk factors), have a pelvic examination, and be examined for cancers

CANCER'S SEVEN WARNING SIGNALS
Change in bowel or bladder habits
A sore that does not heal
Unusual bleeding or discharge
Thickening or lump in breast or elsewhere
Indigestion or difficulty in swallowing
Obvious change in wart or mole
Nagging cough or hoarseness

of the thyroid, testicles, prostate, lymph nodes, oral region, and skin, as well as for some nonmalignant diseases. It is important to begin having periodic consultations at an early age because this is when many personal health habits are established.

The ACS stresses that their guidelines have been developed for people *without* symptoms and that those who have symptoms or signs suggestive of cancer should immediately seek medical help. As a reminder, the American Cancer Society's warning signals and safeguards are included here.

THE SEVEN SAFEGUARDS URGED BY ACS

Lung: Don't smoke cigarettes.
Colon-rectum: Have a proctoscopic exam as part of a regular checkup, after age 40.
Breast: Practice monthly breast self-examination.
Uterus: Have a Pap test as part of a regular checkup.
Skin: Avoid overexposure to the sun.
Oral: Have a regular mouth examination by your physician or dentist.
Complete body: Have an overall physical checkup annually or at 3-year intervals depending on your age.

4

Cancer and nutrition

Research is being conducted worldwide on the links between diet, nutrition, and cancer. As of 1982, there are no proven ways to prevent or cure cancer by a special diet or any particular vitamins or minerals. However, current evidence suggests that if we modify our diets as well as our way of life, we can reduce our cancer risk.

For instance, there is a high correlation in the United States between consumption of meat and fat and a number of diseases, including diabetes, ischemic heart disease (coronary artery disease), and colon cancer. In Japan, the high incidence of stomach cancer is believed to be related to nitrites and salt and smoked and pickled foods—all used as preservatives.

At the same time, the Japanese have a low rate of consumption of milk and milk products. (Attempts are being made in Japan to reduce the risk of stomach cancer by improved refrigeration and a reduction of salt, nitrites, and smoked and pickled foods, with a concurrent increase in the use of milk and milk products.)

We will have to wait many years for research to *prove conclusively* the speculated relationship between many dietary habits and cancer. In the meantime, cancer specialists and researchers should continue their efforts to make the public aware of known contributory causes of cancer in the diet as well as the latest theories on the role of vitamins and other substances in preventing cancer.

In November 1981 a 5-year study was reported from the National Cancer Institute that covered 10% of the American population; it was the most complete review on how cancer affects the average American. Of particular note was the mysterious fact that Hispanics develop one-third fewer cancers than other Americans. Hispanic males had 38% fewer cancers than white males, and females had 27% fewer cancers than white females in New Mexico and 42% fewer in Puerto Rico.

The reason may relate to a possible genetic protection and the known relationship of a diet high in animal and dairy fats which cause an increased number of colon and breast cancers. Poverty and tradition have resulted in a Hispanic diet high in legume proteins (beans) and low in meat. Hispanics often receive less medical care and thus some cancer may be under-reported.

Cancer incidence among black men is 22% higher than white men, although black women have slightly fewer cancers than white women.

Following are some well-accepted and some speculative theories on the role diet may play in the development of cancer.

ALCOHOL

There is little question that consumption of alcohol, in conjunction with other carcinogens such as tobacco, markedly increases the chances of developing cancer, especially cancer of the mouth, throat, esophagus, and larynx. For the moderate drinker who does not smoke, the risk of head and neck cancers is 2 to 3 times the average incidence rates. For those who drink alcoholic beverages *and* smoke, the risk jumps to 15 times the average rate.

An increased incidence of liver cancer is found in people with cirrhosis of the liver from alcohol. (Viruses—mainly hepatitis—and some drugs also cause cirrhosis of the liver.) Cirrhosis from alcohol develops in 15% of heavy drinkers.

The carcinogenic potential of alcohol—that is, probably some component(s) of the beverage—varies with the region. In France, esophageal cancer is related to hard alcohol, but not to beer or wine. In Southern Africa, esophageal cancer is related to beer made from maize.

Exactly how alcohol promotes the development of cancer is not known. One theory is that a cancer-causing agent may be dissolved in alcohol and thus absorbed into the body through the linings of the mouth and the gastrointestinal tract.

It is recommended that alcohol consumption be limited to one or two alcoholic drinks per day.

AFLATOXINS

Aflatoxins are highly potent carcinogens produced by the fungus *Aspergillus flavus*. They commonly develop in moist carbohydrate foods in hot, humid climates. Therefore, nuts, grains, seeds, and rice should be kept dry after being harvested and stored. In the United States, peanut and grain storage are carefully checked during the drying process. However, the drying procedure is not always as strictly monitored in Southeast Asia and Africa. In these areas, hepatitis B virus is common and may act together with aflatoxins to produce liver cancer. Aflatoxins have been proven to produce liver cancers in rats and in zoo bears fed stale peanuts. Males seem to have a greater predilection for this cancer than females.

It is recommended that when in areas such as Thailand, Southeast Asia, China, and Africa, one try to avoid eating nuts, rice, grains, and seeds that are not properly dried—that show signs of mold. Moldy breads should also be avoided.

FIBER

Fiber is found in plant foods and is important in providing bulk stools. In 1969, Dr. Dennis Burkitt, working in Africa, said that he became "acutely conscious that a high proportion of the beds in Western hospitals are filled with patients suffering from diseases that are rare or unknown in the rest of the world." He postulated that the high incidence of colon cancer (the second and third most common cancer in men and women, respectively) was related to the lack of fiber in the Western diet. In Africa, where fiber is a major part of the diet, colon cancer is almost nonexistent.

Burkitt's theory was based on the fact that fiber absorbs liquids, is not digestible, and passes rapidly through the gastrointestinal tract. He suggested that by increasing bulk and hastening bowel movements, fiber reduces the exposure time of gut lining to waste products (bile metabolites) that may act as carcinogens.

Preliminary studies in Norway and the United States may corroborate Burkitt's findings, where an estimated 25% decrease in colon cancer risk was noted when large amounts of vegetables were consumed.

The process by which colon cancer may develop is as follows: Diets high in cholesterol cause an increase in bile excretion from the gallbladder into the intestines. Gastrointestinal bacteria then degrade (digest) the bile into metabolites, some of which are carcinogenic and have been implicated in the causation of colon cancer.

Low concentrations of blood cholesterol are also implicated in increased incidences of colon cancer and may be related to the increased excretion of bile in the gastrointestinal tract.

One ounce of fiber a day may be all that is needed to produce a soft, bulky, easily expelled stool. A simple way to provide fiber is to use Miller's Bran, which is a dry wheat powder that is convenient, inexpensive, and available in supermarkets. One level teaspoon of Miller's Bran contains 2 grams of fiber. Start with small doses (1-3 teaspoons) and increase intake to 3 tablespoons (9 teaspoons) of Miller's Bran per day. This will help improve bowel function for most adults. The daily recommended dose is 25 grams of fiber. Also, a diet that includes the following fiber sources is recommended: nuts, legumes, grains (whole wheat bread), cereals (bran, shredded wheat, oatmeal), fresh fruits, vegetables, brown rice, bulgur (cracked wheat), kasha (buckwheat groats), seeds, and popcorn (without butter).

CONSTIPATION

Constipation may be associated with the development of breast cancer. For centuries physicians have believed that large bowel bacterial fermentation occurs in populations that consume large amounts of meat and refined carbohydrates. The type of meats (fattier ones) may be important as well. Bacteria in the large intestine can change steroid and fatty acids, which linger due to constipation, into active carcinogenic estrogen metabolites.

Vegetarian women excrete estrogens in their stools. Nonvegetarian women have more estrogen metabolites because they eat meat. These estrogen metabolites are absorbed to a greater extent in the gastrointestinal tract instead of being excreted.

Meat-eating women who consume large amounts of coffee, tea, or cocoa and also suffer from chronic constipation have shown a higher incidence of lumpy breasts (chronic cystic mastitis). Often the benign breast lumps resolve when dietary habits are altered.

Drs. Nicholas Petrakis and Eileen King at the University of California have studied breast fluids of women with chronic constipation (two or fewer bowel movements per week). Their breast fluid was four and one-half times more likely than the average female (women who have one bowel movement per day) to contain abnormal cells, which showed severe atypical cytological changes. These authors have associated these atypical cytological changes with severe benign breast disease and breast cancer. Further studies will be needed to determine the meaning of this relationship.

Of interest is that vegetarians have been shown to have lower estrogen levels in their blood than meat eaters. The reason may be that a different gastrointestinal flora separates estrogens in the gut, allowing higher estrogen reabsorption in meat eaters. Constipated people also have a longer period of time for possible absorption.

It is recommended that fiber intake be increased to reduce constipation and that meat, coffee, tea, and cocoa consumption be decreased.

NITRITES AND NITRATES

Nitrites and nitrates, both of which occur in nature, interact in the gastrointestinal tract with amines, which are by-products from the breakdown of proteins, to form nitrosamines. Nitrosamine compounds are highly carcinogenic in animals.

Sodium nitrites and nitrates are found in vegetables and other foods. Sodium nitrite is also used to preserve foods that cannot be exposed to high temperatures. Thus frankfurters, salami, bacon, ham, and cured fish are treated with nitrites to prevent botulism, a deadly bacterial poison.

Astonishingly, cured meats are the source of only about 5 to 10% of the nitrites we consume. Over 90% of the nitrites and nitrates in our bodies are from the ingestion of vegetables and other foods. The nitrites and nitrates from all these sources are absorbed from the stomach and the intestine into the bloodstream. When these nitrates reach the mouth, they are reconverted, in a recycling process, to nitrites and again ingested in the gastrointestinal tract. The stomach fluids are acidic and at each stage in the cycle enhance the transformation of the nitrites into nitrosamines, the carcinogens that ultimately form stomach cancer.

Nitrosamines are also involved in an association between beer and stomach cancer. Many beers form nitrosamines during the heat-drying process of green barley. Beer companies have now reduced the level of nitrosamines by improving the drying process and by the use of sulfur (sulfur interferes with the formation of nitrosamines).

Vitamin C may neutralize the carcinogenic effect of nitrosamines; therefore, vitamin C has been added to cured meats or can be taken orally after ingestion of cured meats. If vitamin C has been added to a cured meat, it will be so stated on the label.

In 1978, the federal Food and Drug Administration (FDA) published a warning that nitrites might be a risk factor in the development of cancer. Rats fed high doses of sodium nitrite had a 10% incidence of cancer (lymphoma) compared with a 5% incidence in control animals who did not receive sodium nitrite. After intensive review of the data, the FDA ruled that this difference in the incidence of lymphoma was not significant, and it reversed its stand.

In a risk-benefit analysis, the FDA also calculated that of 135 cases of cancer a year related to nitrites, only 6 of these cases would be the result of nitrites in cured meats. Moreover, if these meats were not cured with nitrites, 22 cases of fatal botulism would occur, even with an intensive public education program. Without a public education program, the occurrence of botulism would be even higher. The 6 cases of cancer that result from the use of nitrites seem insignificant in comparison with not only 22+ cases of botulism but 100,000 new cases of lung cancer, primarily caused by cigarette smoking, such as developed in 1979. Paradoxically, the amount of nitrosamines in a 3-ounce portion of nitrite-preserved bacon is roughly the same as that absorbed in smoking a pack of cigarettes.

Although the risk of cancer from nitrites in cured meat is low, consumption of fresh meats, poultry, and seafood is recommended over that of ham, bacon, sausage, frankfurters, corned beef, and smoked seafoods.

FATS AND OBESITY

Research studies have linked a high consumption of saturated and unsaturated fats with cancer of the colon, breast, rectum, and endometrium. For example, in the West, where 40% of our daily caloric intake is from fats (meat, cheese, butter, margarine, and whole milk products), the incidence of colon and breast cancer is high. In Japan, Thailand, and India, where fat comprises only 12% of daily caloric intake, the incidence of these two cancers is low.

One of the most interesting pieces of evidence of the link between fat consumption and cancer is found in a study of Japanese who migrated to Hawaii. When they began to adopt Western dietary habits, they developed a higher incidence of both breast and colon cancer. Those who became completely westernized in Hawaii and Los Angeles developed an even higher incidence of the disease. Conversely, colon and breast cancer is about one-half as common among Seventh Day Adventists (who are vegetarians and avoid coffee and alcohol) as it is among the general population in the United States, despite a "normal" intake of fats among these people.

No one knows how fat intake results in higher rates of cancer, but evidence shows that a diet high in fat stimulates the production of two female hormones, estrogen and prolactin, both of which can initiate the growth of breast cancer.

Women with large body mass (obesity), high fat intake, and a high cholesterol level have a greater risk of developing breast cancer and an increased rate of cancer recurrence than the general population. Of interest is new information on cholesterol that suggests an inverse relationship between cholesterol and cancer. Two studies reported that a lower blood cholesterol is related to an increased incidence of colon cancer only in men and to total mortality from cancer.

It is recommended that fat intake be reduced from 40% to 20-30%. Foods high in fat are Crisco, lard, butter, margarine, all oils, cream, whole milk, sour cream, high-fat cheeses, fatty meats (such as pork, duck, bacon, and sausage), and foods cooked in grease or fats such as potato chips and bakery products. Foods low in fat are skimmed milk and low-fat cheeses, lean meats, vegetables, fruits, cereals, and unbuttered popcorn. Tofu (soybean curd), peas, nuts, beans, and seeds are good protein substitutes. Iced milk or sherbet can substitute for ice cream.

ADDITIONAL DIETARY TIPS

Smoked and barbecued foods contain a strong carcinogen called benzpyrene, a product of the burning wood or charcoal that penetrates the meat, poultry, fish, or shellfish via the fumes and smoke.

The infusion of carcinogens into barbecued food can be reduced by using leaner meats and reducing the fat drippings that cause additional flame and smoke, which increase the concentration of benzpyrene. Keeping the food further away from the flames and coals, using lower temperatures, or wrapping the food in tinfoil are also ways of reducing the infiltration of this carcinogen.

Frying food on top of the stove at a temperature higher than 300° F also increases the risk of producing benzpyrene. It is safer to broil food or to use a microwave oven (without the browning plate). No radiation, nitrosamines, or benzpyrene are produced by cooking in microwave ovens. Other safe methods of cooking are baking, crock pot slow cooking, and stewing.

COFFEE

In 1981 Dr. Brian MacMahon of the Harvard School of Public Health studied the alcohol, tea, and coffee consumption habits of 369 people with cancer of the pancreas and 644 people who were free of the disease. Pancreatic cancer was higher among coffee drinkers than among non-coffee drinkers, and the more coffee that was consumed, the higher was the incidence of cancer. There was a weak positive association between pancreatic cancer and cigarette smoking. This may reflect a causal relationship. Consumption of one to two cups of coffee doubled the likelihood of developing pancreatic cancer whereas consumption of five or more cups *tripled* the risk. Alcohol and tea were not implicated as causative factors in the development of pancreatic cancer.

Drs. Hershel Jick and Barbara Dinan reported similar results but could not confirm a positive association between coffee consumption and cancer of the pancreas.

In the United States over one-half the population over the age of 10 drinks coffee daily. We will have to await further studies and analyses before we can confirm this possible association.

FOOD ADDITIVES

More than 2500 different additives have been used in foods as preservatives, stabilizers, thickeners, emulsifiers, antioxidants, color enhancers, and nutritional supplements. Those additives that are carcinogenic have been banned by the FDA. Currently nitrates, nitrites, and saccharin, which have known cancer links, are widely used and are still under review.

In 1977, a ban on saccharin was proposed. Canadian researchers have reported that 3 of 100 rats fed huge saccharin diets (5% of their total diet) developed bladder cancer. In another study, the habits of 632 people with bladder cancer were compared with those of people without cancer, and those with bladder cancer had a high intake of saccharin.

The ban on saccharin has been deferred, but its use by pregnant women is discouraged because we do not know whether it poses a risk to the fetus. The use of saccharin by young people is also discouraged to avoid prolonged exposure over a lifetime.

Cyclamates were introduced in the United States in the 1950s. In a study done in the 1960s, 4 of 240 rats on a high cyclamate diet developed cancer. Cyclamates were banned in 1969. Subsequent tests have failed to produce the same results as the first study, which is now considered to have been an experimental error. Thus cyclamates with no evidence of cancer risk are banned in the United States, whereas saccharin, which presents a low cancer risk, is used in the United States and banned in Canada. However, the risk of developing cancer from saccharin is minimal so long as the exposure is limited. A 12-ounce bottle of diet soda contains 0.005 ounce of saccharin, which is only of importance if diet soda is consumed in large amounts.

SELENIUM

Trace metals, of which selenium and zinc are the most common, are important in maintaining good health. Seafoods and organ meats can be rich in selenium, depending on the soil/selenium content where the animals feed.

Selenium acts as an antioxidant and helps protect DNA from toxic lipid peroxides and free radicals, and there is some speculation that it may prevent the production of active carcinogens. However, there is no final proof that selenium will be effective in the prevention or treatment of cancer. The studies are just beginning. For example, recent studies in mice show that the addition of selenium to the drinking water reduced the incidence of breast cancer and preneoplastic (precancerous) tumors such as colon cancer. Thus selenium given to an animal before inducing the development of cancer cells by viral or chemical means appears to prevent the formation of cancer.

The results of two Canadian studies have shown a correlation between increased selenium levels and decreases in cancer mortality. However, similar studies in 22 countries do not corroborate these results.

Clinical trials are now under way in the United States, China, and Finland on the use of selenium supplements in the prevention and treatment of cancer. These trials will require many years of research because the mechanism of the metabolic interactions for selenium are not yet understood. At this time there is no evidence that selenium has any effect on a cancer that has already developed.

Another problem is that selenium can be harmful in large quantities. The current recommended daily dosage of selenium is 200 micrograms. Toxicity, or chronic selenosis, has resulted from doses as high as 2400 micrograms a day, and data from research with animals show that high intake of selenium can result in weight loss and death.

ZINC

Zinc is one of the essential elements in 95 of the enzymes involved in cell division. A zinc deficiency is found in most patients with advanced cancer, but this is related to the immune deficiency of other vitamins and minerals that occurs with advanced disease.

Clinical trials suggest that zinc may help restore the normal functioning of the immune system and the sense of taste, but more research is needed before this is known for certain. The current recommended level of zinc for cancer patients is 10 to 15 milligrams a day. Some patients have elected to take as many as 50 milligrams a day to help improve their sense of taste and therefore their appetite. If there is toxicity or another side effect from taking large amounts of zinc, it is hard to detect. Caution should be exercised.

VITAMINS A, C, AND E

During the last decade, data from research on both animals and humans suggest that vitamins A, C, and E may play a role in prevention and treatment of some forms of cancer. However, it will take many years to determine the nature and extent of this relationship, and to attempt to provide guidelines on doses of these vitamins with respect to cancer. In spite of all the publicity they have received, vitamins will probably not be found to be the sole agents that can prevent or cure cancer.

Because the evidence is inconclusive, the traditional physician rejects the need for high doses and megadoses of vitamins in cancer prevention and treatment. Moreover, there is evidence that such doses are both wasteful and potentially toxic. Many of my patients take high doses of vitamins. I do not discourage them, but I always advise them of toxicity and other side effects. My main concern is that they continue to receive standard medical therapy.

Vitamin A

Vitamin A is a fat-soluble organic compound derived from vegetable and fruit carotenoid pigments called beta-carotene. It is a 20-car-on retinal.

β-carotene is converted to vitamin A primarily in the intestinal mucosa (lining), but some β-carotene is absorbed intact, stored in the liver, and requires an enzyme called β-carotene dioxygenase to convert it to vitamin A. We may ingest vitamin A directly in animal foods such as milk or liver, or in capsules.

Vitamin A may play a role in preventing cancer. The results of one animal study showed less in animals fed a normal level of vitamin A, relative to paired animals on a vitamin A–deficient routine. A second study looking at possible mechanisms of action found that vitamin A as β-carotene has a hormone-like action that affects cell differentiation—the maturing process of cells. Therefore, vitamin A may prevent or retard the formation of tumor cells. The results of one epidemiological human study—whereby blood levels of vitamin A were measured, and the people were then observed for changes—suggest that people with higher vitamin A levels are less likely to develop cancer years later. However, one could also conclude that higher dietary vitamin A intake is associated generally with better self-care, and that other factors may be responsible for the decreased cancer incidence.

Moreover, in several areas of the world—India, the Middle East, and Africa—there is no increase in the number of cases of cancer in general, or of squamous lung cancer in particular, in spite of a diet deficient in vitamin A.

Thus under no circumstances can studies such as those just cited be accepted as definitive. Many years will pass before current research on humans confirms or denies the results of these studies and answers the question, "Can vitamin A help prevent or cure cancer?"

Large doses of carrot juice (high in β-carotene) are consumed by many people in the hope of preventing or curing cancer. I have not witnessed any preventive effect from this practice. Our bodies prevent vitamin A toxicity by storing carotene and converting it to vitamin A only as needed. Hence higher carotene intake does not result in huge increases in vitamin A. People who have taken high doses of vitamin A still receive diagnoses of cancer. As far as the curative potential of vitamin A is concerned, it is not possible to judge the effects of any vitamin supplements or any other substance when a person is also receiving standard cancer therapy. It would be helpful if one could devise a human experiment with people afflicted with one type of cancer, some receiving vitamins and others not, but many variable circumstances tend to prevent this.

At this time, β-carotene and vitamin A are considered safe for humans at doses of 30 milligrams and 10,000 I.U. per day, respectively. However, large doses of β-carotene from vegetables and fruits turn the skin yellow (called carotenemia), and preformed vitamin A in high doses can cause toxic side effects such as blurred vision or blindness and liver and bone damage. Therefore, when doses of vitamin A in experimental programs average as high as 100,000 I.U., periodic chemical analyses of the blood are performed to monitor these toxic side effects.

A deficiency of vitamin A can impair the eyes' ability to adapt to the dark. It can also lower sperm production.

Until the results of research tell us otherwise, consumption of vitamin A in the foods in which it naturally occurs is recommended. These foods include butter, margarine, liver, liver oil, green leafy vegetables (especially spinach and swiss chard), green peppers, carrots, sweet potatoes, pumpkins, yellow squashes, and yellow-orange fruits.

Vitamin C

Vitamin C is an organic compound called ascorbic acid. As mentioned in the discussion on nitrites and nitrates, vitamin C helps prevent the transformation of nitrites, nitrates, and amines into carcinogenic nitrosamines.

Vitamin C is also being studied for a possible role in the cure of cancer, but the data from studies to date are conflicting and inconclusive.

In 1974, Drs. Linus Pauling and Ewan Cameron reported on a study of 1100 patients who were dying of cancer. Of these patients, 110 received massive doses of Vitamin C. Although all the patients ultimately died of cancer, Drs. Pauling and Cameron reported that those patients who received vitamin C lived longer.

However, carefully controlled studies at the Mayo Clinic by Dr. Charles Moertel have failed to confirm the findings of Drs. Pauling and Cameron. Dr. Pauling is now expanding his research to try to reaffirm the results of his prior study and to learn more about the role of vitamin C in the prevention and treatment of cancer.

My own experience tends to confirm the results of the Mayo Clinic studies. However, as with vitamin A, it is impossible to make an honest evaluation of the role of a specific vitamin when a patient is on a basic nutritional program or receiving radiotherapy or chemotherapy. I am not currently prescribing high doses of vitamin C for my patients.

The megadoses of vitamin C taken by cancer patients range from 2 to 30 g daily, although the usual megadose is from 4 to 10 g daily. The side effects from vitamin C are many, including gastrointestinal distress such as diarrhea, kidney oxylate stones, and increased iron absorption, which produces iron toxicity in some people. Vitamin B_{12} can be destroyed. Furthermore, the body becomes acclimatized to higher doses of the vitamin, destroys it at a very rapid rate, and may become relatively ascorbic acid-deficient if these high levels are abruptly stopped for some reason.

When inhaled, cigarette smoke destroys vitamin C. Therefore, vitamin C supplements have been recommended for smokers.

Confirming our knowledge of the role of vitamin C in preventing the formation of nitrosamines, epidemiological studies conducted internationally suggest that fresh vegetables and fruits containing ascorbic acid reduce the gastrointestinal cancer rate—that is, cancer of the stomach and esophagus.

Action should therefore be taken to change our eating habits (especially those of children) by reducing the consumption of salted and pickled products and to consider the use of small doses (100 to 200 milligrams) of vitamin C after eating these foods or foods containing nitrites or nitrates.

Foods high in vitamin C are recommended for inclusion in a well-balanced

diet. Fruits such as oranges, grapefruits, lemons, cantaloupe, and straw-
berries, and vegetables such as broccoli, asparagus, cabbage, and leafy greens
are high in vitamin C.

Vitamin E

Vitamin E, also known as alpha tocopherol, is a fat-soluble organic compound. Like vitamin C, vitamin E helps block the production of nitrosamines
in the gastrointestinal tract.

Certain free radicals, such as superoxides, affect metabolic changes in the
body; they also can induce genetic DNA mutations, which may lead to cancer.
Vitamin E is an antioxidant, which may help retard the action of these free
radicals.

Because vitamin E has been considered safe and might have some value, it
has been used in experimental clinical trials. In one study, it was given in
600-I.U./day doses for cystic mastitis, which consists of aching and tenderness
in heavy breasts. The symptoms cleared up in 10 of 26 cases. Fibrocystic
breast disease, as it is called, has been shown to precede the later development of breast cancer in some women. It is not yet known whether improvement of the fibrocystic condition alters the later incidence of breast cancer.

Few other data are available on the role of vitamin E in the prevention and
cure of cancer. There is no evidence that megadoses of vitamin E can prevent
or cure *any* disease, but research is being conducted to try to obtain more
information about this vitamin. New information considers over 600 I.U./day
as a possible megadose. Toxicity, although rare, has been reported, including
phlebitis, hypertension, blood clots, muscle pains, itching, hormonal alterations, and altered immune system in high doses.

Fats such as vegetable oils that contain vitamin E are one of the richest
dietary sources. Fats and vitamin E are absorbed together in the intestines.
When megadoses of vitamin E are taken, the amount absorbed in the intestines
does not increase proportionately. Excess vitamin E is excreted in the stool.

Normal nutritional intake of vitamin E is recommended. Vitamin E is
found in cereals, nuts, seeds, whole-grain germ, such as wheat germ, and
whole-grain breads and cereals, unsaturated vegetable oils (especially
corn and safflower oils), and soybean oil. White bread, refined grains, saturated fats (lard, coconut oil, olive oil, butter, and shortening) should be
avoided.

It is clear from the foregoing discussion that the issue of cancer and
nutrition contains some certainties, much disagreement, and continuing research worldwide.

Measures that can be taken to reduce the risk of cancer are the following:
- Reduce alcohol consumption.
- Stop smoking.
- Reduce fat, meat, and caloric intake to avoid obesity and achieve ideal
  weight. Substitute low-fat for high-fat meat and dairy products. Total
  daily fat intake should not exceed more than one-third of the total daily
  caloric intake.

- Increase fiber intake: nuts, cereals (bran, shredded wheat, oatmeal), fresh fruits, vegetables, brown rice, bulgur (cracked wheat), kasha (buckwheat groats), seeds, popcorn (without butter), dried beans, and unrefined whole-grain products (oats, rice, wheat).
- Avoid excessive intake of nitrites and nitrates: barbecued and charcoal broiled foods; frankfurters, salami, bacon, ham, and cured fish.
- Avoid heavily salted and/or marinated foods, including pickles and salty snacks. Use less table salt.
- Avoid excessive sugar from all sources: white sugar, brown sugar, honey, syrups, candy, soft drinks, and ice cream.

5

Cancer and the environment

Cancer is universal. There is no place or country on this planet that has been free of cancer, although there are marked variations geographically in the incidence of cancer. In Chile the rate is less than 100 cases of cancer per 100,000 people; the United States is average, with 175 cases per 100,000; and Great Britain has the highest rate with more than 250 cases per 100,000 population. Scotland has the highest cancer death rate—more than five and one-half times higher than in Thailand, the country with the lowest death rate.

These geographic differences reflect a number of factors: smoking, exposure to cancer-causing chemicals, heredity, and dietary pattern. These factors apply to populations in dense urbanized countries as well as in underdeveloped countries where life expectancy is short.

One of the first scientists to note the frequency of cancer cases among a particular group and to make the association between environmental carcinogens and cancer was Dr. Percivall Pott. In 1775, he studied the incidence of scrotal cancer in chimney sweeps. Pott described young men and boys as "thrust up narrow, and sometimes hot chimneys, where they are bruised, burned, and almost suffocated; and when they get to puberty, become peculiarly liable to a noisome, painful and fatal disease." These boys often worked naked, rarely bathed, and were full of soot, especially in their groin areas. He postulated that soot was the cause of their scrotal cancer.

In 1915, 140 years after Pott's publication, Drs. Katsasaburo Yamagiwa and Koichi Ichikawa at the Imperial University of Tokyo tested coal tar from soot by painting tar on rabbit ears. Cancer developed on the painted area as it had in the sooty scrotums of the London chimney sweeps.

Even if the world were free of such carcinogens, cancer would still occur, in part because of other environmental factors such as sunlight, x-rays, pesticides, asbestos, and industrial products.

In a rapidly developing world, studies on the incidence and types of cancer have given us clues to the causes of cancer. In Singapore, cancer was relatively unimportant as a cause of death in 1950 but became the number one cause of death by 1965, later to be replaced by heart disease. Changes in life-style as well as prolongation of life are contributing causes.

We often hear of a "cancer epidemic," but if one analyzes the data, the only epidemic is that of lung cancer.

34

In a country such as the United States where one-fourth of the population develops cancer, many people have cancerphobia. Cancerphobia is due in part to a misunderstanding of the statistics and the disease process, as well as disappointment that the promised cure of the "Crusade Against Cancer" has not happened, even with modern research. The Nixon concept that cancer was to be cured by 1976 with an infusion of money was not reasonable. Although great advances are occurring in diagnosis and therapy, we will be doing well if we achieve this goal by the year 2000.

The effort to learn the secrets of cancer continues. An unusual phenomenon is the high frequency of specific types of cancer in certain locations around the world. In Central Africa where there is a moist climate, a tumor of the jaw and neck, known as Burkitt's lymphoma, is common in children. In Egypt and along the Nile River, a common parasitic infection (schistosomiasis) often develops into bladder and urinary tract cancer. For unknown reasons, incidence rates of breast and intestinal cancer are higher than the national average in the Great Lakes area. In countries like Britain and the southern United States where cigarette smoking and industrial pollutants are excessive, lung cancer statistics are higher. In Queensland, Australia, and in Arizona where the sun shines intensely, an increase in skin cancer and melanoma is noted. In India, a local food, the betel nut mixed with lime paste, causes a high incidence of mouth cancer. Japan has the world's highest incidence of stomach cancer, and in Lin Xian, China, there is a high incidence of esophageal cancer related to a mold or fungus that grows in moist, poorly dried food. Thus clues to the causes of certain types of cancer may be discovered by studying the environmental and social customs of people in areas where these cancers occur.

SMOKING AND CANCER

Lung cancer was a rare occurrence in the first decade of this century. Prior to World War II, it was believed to be hereditary. This inaccurate belief has been replaced by an environmental cause—cigarettes. There is no longer any question that the worldwide rise in lung cancer during the past 70 years can be attributed to the increased use of cigarettes.

Of 4000 autopsies performed at the University of Wisconsin between 1899 and 1919, only 4 revealed lung cancer. Lung cancer now comprises one-fourth of male cancer deaths in the United States; within 2 years it will replace breast cancer as the leading cause of female cancer deaths. Several surveys show that over 90% of lung cancer patients are smokers or former smokers. Smokers in the United States consume 600 billion cigarettes (one-half of these being the filter variety) annually. Each cigarette contains 6800 different chemicals, many carcinogenic.

Each year cigarettes are made less harmful with better filters to reduce tar and nicotine. However, this only means that many people smoke *more* of these cigarettes to satisfy their nicotine addiction, with the result that their lung cancer risk remains the same.

Switching to a pipe or cigar may in part reduce the risk of cancer of the lung, but there is still a high risk for cancer of the lips, pharynx, and esophagus because the smoke from pipes and cigars contains the same amount of tar and nicotine as smoke from cigarettes. It is merely not inhaled.

Smoking cigarettes is one of the most popular habits in the United States. The nicotine high and the feeling of well-being derived from smoking cigarettes make people disregard common sense. Even the warning *Cigarettes are hazardous to your health* on each package of cigarettes has not deterred many people from smoking.

In a 20-year study of smoking and deaths in British physicians, Doll and Petro found that 25 or more cigarettes a day for life resulted in an increase in death from lung cancer 25 times that for nonsmokers. The increase in chronic lung disease was 46 times, as well as an increase in coronary disease.

Some people do stop smoking and succeed, but others fail. To succeed, you need motivation, the support of friends and family, and sheer determination. If you succeed, you can save your own life as well as someone else's.

Alcohol functions as a co-carcinogen with smoking. Oral and neck cancer occur 15 times more frequently in people who drink as well as smoke than in those who do neither. Cigarettes are the primary environmental cause of cancer.

For those who stop smoking, every day, month, and year that passes reduces the risk of lung cancer. Not smoking for 10 to 15 years reduces the risk of cancer to equal that of a person who has never smoked.

SUNLIGHT

Many forms of environmental pollution can be avoided, but low-level sunburning rays are always present. Approximately 60% of each day's carcinogenic radiation is received between 10AM and 2PM. By avoiding sun for the two noontime hours, one can reduce ultraviolet exposure 35 to 50%. Seasonal changes are also significant. The sun's rays are stronger in summer than in winter. The radiation that produces sunburn constitutes less than 0.2% of total sunlight and is its most variable part.

The ultraviolet rays of sunshine penetrate the skin and can cause damage ranging from premature aging of the skin to wrinkles and dryness. This includes keratoses and skin cancers, the most virulent being malignant melanoma. The risk and range of susceptibility depends on several factors: where you live, the length of exposure and strength of the rays, the thickness of your skin, the parts of the body exposed, and the color of your skin. Darker skin pigments contain melanin, which is a natural filter against the sun's rays. Blond- or red-haired people with blue eyes and light-colored skin have less melanin. Thus melanoma is rare in blacks and most prevalent in fair-skinned whites.

Superficial skin cancers, primarily basal cell and squamous cell cancers, are over 95% curable. They relate directly to sun exposure.

However, melanomas are now becoming more common, especially in areas of the world with intense sunlight, such as Arizona and Queensland (Australia), where the death rate is 14 per 100,000 for skin melanoma. These populations also show a genetic predisposition to skin melanoma.

To avoid skin cancer, the following recommendations are made:

- Avoid the sun during midday when the rays are strongest.
- Remember that burning ultraviolet rays occur on overcast days. They are invisible and not screened by clouds.
- Cover exposed areas of the body when feasible; wear a hat and a long-sleeved shirt.
- Don't depend on beach umbrellas. They offer little protection from sun rays reflected by sand, water, or snow.
- Use a sunscreen (PABA—para-aminobenzoic acid). Sunscreens are numbered 2 to 15, the higher number giving better protection. These ratings represent the sun-protection factor, a multiple of the time required by the sun to produce any given effect on an individual's skin. Thus a factor of 3 means it will take three times as long for skin to redden. Most sunscreens are rated 8 or more, but I recommend a 12 to 15 sun-protection factor. The more expensive sunscreens offer no advantages over inexpensive ones. Only the rating matters. The ideal sunscreen should penetrate the skin's outer layer and not be lost in perspiration or easily washed or rubbed off. However, no preparation remains effective during prolonged swimming. Therefore, sunscreens should be reapplied after bathing or swimming.
- Avoid mineral, olive, or baby oil, because oils magnify and increase the sun's burning effect.

RADIATION

Following its discovery at the turn of the century, radiation quickly became an effective tool to help diagnose diseases (the x-ray picture) and to treat cancer. The deleterious side effects also became apparent. Marie Curie, who won a Nobel Prize for research on radium, died of aplastic anemia from exposure to radium.

Women who worked in watch factories painting radium onto luminous watch dials died of cancer—of the jawbones, primarily. They would use their lips to point their brush, leaving residual radioactive materials on their lips.

We are all exposed to radiation throughout our lives. There are three main sources of radiation: natural background, medical, and miscellaneous.

Natural background radiation includes cosmic rays from outer space and radiation from naturally occurring radioisotopes in our bodies and our surroundings. The amount we receive varies according to such factors as the altitude at which we live. The natural background radiation in the United States averages about 0.08 rem per year (a rem is a unit of radiation).

The main contribution to medical radiation exposure is from diagnostic radiology. The amount of radiation given for one x-ray film may be quite large (e.g., 2 rem for a lateral lumbar spine film), but the average for the whole body and the whole population for routine diagnostic tests is about 0.1 rem per year.

Miscellaneous sources of radiation include such diverse items as color TV sets, airport baggage-inspection systems, luminous watches, tobacco, and some types of glass and ceramics—all of which may contribute small amounts of radiation, with an average exposure for the whole population of about 0.002 rem.

We have some degree of control over the amounts of radiation we receive. Those who choose to live in Denver receive 0.06 rem more from natural background radiation than those who live in San Francisco. People who work with x-rays—radiologists and x-ray technicians—may typically receive 0.2 to 0.4 rem per year from occupational exposure. Even when a medical or dental x-ray examination is necessary, we can insist that exposure be limited to what is necessary and useful. Sometimes it is possible to use a lead apron to protect the rest of the body.

Observations of irradiated animals and survivors of atomic bomb attacks show that radiation can cause cancer and that the developing fetus in the womb is much more sensitive than the adult.

The probabilities of getting cancer from radiation sources in everyday life (excluding atomic bomb attacks) are slight. The results of many studies now agree that if a woman receives abdominal x-rays during pregnancy, the subsequent child's risk of developing leukemia is increased from 4 cases per 10,000 children to about 6 cases. Although this additional risk is very small, present practice is to avoid x-rays during pregnancy except for emergencies.

Nuclear plants release radiation waste into air and water, and although the carcinogenic effect is believed to be minimal—less than the contamination from a coal-burning power plant—we again will have to await the test of time. Nuclear accidents have occurred and have led to deaths. Therefore, great caution must be instituted. The tragedy at Three Mile Island in Pennsylvania, where there was an accidental spill, has yet to be resolved 3 years later.

The maximum dose received by anyone living near the Three Mile Island power station was 0.04 rem, one-half the average person's annual dose. The potential risk of fatal cancer from this dose is 1/100,000, or one additional death from cancer in the Three Mile Island vicinity. This should be compared to the normal risk of fatal cancer of 1 in 7.

ASBESTOS

There are reports from as long ago as 1940 that workers who spun asbestos cloth died of lung disease before age 50. The asbestos fibers (20–50 microns) accumulate in the lungs and can cause cancer in susceptible people, person, especially if they are smokers. The fibers affect the mouth, larynx, esophagus, stomach, and large intestines. Two major diseases can develop: asbestosis and mesothelioma. Asbestosis is a disease that causes progressive lung obstruction and fibrosis, which subsequently develops into lung cancer in 40% of patients. Mesothelioma is a rare form of cancer of the lining of the lungs caused by asbestos inhalation and smoking. There is a long latency period of 10 to 30 or more years before either disease occurs.

The risk of asbestosis and mesothelioma is high for those who have worked in the shipyards with asbestos pipe or boilers, in asbestos mines, or in factories with ceiling tiles or other products containing asbestos.

There is a synergistic relationship between asbestos and smoking. The risk of cancer in people exposed to asbestos fibers is 10 times greater in smokers than in nonsmokers.

VINYL CHLORIDE

Recently, vinyl chloride (a chemical used in aerosol sprays and the manufacture of plastics) became implicated when in May 1970 Dr. P. L. Viola at the Cancer Institute in Rome reported that high doses of aerosol sprays caused cancer in animals.

Epidemiological studies were initiated in 1972; in 1973 and 1974, three cases of liver cancer (a rare form) were found in a vinyl chloride plant in Louisville, Kentucky.

Vinyl chloride is an important ingredient in plastics, records, plastic packaging, and medical tubing. The plastic product is of *no* danger, but workers in a vinyl chloride factory have a 200 times greater risk than the general public of developing liver cancer.

Vinyl chloride has been banned from aerosols, and plastic manufacturers have altered their manufacturing procedures to avoid the exposure of workers.

SOME OTHER INDUSTRIAL HAZARDS

Dangerous chemicals used in manufacturing spread far beyond the site of the factory. Tons of wastes are spewed into the air, drained into waters, or buried underground. Farmers use pesticides to protect their crops and animals, but the chemicals (by definition deadly) penetrate water supplies, forage, and eventually the humans who consume the animals and vegetables produced on the farm.

Here are just a few of the results of ignorance and carelessness. Iron miners have a higher incidence of lung and laryngeal cancer related to iron oxide from the iron ore. Gold miners, hard rock miners, and vintners are exposed to arsenic, a contaminant in the ores and in the insecticides used to grow grapes for wine production. Textile workers exposed to aniline dyes such as aromatic amines, beta-naphthylamine, and magenta have an increased incidence of bladder cancer. Textile printers working with cadmium-containing dyes have an increased incidence of kidney cancer.

People who live in areas of heavy pollution—near copper, zinc, or lead smelters, or in industrial cities such as Liverpool—have higher lung cancer rates than people in comparable cities with clean air. (As always, the rate is doubled in smokers.) The relationship between pollution and cancer is apparent, and arsenic in the air is one of the suspected agents.

MEDICATIONS

Cancers have been related to drugs prescribed to treat diseases, even cancer. Concerns are currently being expressed about the role of hormones—both synthetic and natural—used as medication.

Two million women took diethylstilbestrol (DES) to prevent miscarriages. It is no longer considered an effective therapy for this purpose. In 1966 a few cases of an unusual form of vaginal cancer were diagnosed in the daughters of women who took DES during pregnancy; seven such cases were found in the next 4 years. In addition, the several sons born of mothers who took DES were found to have deficient sperm counts (possible sterility).

Every day hormones are used for menopausal symptoms such as hot flashes and palpitations. A study at the University of Southern California reported that taking hormone supplements at age 50 for menopause doubles the risk of breast cancer by age 75. An increase in uterine endometrial cancer of from five to eight times the average has also been noted after taking hormones.

Eighty million women around the world take contraceptive pills, which also contain hormones, and studies are being conducted to determine the long-term risk of these women in developing cancer. Thus far, no association has been found. However, researchers agree that it is still too early to predict long-term risk, because large numbers of women have only been on the pill for 15 years and in many cases it takes from 10 to 30 years for cancer to evolve and be detected. One such study was conducted at the Kaiser Permanente Medical Center in California, of 16,000 women who took the pill for 10 or more years. The study concluded that the risk of developing cancer as a result of taking the pill is minimal when compared to the cancer risks of smoking or overexposure to the sun.

There is some evidence that the pill may offer protection against cancer; or it may play a varied role, providing protection for certain groups at certain ages and promoting cancer at another time. The decision whether to take the pill is a personal one. The minimal risks must be weighed against the benefits.

The relationship of drugs to human cancer is still under investigation. Much of the work obviously has to be done on animals, and it is difficult to translate the results to human cancer risks. However, drugs that show a potential danger are removed from the market by the FDA.

The relationship between toxic environmental hazards and cancer is becoming more apparent. Unfortunately, the latency period between exposure and development of the disease is at least 20 to 30 years, which means that substances we now believe to be safe may not be so, and vice versa. But we have to live, and we will always be exposed to environmental elements that have the potential to cause cancer. We must therefore be our own guardians and protect ourselves with the latest scientific knowledge and with common sense.

PART THREE

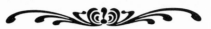

Treating cancer

6

A diagnosis of cancer: the unwritten contract

The day I found out I had cancer was
the worst day of my life.

HUBERT H. HUMPHREY

A young man once came to me after knowing for 9 months that he had a testicular mass. He had postponed consulting a doctor because he suspected he had cancer and feared that undergoing treatment would prevent him from providing for the financial future of his family. By this delay, he forfeited the possibility of a cure.

A person may put off consulting a physician for many reasons, chief among them the fear that his or her suspicions will be confirmed. But whatever the reasons for postponement, recriminations from the doctor only increase remorse. When physician and patient meet, it is time to get to know each other and to discuss the procedures to be followed in obtaining a medical evaluation of the illness. It is time to forget past omissions and to concentrate on the present and the future.

Of course, not every person who consults a doctor about a perplexing ailment suspects or assumes that cancer is present; nor does every person who suspects cancer actually have it. However, because I am a hematologist and an oncologist (a specialist in blood and tumor problems), my patients are referred to me by other doctors and usually are aware of the reason for the consultation. Some people are referred to me by their family physicians for a second or third opinion to confirm a diagnosis; others are referred by internists, surgeons, or cancer specialists for further evaluation or to reassess a treatment program.

If I am to treat a person for cancer, it is important that we have a candid exchange of information in our first meetings. Because new patients are always apprehensive, I give them the basic facts about cancer and its treatment, and I ask them to describe their symptoms and to tell me some of the personal facts that I need to know as their physician or consultant. Little can be said to the average person to hide a diagnosis of cancer. Knowledge is not only readily available but useful to a person who will undergo treatment and live with the disease. Informed patients will be more receptive to treatment and thereby improve their chances of combating the disease. Moreover, the attitudes they acquire in these initial interviews may well affect the quality of life they are able to maintain for the duration of the illness.

THE DIAGNOSIS

A familiarity with the basic diagnostic terms and procedures is useful to a cancer patient. After I have discussed the history of a person's complaint—where the pain or lump or other symptom is located, whether it hurts, what relieves it, whether there has been fever or weight loss—I perform a physical examination. An external examination is performed of the ears, nose, throat, lymph glands, skin, chest, heart, abdomen, extremities, and nervous system. An internal examination is made of the pelvic region in women and the rectum in men and women.

Based on the nature of the complaint and the results of the physical examination, I arrange for the specific diagnostic tests that appear warranted by the problem. The problem could be a mass or an enlarged organ, a heart murmur, the presence of abdominal or chest fluid, or a change in reactions in the nervous system. A brief discussion of some of the most common diagnostic procedures is given in the following paragraphs.

Endoscopy

An endoscope is a general term for a telescope-like optical instrument used to look at the internal organs of the body. By directly viewing an organ through one of the instruments listed here, cancer can be seen, biopsies arranged or performed, and diagnoses made.

- Bronchoscope for the lungs
- Laparoscope for the abdomen
- Cystoscope for the bladder
- Gastroscope for the stomach or duodenum
- Colonoscope for the upper colon
- Sigmoidoscope for the lower colon
- Proctoscope for the end of the gastrointestinal tract (anus and rectum)

The tube used for endoscopies was formerly made of metal and therefore rigid. It is now made of minute flexible plastic fibers that allow it to bend easily, limiting discomfort to the patient and often giving the examiner a better view of the organ or cavity. During certain endoscopies, an x-ray may be taken simultaneously to help in the evaluation.

As an example of an endoscopic procedure, a physician may discover by finger examination a tumor mass in the rectum. A sigmoidoscope is then used to see directly into the rectum and lower colon, make an assessment of the nature of the mass, and—if there is suspicion that it may be cancerous—remove a piece of the tissue (perform a biopsy) for examination by a pathologist.

Urinalysis

This test of the composition of the urine reveals abnormalities in the kidney or the bladder. For instance, a protein loss is an indication of kidney disease; the presence of sugar may indicate diabetes, whereas the presence of crystals could be the result of gout. An overabundance of white blood cells could indicate an infection; too many red cells are an indication of bleeding; tumor cells might mean cancer, for which further tests would be scheduled.

The hemocult stool test

The Hemocult Stool Test is a simple procedure to detect the presence of blood in the stool. The physician or patient smears a small amount of stool on a specially treated paper and adds chemicals that reveal the presence of blood. The most common cause of blood loss is hemorrhoids or a polyp (a benign tumor or a premalignant growth); however, the presence of blood can also indicate a hidden cancer. To diagnose the source and cause of the blood, a further examination is made with a proctoscope, sigmoidoscope or colonoscope if examination of the lower colon is deemed necessary, or a barium enema. In the event that an area appears suspicious, the physician removes a sample of tissue for pathological examination.

To obtain the most accurate results, a person who is to have a Hemocult Stool Test should be on a meat-free, aspirin-free, high-roughage diet because meat contains blood and aspirin can cause gastric bleeding.

Analysis of body fluids

Sometimes physical or x-ray examination will reveal the presence of fluid in the abdomen or chest cavity. Fluid can also occur in the joints, such as the elbow, knee, or hip. This fluid can be extracted by the insertion of a needle and examined to determine the presence or absence of cancer cells.

The removal of the fluid in the chest or abdomen also relieves the discomfort caused by the pressure.

Lumbar puncture

A lumbar puncture is a procedure through which fluid is removed from the spinal canal (sometimes called a spinal tap) by insertion of a needle between the lumbar vertebrae. Chemical tests, bacterial cultures, or cytological tests are then performed on the fluid to determine whether there is an infection, inflammation, or cancer.

Blood count and chemistries

A sample of blood is taken and examined for the amount of red and white blood cells present. An analysis of the composition of the blood is usually ordered to assess the amount of the most common blood enzymes, proteins, and minerals (chemicals), because increased amounts of these substances are often an indication of abnormalities in the liver, kidney, or bone, or in metabolic functions of the body. Such abnormalities may be the result of a simple inflammation or of a malignant process.

Pap smear

The Pap smear, named for George Nicolas Papanicolaou, is most often associated with a screening test to detect abnormal or cancerous cells in the cervix. The test is also used in evaluating endocrine functions and in the diagnosis of malignancies of the organs such as the respiratory tract and lungs, gastrointestinal tract, and urinary tract. In this process a smear of tissue or cells is sent to the cytologist, a specialized technician, who stains the slide with dyes and evaluates the smear for abnormal cells or cancer cells. A pathologist also examines the slide after it has been screened by the cytologist to confirm whether a malignant or benign process is present. If the tests are inconclusive, a biopsy is performed to establish a firm diagnosis.

Body imaging

We are in a new era of body imaging. X-rays are no longer the sole means of producing an image of the body. Nuclear scans (radioisotopes) of many elements can now be injected into patients for diagnostic purposes; moreover, the computer has greatly increased the accuracy of diagnoses. Ultrasound, previously available only at research centers and of limited usefulness, is also a new dimension developed over the last 10 years.

X-rays. The traditional x-ray examination of a patient is still the backbone of diagnostic evaluation in terms of body imaging. X-radiation is produced by an x-ray tube, a device built like a large vacuum tube in which a high-speed stream of electrons strikes a metal target, producing a spray of x-rays that are then focused into a useful beam. It is much like a light beam except that its energy is much more intense and it is invisible to the eye. This intense beam of x-rays passes through an object or a patient and, via phosphor screens, casts light upon an x-ray film.

X-ray film is much like the film used in a camera for normal photographic work. Once exposed by the radiation of the x-ray source passing through the patient, the film is processed in a film processor and a standard black and white image is produced. Various portions of the body produce different densities to the x-ray beam: the image on the film demonstrates bone as white; air, such as in lungs, as black; and most soft tissues of the body as varying shades of gray.

Not only is x-ray film used to visualize the image, but a fluoroscope may allow us to see a continuous image by allowing the x-ray beam to strike a small fluorescent screen, the image from which is electronically amplified through a television system. Moving pictures or videotape images of moving objects such as the heart may be made in this manner. X-ray pictures may also be taken during the fluoroscopic procedure.

Instead of using regular silver-coated film, a special technique called xerography has been developed in recent years. This technique uses a specially charged plate of selenium, small electrically charged particles that change their electrical polarity in response to differing intensities of x-ray exposure. X-rays passing through a patient then fall upon this specially charged selenium plate, causing a useful image to be produced. This image has very special characteristics and is extremely high (clear) in contrast to an image produced with the normal silver-coated film. Xerograms are most useful in breast and other soft-tissue examinations.

The most exciting change in imaging has been computer-aided tomography. A CAT scan or CT scan is a newcomer to the field of x-ray diagnosis. It consists of the use of an expensive and complex computer program to create an image by processing the x-ray image created when x-rays pass through the body and strike specially designed sensing devices. The CT-scanning technique has increased the ability to see small parts deep in the body fantastically well without the necessity in many instances of the complicated and sometimes hazardous techniques used in the past.

To enhance even further the image produced by passing the x-ray beam through a patient onto an x-ray film, onto a fluoroscopic screen to produce a television image, or into a computer to produce a computer-assisted image, "contrast materials" can be added. For example, a patient may swallow a barium preparation, a chalky-tasting liquid (described with varying degrees of distaste by patients) designed to coat the inside of the stomach and intestines to make them more visible on the x-ray image. Colon examinations, or barium enemas, employ the same technique except that barium is delivered into the opposite end of the bowel, a procedure found somewhat embarrassing to patients but thoroughly accepted as an everyday occurrence in a radiology department. In these tests both the large bowel and the small bowel can be examined.

Kidney x-ray films or an IVP (intravenous pyelogram) are obtained by injecting a water-soluble contrast material containing iodine into the patient's bloodstream. This material is excreted by the kidney, allowing the image of the kidneys, the ureters, and the bladder to be seen on the x-ray film. Sometimes a contrast material is injected into the bloodstream to improve the image seen on a CT scan of either the brain or the whole body. Contrast material may be injected into other sites of the body such as the arteries, veins, joints, or spinal canal, all for the purpose of enhancing the image of the part to be examined.

Another contrast examination of some importance in cancer work is lymphangiography, a technique wherein minute needles are placed in very small lymph vessels in the feet and the contrast material injected very slowly. Films of the legs and the abdomen are then exposed to evaluate the status of the lymph system. CT examinations have, in some cases, made the lymphangiogram unnecessary.

An x-ray examination discussion is not complete without mentioning the chest roentgenogram, still one of the most useful examinations both in general medical work and in cancer work. The chest film may show tumors arising in the lungs or may sometimes demonstrate evidence of tumors that travel in the bloodstream from other sites and are deposited in the lungs. Bone surveys are also very important examinations. Their purpose is to see most of the bones in the body to allow a determination as to whether any tumors are present in the skeleton.

Safety is an issue that worries many patients. The radiation received by a patient undergoing an x-ray test for diagnosis is not in itself harmful. However, x-ray tests should be avoided, if possible, when patients are in an early phase of pregnancy; and repeated x-ray tests of the facial area in younger patients or repeated examinations of the genital area should be avoided for all patients, if possible, because of potential harm to the ovaries and testicles. Radiation doses are carefully worked out and monitored in accordance with medically established safety standards and procedures.

Nuclear scans (radioactive isotopes). A second kind of examination consists of the use of radioactive isotopes, which are generally given intravenously. Many of these radioisotopes are organ-specific. These substances emit gamma rays that travel to the organ and exit from the body, with minimal radiation to tissues, to create an image on a scintillation detector or on photographic film. The radioisotopes have a short half-life, meaning that they remain in the body only a short time—hours or, at the most, days.

The radioisotope bone-scan test best illustrates what isotope studies can do for tumor patients. Radioactive isotopes are injected into the blood. When these radioactive isotopes have dispersed to the bones, special recording devices can "photograph" the skeleton, seeing only the special kind of radiation given off by the radioisotope. The basic principle behind this procedure is that cancer cells make the bone react to the radioactive isotope to a greater degree than normal bone. Thus an image is made that differentiates cancer masses in the skeleton from normal bone. The cancerous areas light up as "hot spots." This procedure is far more effective than conventional x-ray examinations in finding early tumors. Other radioactive isotopes such as gallium 67 atrote are taken up by some tumors.

Other substances reveal the presence of cancer in just the opposite way. For example, radioisotopes for liver scanning concentrate in normal tissue in the liver but are not taken up by cancer cells. Therefore, radioisotopes concentrate in normal liver tissue; the cancerous areas that show no image on the photograph are referred to as "cold spots."

Radioactive isotopes are also used to monitor a patient's response to therapy and to determine whether a tumor has spread to other organ systems.

Of all the diagnostic examinations done in the isotope laboratory, none carries a significant risk to health. The diagnostic isotope tests are very safe, even for children. Children can be imaged safely with the dose being scaled down from the larger adult doses. Pregnant women are not studied unless absolutely essential for proper diagnosis and treatment.

Ultrasound. Ultrasound examination is a new technique that avoids the delivery of any potentially harmful radiation to the patient. Ultrasound is a cousin of sonar, the device used to seek submarines beneath the water. A high-frequency inaudible sound that passes through the patient is generated, causing reflections like a voice echoing against a canyon wall. These are then electronically processed into a sectional anatomic image. The ultrasound examination is useful in only certain parts of the body. It is not useful at this time for lungs or for the stomach. It is useful in examining the pregnant uterus, the liver, the pancreas, and the kidneys. It is also an extremely effective tool for imaging the heart.

All of the aforementioned imaging devices—x-ray films, xerograms, CT scans, isotope studies, and ultrasound examinations—serve only to help doctors detect the presence, extent, and location of any structural abnormality, such as a cancer. It frequently remains for the endoscopist, pathologist, or surgeon to diagnose the problem.

The final answer to the question, "Is it cancer?" is made by the pathologist. After the preliminary diagnosis is completed as described, surgery (biopsy) is often required to obtain a piece of the tumor for pathological evaluation. A biopsy can be performed on almost any part of the body, including bone, liver, breast, pancreas, cervix, and brain. In a biopsy, an incision is made to remove a piece of the tumor or—if feasible—the entire tumor. Pieces of tumor can also be obtained by using a special surgical cutting needle or a needle with a syringe that can aspirate (withdraw by suction) the specimen. Frequently a radiologist or specialist in nuclear medicine may be called on to locate the tumor and perform a needle biopsy.

In some cases a more extensive surgical procedure, such as a laparotomy (opening of the abdomen), is required to obtain a sample of tumor. Having thus gained access to the body, the surgeon conducts a thorough examination. If a benign or malignant tumor is evident, the surgeon may remove it immediately; if there is a question about the diagnosis, a specimen is taken from the mass and immediately sent to a pathologist. The pathologist freezes the tissue with liquid nitrogen and cuts microscopically thin slices that can be examined under the microscope. In a matter of minutes a diagnosis of a benign or cancerous tumor may be made, enabling the surgeon to take the appropriate action.

Sometimes the pathologist reports that the results of the frozen section are in question. In such a case, the operation is terminated. A more thorough examination of the tissue is made by the pathologist, a process that usually takes 1 or 2 days. If necessary, a second operation is then scheduled.

STAGING

The initial objective in making a diagnosis is to "stage" the disease—that is, to determine the extent of the particular type of cancer so that the oncologist can plan a therapeutic program with the patient. In planning such a program, an oncologist has access to the latest information on treatments. The staging of the disease also provides a baseline for comparison after treatment.

THE DIAGNOSIS AND PATIENTS' RIGHTS

Except in the rare circumstance of a psychiatric disorder or advanced senility, a patient is kept informed as to why a particular test is being performed and what the results could mean. False hope and disappointment only lead to distrust of the medical profession and wariness of any future treatment.

Patients should be aware that they are entitled to all information about testing, test results, and therapeutic procedures. Patients in California now read and sign in the presence of their doctors an "informed consent" for special diagnostic procedures (such as angiograms), surgery, radiotherapy, and experimental chemotherapy and immunotherapy. Although each state has its own legal definition of informed consent, legislative changes such as those in California are occurring throughout the United States. For example, in Massachusetts, and again in California, the law now specifies that patients with breast cancer must be fully informed by their physicians of all alternative forms of treatment.

Appendix I contains a Patient's Bill of Rights approved by the American Hospital Association in February 1973, and Appendix II shows a copy of an informed consent form that I use in my practice. This provides the minimal necessary consent, and of course it protects the patient as well as the physician.

A full evaluation usually takes several days because of the necessity for diagnostic procedures, additional consultations, and possibly surgery. Occasionally it may even take several weeks to establish a diagnosis. Of course the slightest delay will seem interminable to a person who has been worrying alone for weeks or months.

In rare instances, a medical evaluation may be inconclusive. One of my patients had had fever and enlarged lymph nodes. Three biopsies had been performed before he was referred for consultation for a possible lymphoma. A fourth biopsy was performed and reported as a lymphoma, but additional tests and exploratory surgery had negative results. A dozen pathologists who specialize in diagnosing lymphomas at different medical centers reviewed his slides without arriving at a unanimous conclusion. The patient has been observed closely since that time (6 years) and has not shown any sign of disease.

Misdiagnoses are also rare. In Mort Segal's case (see Chapter 11), a rare malignancy was misdiagnosed as benign until, 9 months later, what was thought to be a cyst was excised and proved to be malignant. Misdiagnoses do not often occur because questionable slides are routinely sent to pathology consultants around the country, a procedure that represents an additional safeguard for the patient. It was only the extremely rare nature and the difficulty of pathological interpretation of Mort Segal's malignancy that led to the delay in diagnosis. Most cases are not complex.

DISCUSSING THE DIAGNOSIS

Although most of my patients are aware that they have, or may have, a malignancy, I am sometimes in the position of having to break the news or confirm a suspicion that cancer has been found. What I tell a patient depends in part on how many previous conversations we have had and on whether the patient has just undergone surgery. If we are not well acquainted, I may begin by asking what the patient knows about his or her condition or what other doctors may have said about it.

Knowing that what I say may affect the rest of a life, I proceed slowly and carefully, ready to temper my approach as the person reveals how much he or she wants to know at that moment. It is, after all, a patient's prerogative to determine how much he or she wants to hear. I, on the other hand, must be sure to provide an opportunity for someone to find out everything he or she wants to know. Many patients now bluntly ask the question, "Do I have cancer?" In such circumstances I can be totally frank. But if patients tell me to take over, that they do not wish to know the details of the disease or the treatments, I usually do not press the issue. Each person knows how he or she is best able to function. The only people whom I believe must be informed are those who are financially responsible for others.

Most discussions of diagnoses and recommendations of treatment take place in my office, although some discussions take place in the hospital. To avoid the many interruptions that can occur during the daytime, I try to plan serious hospital talks for late afternoon or early evening when there is adequate time to reply to a patient's questions. Naturally, when someone has just undergone surgery, I postpone a discussion of the diagnosis until he or she is strong and lucid enough to deal with any potentially shocking news. I usually sit beside the bed so that we both feel unrushed and informal. Similarly, in the office, I close the door and ask that no telephone calls be put through except for emergencies. Doctors often seem so busy that a patient feels guilty and apologetic for taking up their time.

Whether in the office or the hospital, I prefer, when possible, to have the closest family members present during the explanation. This eliminates the need for repetition and reduces the possibility of misunderstanding. Sometimes, too, the inclusion of the loved ones lessens a patient's fear of abandonment and provides reassurance that the family is not concealing any facts from him or her. Together the family and the patient can ask questions and consider problems that may arise in the future, for, ideally, the long-term treatment of cancer involves the cooperation of the whole family. The benefits to a patient of such a supportive family are apparent in the chapters on Darrell Ansbacher and Magdalena Matunan.

During the initial explanatory process, patients can be helpful—and ultimately better informed—if they respond to leading questions such as "Do you have any questions about your diagnosis?" A doctor is not helped by a reply of "No," or "You're the doctor. You should know." As I mentioned in Chapter 1, the doctor-patient relationship works best when both participants are responsive, as in the following dialogue.

"What do you think is wrong?"

"I'm not sure."

"Well, there are several possibilities. Acute infection or arthritic or systemic disease—or some other type, an ulcer or a malignancy. What do you think is causing your problem?"

"I really don't know. Can you tell me?" or "Do I have cancer?"

When the reply is, "Yes, you have cancer," or "Yes, you have a tumor," a detailed explanation should be given, repeating much of the basic information the patient may have received during the diagnostic procedures. The doctor should explain the type and extent of malignancy, although not necessarily all at one time; and, most important, one should make the patient aware of the treatments that are available to combat the disease. I always explain that we will begin with the mode of therapy prescribed for this particular form and stage of cancer but that there are others that may be equally good or provide a backup if the first one is not effective.

In spite of my effort to give a clear explanation, I have found that a lot of misunderstanding results from the initial discussion of a diagnosis and treatment. Patients are usually too stunned to think clearly and need time to assimilate bad news. Often they cannot respond to my final question, "Is there anything you don't understand about your problem?" They may have understood nothing because they have heard nothing since the word cancer was uttered. Several years ago a patient left my office after an extensive 30-minute discussion of her cancer and was met at the office door by her cousin, who asked, "What did the doctor tell you?" Although only 90 seconds had elapsed since our talk, she replied, "I forgot." It was obvious that my explanation had fallen on deaf ears. She was still in a daze from the first few sentences of our conversation.

When such a situation occurs, I suggest that we speak again later that day or the next day. Someone who has just received a diagnosis of cancer needs time to absorb the information, to reflect, and to make plans. For this reason, I usually ask patients if they would like to have a record of our initial conversations concerning diagnosis and treatment on a cassette tape. The patient, and whomever else (family or friend) the patient wishes to have present for the explanation, can listen to the tape later at home in a less stressful environment.

The patient, family members, and friends may have misconceptions before they learn the facts about the illness and treatment. They undoubtedly have fears and anxieties that should be aired. The tape helps to defuse these emotions and enables those close to the patient to talk with him or her openly.

Also, patients and their families or friends may have left my office with different ideas as to what has been said. By listening to the tape, they can clear up misrepresentations and misunderstandings or produce further questions for the next visit. The cassette recording can also help maintain vital communication between the cancer patient and those close to him or her when the latter are unable to be present during a consultation, because they can listen to the tape later. Some patients have sent the recording to concerned relatives in other parts of the country to keep them informed of their current medical status.

The presence of the tape recorder makes me more conscious of the need for clarity, and I therefore tend to present my explanations in a more concise and organized manner. At the same time, the tape recorder tends to make patients more conscious of their right to ask questions and of their responsibility for exercising that right.

Whether or not patients exercise their option to use the tape cassette, I encourage them to write down questions raised during our consultations. In effect, I ask them to make what I call a "shopping list" of all the questions that occur to them about their form of cancer, future treatments, or anything else that worries them, no matter how unrelated or trivial it may seem to them. This process will help them to include worries they might otherwise suppress or might just forget to ask me during our next talk. Questions and concerns run the gamut: "Please explain the whole thing again. What is happening inside my body?" "If I lose my hair will it grow back?" "Is there anything I can take if I get nausea from chemotherapy? I have to go to work every day." "I've had no medical insurance since I left my job 2 months ago. I can't afford to be sick. Are there any sources of financial aid?" "Can I still play tennis while having chemotherapy?" "I know this is going to take a lot out of me. What can I do to make up for the extra nutrition my body will need?" "I have to be able to do housework soon after I get home from the hospital. What can I do to keep my muscles strong while I'm hospitalized?" "I know cancer isn't catching, but I can't quite rid myself of the notion. Is it really all right if I sleep with my husband?" Any facts that I can give patients that will relieve their worries will also free them to devote their energies to self-care and living.

THE FAMILY AND THE DIAGNOSIS

Occasionally a family member will take me aside when a patient is still undergoing diagnosis and request that the patient not be told the real diagnosis if it turns out to be cancer. My feeling is that any agreement concerning a patient should be between the patient and the physician. When someone comes to me for medical help, it is with that person that I make the "unwritten contract" for mutual candor and trust, although I do, as I have indicated, welcome the support of family or friends.

The wife of one of my patients made a request for secrecy. She eventually admitted that she felt guilty toward her husband and might subconsciously have assumed responsibility for causing his disease. With another patient, I suspected that his wife wanted to play a dominant role in her husband's illness. She offered as an excuse for withholding information her belief that her husband was psychologically incapable of handling the truth. Such a supposedly weak patient is usually stronger than anyone thinks and is quite capable of dealing openly with his or her cancer. In both cases I convinced the wives that their husbands would cooperate more fully in their therapy if they knew about their disease. (Only when patients have a psychological impairment do I agree to give them limited information.)

The reverse situation has also arisen. I have had patients request that their disease be kept secret to protect a spouse or other family member. In these cases I try to explain to the patient the therapeutic advantages of treating a family as a unit. For instance, a husband who joins his wife during an office visit will share her problems, know her fears and the routine of her therapy, and therefore be able to give invaluable backup support. I had one patient who would always tell me she felt great until her husband would interrupt with "That's not true. You felt nauseous last night . . . " and so on. I could then prescribe an appropriate antinausea medicine.

Of course, everyone has heard of instances when a family member and the patient each thought he or she was alone in knowing the truth. Generally, this protective attitude is self-defeating, not only because precious energy is expended but, the longer the facade is carried out, the greater the fear and anxiety for both people. Therefore, when possible, I try to play a positive role by bringing two such people together.

Sometimes the circumstances are even more difficult. I am occasionally brought in on a case in which the deception of a patient has been going on for some time. The family or the primary physician made an early decision not to tell the patient the truth, so the question arises of the wisdom of intervening in an established relationship. My policy in such cases is that if patients have no psychiatric problem, and if they ask me directly, I explain the nature of the disease in as much detail as they wish. If they show no inclination to know about their illness, I tend to comply with the wishes of the family and the primary physician, even though such a policy has many times brought unfortunate results.

In one such case I had a patient who had advanced cancer with lung involvement. Her husband, a powerful, domineering man, was adamant about not telling her about her illness. Throughout their marriage he had protected her from every unpleasantness; now he would protect her from the knowledge of her cancer. Against my own judgment and advice, I deferred to his wishes because I was afraid my interference would create a situation that could be emotionally damaging to the established structure of a 30-year marriage.

In accordance with instructions from her physician, who had known her for many years, and the concurrence of her husband, I told the woman she had an inflammation and instructed the hospital staff to be discreet in her presence. After exploratory surgery and chemotherapy she was released and went home. As her disease progressed, she gradually deteriorated and naturally wondered why, although her husband repeatedly assured her everything would be all right.

One evening she was admitted to another hospital for further therapy. Her husband was sitting with her when the medical resident visited her room to obtain a routine history and physical examination. She was frightened and in pain. In an effort to reassure her the doctor said, "Don't worry. You're in the hands of one of the best cancer doctors in San Francisco." The woman screamed and burst into tears. Her husband collapsed in his chair with chest pains. Fortunately, an emergency electrocardiogram and medical evaluation did not reveal the suspected heart attack, but the woman lost confidence in me and subsequently would believe only a part of anything I or her husband told her. She became depressed and angry, even more distrustful of her husband than she was of me. She died several weeks later.

We betrayed this patient, first by concealing the truth and then by failing to provide adequate protection from the truth—although I always felt she suspected she had cancer, as most patients do. If she had guessed her real condition before she died, she could not then have avoided feeling the same resentment and hurt she had felt on hearing it from a stranger. More significantly, however, she might perhaps have planned her final months differently if she had known she was going to die. The ambivalence of my feelings in this situation is obvious; but I do not feel that I as a consulting physician have a right to reverse such a critical decision unless the patient brings the matter up with me.

Of course, a patient who is not aware of the diagnosis of cancer presents other practical problems to a physician. The diagnostic and therapeutic procedures involved in most types of cancer are usually so complex that such a patient is bound to worry why such procedures are necessary for what he or she has been told is a simple infection. One does not easily explain away the need for radiation or drugs. (Fortunately, patients almost always know the truth. They have observed cancer in their friends, read about cancer in magazines and newspapers, and seen fictional and documentary television programs on the subject. Moreover, the public is constantly being urged to perform self-examinations for early detection, to avoid foods with certain additives, and to refrain from cigarette smoking.) I have found it is easier to take care of patients who know they have cancer, understand its implications, and are willing to make compromises and endure the side effects of therapy in the hope of attaining improved health.

PLANNING TREATMENT

In accordance with the terms of the unwritten contract, I try not to make any medical decisions without taking into consideration the emotional needs of patients. The more we talk about their family, work, religious views, hobbies, moods, and general life-style, the more I learn what those needs are. At the same time, I have to tell them that our choice of therapy, or combination of therapies, will be limited at any given time by their type of cancer and its stage of development. I describe the risks, side effects, and anticipated results of the most current, appropriate therapies, so that there will be no unnecessary shocks in the present or the future.

A therapy that is new to a patient must be given time to work so that the effects can be properly assessed. I try to explain to patients that when they buy a new car, they have no idea how well it is going to function until they have driven it for a few weeks or months. They then will know how it functions in terms of gas mileage and economy, how often it needs repairs, and so on. The same analogy applies to an analysis of the effects of a given therapy. Although the treatment differs for each type and stage of cancer, one must usually wait 6 to 12 weeks after a treatment has been instituted to appropriately assess the early results through laboratory tests, x-ray films, and scans.

Many people are concerned when changes are made in their therapeutic program, but a change does not always mean that cancer has progressed or that a new problem has appeared. It is not uncommon to change from one mode of therapy to another, to alter the dosage or content of a therapy, or even to cease treatment for limited periods. Sometimes such a change is made because a given therapy is not effective; at other times a new concept of treatment has proved valid, or a new treatment shows promise. Sometimes an unrelated medical problem or the patient's desire necessitates a change in, or cessation of, a particular therapy.

Fortunately, there are alternative therapies for most forms of cancer. I was told by one of my patients that I sometimes sound like a sorcerer with a magical bag of tricks, an indefinite number of therapies. Yet it is amazing how often a person who has been successfully treated on a given program and has subsequently relapsed can achieve another remission with a change in therapy. I am not saying that just because a patient accepts treatment, success is guaranteed. We all know there are limits to the possibilities of therapy. But a patient will never know what might have happened unless he or she is willing to try another therapy, assume the risks, and undergo assessment of the results. This is the commonsense approach to the treatment of cancer.

Oncologists must know what is current and available with regard to cancer therapy, as well as what may be forthcoming from cancer research, so that they can send their patients to specialized centers for treatment unavailable elsewhere. Nevertheless, despite assurances that they are receiving the most up-to-date and effective treatment known, some patients are so terrified that they will not accept standard therapy. This pattern is seen most frequently in patients who have been told that the currently available therapy for this disease will contain the rate of spread but holds little promise for cure. Unable to accept the fact that modern medicine cannot effect a cure, they spend much of their remaining life running in desperation to distant clinics or other countries seeking a miracle cure.

One patient who came to me for consultation and therapy had previously traveled to both Germany and Mexico with her husband because they had been unwilling to accept the therapy recommended at a major university cancer center in California. Instead, she took at least 20 different types of vitamins, plus carrot juice, various enzymes, and Laetrile. I recommended certain alternative medical therapies to this couple, but they were unable to make a choice. Finally, because valuable time was passing, I said to them, "There is no sense in my discussing this with you any further until you are willing to come to a decision. If you want me to decide for you, I'll be happy to do so. You have two choices at this time: surgery plus radiotherapy or, should you not want surgery, radiotherapy plus medical therapy—hormones and/or chemotherapy. I've explained the pros and cons of both approaches, and although I have a preference, I am not absolutely certain which is the better treatment. That can be assessed only after a therapy has been tried and the results graded. If you don't wish to try either one because of your own fears, that's your business. As far as I'm concerned, I'll wait to hear from you." This may sound like a tough approach after my description of the benefits of a reciprocal exchange between patient and physician, but a decision had to be made. Subsequently, it was made, and it resulted in a dramatic medical improvement with radiotherapy and chemotherapy.

Another patient, Louise Milner, whose story appears in this book, told me she was taking a 2-week vacation in Hawaii when she was actually darting off to Tijuana, Mexico for Laetrile treatments. The results of her flight were unfortunate.

Panic and flight are one kind of response. There are other reactions—anger, frustration, depression—for which I must be watchful. The most gallant ones among us may begin to lose their will and feel increasingly fearful after a long period of physical distress. A woman who had been cheerful under the most trying conditions became bitter and morose after repeated nausea during chemotherapy. A man who had fought in two wars, been wounded several times, and endured 15 months of bone cancer without complaint, was suddenly unable to discuss his case without falling asleep. I try to deal with these changes by altering medication, by visiting patients more frequently to discuss their problems and feelings, and by any other method I can think of that seems appropriate. Obviously some problems are resolvable whereas others are chronic with no satisfactory solution. In the latter cases, I believe it is good medical practice to consult another physician. Second and third opinions are becoming increasingly acceptable to both patients and physicians because they realize that no one has all the answers and that another point of view can be helpful, both psychologically and therapeutically.

No matter what a patient's anxieties may be, they should be brought to the attention of the doctor during regular office visits. Many of my patients continue to use the shopping list method that I suggested in our first talks. A person can be so anxious during an office visit, so fearful of receiving a poor medical report, that other troubling thoughts and questions that have arisen since the last visit are forgotten. The shopping list reminds the patient of these concerns, and discussion of them relieves many anxieties. Having a list of questions at hand also makes the most efficient use of the often limited time of an office visit.

OTHER SOURCES OF ANXIETY

Anxiety does not always originate in patients' concern with the medical aspects of their cancer. Sometimes it is related to the ordinary pressures of life—the fear of losing a job, or a misunderstanding with a relative or a friend—and compounded by having to cope with cancer. One of my patients holds a responsible, demanding job that could be jeopardized by the limitations on her energy resulting from her cancer and the therapy required. Her teenage children are always in trouble, and her former husband is unable to help emotionally or even to take care of the children when she is hospitalized. As a result of all these worries, she continued to be depressed even after she obtained a remission from anemia and advanced involvement of the liver and bone from breast cancer. However, because she shared her concerns with me, I was able to offer her extra emotional support. My wife, Isadora, the nurses in the office, and the social workers from Mt. Zion Hospital and Medical Center are also available to chat or make a referral to such services as group therapy, family counseling, or extra help at home.

Because it is not always possible to tell solely from office visits what extra burdens patients must endure in addition to their cancer, I try, if requested, to make a house call early in a relationship. A very well-dressed patient may actually live in minimal circumstances or suffer from tension caused by another family member. One of my patients, a young man with lung cancer, became desperately ill one evening and finally telephoned me. I found him in a rooming house in a deteriorating part of town. He lived in one small room and shared a bathroom at the end of the hall with several other people. When he suffered side effects from radiation he had to depend on the manager of the rooming house to bring him his meals. He had been too proud to ask for help, but, having discovered his true situation, I was able to mobilize nursing care and other assistance. In the home of another patient I found that life was organized around a senile grandparent to the extent that my patient, who had enough problems of her own, could not leave the house without getting a baby-sitter.

I envisage the role of a physician as an adviser and friend and in this capacity try to help patients plan new approaches with the aid of the medical team. This sometimes involves discussions of how a patient's illness, or the knowledge of his or her eventual death, is affecting each member of the family. Sometimes, too, when making a will or arranging insurance or other personal affairs becomes an unwelcome acknowledgment that an illness is terminal, I try to encourage a patient to act for the protection of his or her family. I explain that most people spend their entire working lives planning for the protection and support of their family. They buy insurance and make a will years before illness or death to assure that needed financial support will be available when needed.

I feel that I should become involved in such matters only when a patient indicates receptivity. But at the same time, when it seems to me there is a potential future problem due to a lack of planning, I look for a way to bring this to a patient's attention. I may then be able to provide the proper assistance by introducing my patient to a social worker, an attorney, or some other qualified person. I recently had a patient, Joan (Chap. 12), with terminal cancer, who had little money and was the sole support of a very young child. Arrangements were made for guardianship of the child by a young married relative well in advance of Joan's death. The assurance that her daughter would grow up in happy circumstances relieved Joan of her greatest anxiety.

Listening and talking, an atmosphere of openness and candor, are the means by which an enduring, supportive relationship is developed. If a patient will share emotional, financial, and other concerns with his or her physician, unexpected and welcome interest and help may be forthcoming. What patients tell me guides me in each decision regarding the treatment of their cancer and their general well-being; what I tell them—the knowledge of their disease and its treatment, present and future—hopefully reduces their anxiety and frees them to direct their thoughts toward life. But to make such a relationship a reality, patients must have the wisdom to know their needs and be able to tell their doctor.

REMISSIONS AND RELAPSES

A remission is the goal of every cancer patient. As with any other chronic disease—heart disease, diabetes, arthritis, or kidney disease—a remission can have differing durations and differing potential in terms of a person's long-term health. A complete remission can mean a return to health. No further evidence of the disease is detectable. A partial remission is a more limited medical response where the volume of cancer has been decreased but where the cancer is still detectable.

A person with a partial remission may feel well and enjoy a complete return to health even though significant tumor remains. The reason he or she feels well is that the tumor has been significantly reduced. Even a small reduction in size, as registered on an x-ray film, can bring physical relief.

Some patients remain on therapy indefinitely in the hope of containing or eradicating their disease. We not only encourage them to remain on therapy but to resume the activities of daily living—going to work, doing housework, participating in social events, and taking vacations—even if participation is limited while on therapy. (Usually a patient has a chance to relax between therapeutic programs if one program failed to produce a remission and he or she has agreed to try a new combination of drugs or therapies.)

The completion of a course of therapy is similar to graduating from high school or college. In our office we occasionally have wine or champagne to celebrate a patient's completion of a 12- to 18-month therapeutic program. But in spite of that first feeling of elation, life is not the same as it was before. You cannot go through such an experience without suffering some trauma. The impact of living with cancer affects to a greater or lesser extent your emotional reactions and intellectual approach to life. Every new ache or pain, which we all experience daily and ignore, raises for the former cancer patient the fear of a recurrence. I have been through this myself. Following recent surgery for a chest tumor that proved to be benign, I experienced new symptoms. Only a chest x-ray examination convinced me that the tumor had not recurred.

A recurrence for a person who has been in remission is devastating. But just as when the cancer was first detected, a therapeutic approach will be planned with the goal of a new remission. Anxiety, fear, and depression will again dominate, but they will also be dealt with as they were before. Most people who achieved a first remission and have a recurrence need only minimal encouragement to sustain their determination for a new round of treatment. Others are reluctant to continue. They may have found the side effects of surgery, radiotherapy, or chemotherapy, even when minimal, are more than they can tolerate. For example, an executive who underwent four intensive courses of chemotherapy, combined with immunotherapy, was elated during a period of remission. I warned him his case would have to be followed closely. Now another recurrence is suspected, and although an intensive program of chemotherapy might produce another remission, he insists that treatment be kept to a minimum. Of course, this decision is his prerogative.

When such patients announce that they no longer wish to be treated, or wish to receive only minimal treatment, I must be very convincing. A person with recurrence may have another chance at remission. The potential is there. I believe it is a chance worth taking.

The condition of all cancer patients, whether cured or in remission, should be closely monitored over the years. Patients should also be well informed about the prospects for recurrence of their cancer. With this knowledge they will be more likely to take the preventive measures that may once again save or prolong their lives.

7

Cancer therapy

*The desire to take medicine is perhaps the
greatest feature which distinguishes man
from animals.*

SIR WILLIAM OSLER

Surgery, radiation therapy (x-ray or cobalt), and drugs (chemotherapy) are currently the three mainstays in the treatment of cancer. Using one or a combination of these treatments, physicians are able to cure about 43% of all diagnosed malignancies. (A cure is defined as 5 years, cancer free.) Obviously, the cure rate for some types of cancer is much higher, and for others much lower, than this average. It is important to note here that though treatment fails to cure approximately 57% of those who have cancer, it is rare that vigorous treatment does not *materially* benefit the patient. Even in cases when it is obvious from the onset that cure is unlikely or impossible, adequate therapy can assure a patient not only freedom from pain but many additional months to years of a relatively normal life. A person may even live a normal life span with chronic cancer and die eventually of an unrelated cause.

Nevertheless, it is surprising how often one encounters a nihilistic attitude toward the treatment of cancer, not only among patients and the lay public, but even within the medical community. This attitude can be summed up as, "If it cannot be cured, why bother treating it?" It seems strange that such thinking persists in a society in which the treatment of other incurable diseases, such as heart disease and diabetes, is readily accepted.

Another reason many people refuse treatment for their disease is that they have heard frightening stories about the side effects of treatment. These stories make them more afraid of treatment than they are of cancer. These fears are largely unwarranted, especially today when side effects are increasingly better controlled with improved antinausea drugs, marijuana (which also counteracts nausea), and improved techniques for achieving good nutrition while on chemotherapy. Bleeding and infections are also better controlled, and pain and suffering can be reduced, alleviated, or often prevented altogether.

SURGERY

Surgery offers the ideal primary approach to the cancer problem. If it is possible to "cut it out" without major functional impairment and there is no

60

residual disease, a person may be cured. Surgical excision is appropriate when a tumor is localized and does not involve vital structures. For example, normal function can be maintained after the removal of a kidney or part of a lung.

In some cases, a biopsy is performed at the start of surgery when a small tissue sample is removed and sent to a pathologist for examination. The pathologist immediately reports the findings to the surgeon. If the tumor contains no malignant cells, the surgeon can perform a conservative or limited operation to remove the suspicious mass. If the tumor contains malignant cells, the surgeon can immediately perform an operation designed to eliminate all traces of the malignancy.

Frequently a surgeon is able to remove all visible evidence of the cancer, presumably effecting a cure. However, depending on the type and stage of the tumor, cancer will recur in a certain percentage of cases either adjacent to its original location or at some distant site, such as the liver, lungs, brain, or another organ. This hallmark of cancer—its tendency to metastasize (spread) before the parent tumor is diagnosed and removed—constitutes the single greatest problem in the management of malignant diseases; it is the reason for the importance of having close medical follow-up after treatment for cancer and for the necessity of waiting several months or years after an operation to be certain of cure.

RADIATION THERAPY

The purpose of radiation therapy is to damage the genetic structure (DNA) of tumor cells to make them incapable of further growth and division. In radiation therapy, a beam of x-rays, gamma rays (from cobalt or radium), or electrons is aimed directly at the tumor from the x-ray machine, which is usually located at a specific distance from the body. Newer, still experimental techniques utilize heavy particles—pi mesons (pions) and neutrons—to treat cancers that are less sensitive to conventional radiation.

The x-ray machine is in a special room that is shielded with lead walls to protect x-ray technicians and the radiation therapist, who treat patients daily, from receiving excessive doses of radiation.

The area to be treated is carefully outlined for each patient with a colored marker; this colored outline remains on the body throughout the course of therapy. The marking procedure is usually carried out in a simulation room (a room in which x-rays are taken) by the staff radiotherapist to map out the borders of the tumor. The normal tissues surrounding the tumor receive careful consideration. A lead mold is especially made to protect the normal organs. The mold is placed above the patient on a special tray attached to the machine during radiotherapy so that the beams will only strike the tumor.

It is unlikely that a patient will begin treatment on the same day as the simulation because many of the beam-shaping devices require casting in the form of a mold. This work is usually done by the dosimetrist, a specialist who calculates the dose of radiation to be given.

The tumor and the tolerance of the tissues in the area to be treated, as well as anticipated side effects, are considered when the mathematical calculations for the radiation dose are made for the individual patient. These calculations are based on CT scans and other sophisticated roentgenographic techniques. The development of high-energy machines has markedly reduced the potential for damage to normal cells.

Most major medical centers now have a full range of megavoltage equipment ranging from cobalt to linear accelerators. Depending on the type and location of the tumor, the radiotherapist will select the most appropriate machine to treat the tumor and spare normal tissues.

A patient does not feel any pain or discomfort while receiving radiation therapy. Undergoing treatment is like having a chest x-ray examination (which gives a very minute dose of radiation), the difference being that in radiation therapy the x-ray machine is left on for several minutes to give a therapeutic dose of radiation.

Side effects may occur from radiation therapy as a result of damage to normal tissues. These side effects are determined by the tissues involved. For instance, hair loss may result from radiation to the head, whereas loss of taste and problems in swallowing can occur with head and neck radiation. Nausea, vomiting, and diarrhea are often the result of radiation to the abdomen. Skin in the path of the radiation beam may become red, itchy, and dry. Improved equipment and safety techniques have, for many patients, lessened or eliminated some of these side effects, particularly skin irritation, nausea, vomiting, and diarrhea. Fortunately, radiation therapy is usually limited to 1 to 6 weeks, and most side effects are not permanent.

Sometimes radiation is administered internally, directly into the tumor. This procedure is usually carried out in an operating room under general anesthesia where the radioisotopic material (such as radium) is implanted in small tubes or inserted with needles near or through the tumor. The tubes or needles are allowed to remain in the tumor for a calculated number of hours, allowing the tumor to be treated with a high dose of radiation. Internal radiation can be used in conjunction with external-beam radiation to concentrate the dose to the local area.

Certain tumors, such as cancer of the cervix and the breast, and Hodgkin's disease, may be cured by radiation therapy. Hope for many cancer patients not cured by surgery may lie in this method of treatment. Radiation treatment is not a last resort, as many people think, but a practical method of killing cancer cells, restricting their growth, or reducing a tumor to a size at which surgery becomes practical.

The most likely candidate for radiation is the patient with localized cancer. But even when cancer has spread, radiation may also be used. It can reduce a cancer mass that may be forming an obstruction, causing pain, or presenting a risk of bone fracture.

Radiation therapy is often given in conjunction with another form of cancer treatment such as surgery or chemotherapy. For example, a preoperative dose of radiation may be given to sterilize microscopic tumors a surgeon would be unable to detect when removing the bulk of the disease. Alternatively, chemotherapy such as adriamycin might be administered during the same period radiation therapy is given. The combination of these therapies is potentially more effective in controlling certain tumors, but also may have increased side effects. These side effects can be minimized by monitoring the doses of chemotherapy and radiation therapy.

CHEMOTHERAPY

The word chemotherapy is one of the most misunderstood words in the English language. The meaning is clear: chemo = chemical (or drug) + therapy. When aspirin is used for a headache, penicillin for an infection, digitalis for heart disease, or 5-fluorouracil for colon cancer, it is called chemotherapy—drugs or medications to treat disease.

When mentioned in conjunction with cancer, chemotherapy has bad connotations. Much of this is deserved, but many times it is greatly exaggerated. Not all of the drugs produce serious side effects, and many patients have minimal toxic reactions. There is little publicity concerning the person who comes to the office or clinic, sticks out an arm, takes chemotherapy shots for colon, breast, or ovarian cancer, and then goes to work or home and functions fairly well.

The majority of people can tolerate therapy; some patients have moderate to severe reactions; and a few patients cannot tolerate therapy at all. Fortunately, there are many ways to reduce the side effects, some of which will be discussed in the following.

The purpose of chemotherapy is to treat more advanced or metastatic cancer. It is also used as a cancer preventive by being given as an extra safeguard after surgical removal of a tumor (adjuvant chemotherapy) for cases with a high risk of recurrence. Approximately 50 chemotherapeutic drugs are currently available, although about 30 of these drugs are used to treat the majority of cancers.

Chemotherapy is generally reserved for systemic or invasive cancers, cancers that are spread by the lymph or blood systems to many parts of the body, whereas surgery or radiation therapy is used to treat more localized cancers. Originally used only in cases in which surgery and radiation therapy were no longer effective, chemotherapy is increasingly given after surgical treatment or in conjunction with radiation therapy as an additional safeguard or preventive measure. (See section on Adjuvant Chemotherapy.) In a few diseases, such as Burkitt's lymphoma, choriocarcinoma, ovarian cancer, leukemia, testicular cancer, and some cases of advanced Hodgkin's disease, cures may be achieved by the judicious and aggressive use of chemotherapy alone or in combination with radiotherapy.

Like healthy cells, cancer cells are involved in a continuous process of change, alternately resting and dividing. This is the process a cell undergoes to reproduce and make two daughter cells. However, unlike healthy cells, cancer cells divide in an uncontrollable manner and invade normal tissues. Chemotherapy takes advantage of our knowledge of how cells multiply by dividing. The chemotherapeutic agents are cellular poisons, classified as cell-cycle specific, noncell-cycle specific, and miscellaneous. These classifications refer to the timing of administration of the chemotherapeutic agents.

Because many cells are killed more easily during the process of division than when they are resting, the cell-cycle specific class of drugs (the antimetabolites) is used to attack the cancer cells during the phase of cellular division when they are more vulnerable.

The noncell-cycle specific class of drugs, the alkylating or mustard group, tend to attack all the cells in a tumor, whether they are resting or dividing. These drugs are used to generally reduce the tumor mass. Then the remaining tumor cells (many of which were inactive before administration of the noncell-cycle drug) may become active and start dividing, at which time a cell-cycle drug can be administered. Noncell-cycle and cell-cycle drugs are often used in such a sequence to obtain the maximum therapeutic effect.

As with radiotherapy, it is virtually impossible to attack cancer cells with drugs without affecting normal tissues as well. The normal cells in the body are also dividing, and those that divide the fastest are more susceptible to drug damage. Such fast-dividing normal cells are found in the lining of the digestive tract, in the hair follicles, and in the bone marrow that makes blood cells. Damage to these normal cells from chemotherapeutic agents leads to side effects such as nausea, vomiting, and lowered blood counts (bone marrow). Each drug has its own side effects. Fortunately, these side effects are *not* permanent.

Several different medications are available to combat nausea and vomiting. A few examples are prochlorperazine (Compazine), dimenhydrinate (Dramamine), droperidol (Inapsine), and metoclopramide (Reglan). Marijuana is also effective in counteracting nausea. An experimental program controlled by individual states and the National Cancer Institute provides the active ingredient in marijuana (THC or tetrahydrocannabinol) to be given in cigarettes or pill form. Many patients obtain marijuana from private sources to add to brownies, cookies, or other food or to brew as tea or take in gelatin capsules by mouth or in rectal suppositories.

The amount of hair loss from chemotherapy varies from hair thinning to baldness. Depending on the drug being used, these effects can sometimes be reduced by using a scalp tourniquet or ice cap. In any event, hair loss is temporary, and many patients find that their hair starts growing back while they are still receiving chemotherapy.

When the bone marrow is damaged by chemotherapeutic drugs, red blood cell, platelet, and white blood cell transfusions can be given, based on the need. The need for these transfusions is determined by the blood cell count, which is monitored frequently during a course of treatment. The bone marrow returns to normal with time (2 to 3 weeks).

Tolerance to a particular drug or combination of drugs varies with each individual. Psychological support from family, friends, and medical team during the treatment cycle is always important. One person may experience major toxicity whereas another is minimally affected. I do not like to overemphasize the possibility of side effects because I believe that anxiety about discomfort has produced in some of my patients stronger reactions than they might otherwise have had. Conversely, I am convinced that other patients experience fewer side effects because of their relaxed attitude toward chemotherapy. At one time the philosophy of medical therapy was that to be effective a medicine had to make you sick. There does not appear to be a direct correlation between the degree of discomfort from drug treatment and the degree of medical effectiveness. The most toxic therapy may be ineffective, whereas favorable results may be obtained with minimal side effects.

When severe side effects occur, I try to alter the amount of drugs or the time of application to ease the discomfort of undergoing treatment. For example, working people can often be put on a program that does not interfere with their work schedules. Persons with cancer may receive their therapy just before the weekend so that any side effects will have worn off by Monday. Alternatively, as Mort Segal did, a person can switch from a morning to an evening chemotherapy program so that the work schedule will not be interrupted because of side effects (see Chap. 11). Joan Stansfield's chemotherapy drug program was altered so she could continue to run her household and fulfill her job obligations (see Chap. 12). The aim of these adjustments in treatment is to keep a patient functioning as fully as possible.

Chemotherapeutic drugs may be given in pill or liquid form, or by shots in either a vein or an artery. Single or multiple drugs may also be infused (injected) into certain organs such as the liver, using a small pump to obtain a constant flow of drugs. The method of administration (pill or injections) depends on the drugs. For example, certain drugs are only given intravenously because, when taken orally, they are not readily absorbed in the gastrointestinal tract and/or produce gastrointestinal side effects such as nausea, diarrhea, or other toxic symptoms.

The necessity for frequent office visits can be reduced when chemotherapy is given orally. (Unfortunately, many drugs must be given by injection in the office.) Even when such independence is possible, however, there is still a need for periodic office visits for blood counts and blood chemistry analyses to check the amount of oral chemotherapy needed. The intravenous administration of certain drugs, such as platinum or bleomycin, usually requires hospitalization for a period of 1 to 5 days.

A more complex chemotherapeutic program may require more frequent office visits (often 3 to 5 days in a row) for a cycle of therapy, followed by a rest period. The method by which therapy is given is determined by the physician in consultation with the patient, as well as by the type and stage of malignancy.

There are several ways of evaluating the body's response to therapy, including blood counts, x-ray tests, special isotope scans, blood chemistry panels of liver or kidney function, and other analyses of general body function. These procedures provide a means of detecting toxicity and reducing side effects. They also serve as safeguards before continuing with current therapy or proceeding with a new form of therapy.

Progress is continually being made. An experimental laboratory technique (the clonogenic assay) uses cancer cells grown in culture on a special double-gel layer (a layered gel). Chemotherapeutic drugs are tested on these cells to grade how many colonies of cells survive compared to tumor cells in a control group that are not tested with chemotherapeutic drugs. The tumor cultures are also tested with several different chemotherapeutic drugs and combinations of drugs to determine the most effective treatment for a given patient.

There are a few new chemotherapeutic drugs, but sometimes the same drugs used in a new combination and/or administered on different schedules can make the difference between success and failure in destroying cancer cells. Table 2 lists the most commonly used chemotherapeutic drugs, the diseases they treat, and the possible side effects.

ADJUVANT CHEMOTHERAPY

Adjuvant chemotherapy is a program of additional chemotherapy administered to patients who have a high risk of recurrence of their cancer. It is given after basic treatment by surgery, chemotherapy, or radiation therapy in the hope of eliminating any undetectable microscopic cells that may have traveled to other parts of the body. If such treatment does not produce a cure, it usually will prolong the interval before there is a recurrence.

The most widely used adjuvant chemotherapeutic program is given for breast cancer under three conditions: when cancer cells have been found in the lymph nodes during surgery; when the tumor is large, indicating a possibility of metastasis; and when there are negative hormone receptors. (Receptors are special proteins inside the cell that combine with hormones to take them into the nucleus. When these receptors are found to be absent, they are considered "negative," and the risk of a recurrence of cancer is increased.) Adjuvant therapy for breast cancer is usually administered for 12 to 18 months.

HORMONAL THERAPY

Many cancers are responsive to hormonal therapy, an attempt to reduce a tumor by the administration of hormones, orally or by injection, or by the removal of organs that produce hormones (ovaries, testicles, adrenal glands, or pituitary gland). These hormones are given to reduce the body's production of, or to block the action of, specific hormones that promote the growth of cancer cells. These mechanisms are still only partially understood.

Tumors of the prostate, breast, and kidney have been controlled or significantly reduced by hormonal therapy. Hormonal receptors are important in predicting whether a person will respond to hormonal therapy.

The side effects of hormonal therapy are usually less toxic than those of chemotherapy. However, a small percentage of patients experience nausea, vomiting, and (occasionally) elevated levels of serum calcium. These symptoms are sometimes relieved by the same antinausea drugs used to relieve nausea from chemotherapy.

EXPERIMENTAL THERAPIES

Physicians and other scientists are continually developing new approaches to the treatment of cancer. Such an approach may involve a new combination —or a new technique of administering—the three major anticancer therapies, or it may involve the development of a new drug or combination of drugs.

Experimental approaches to cancer treatment undergo lengthy testing in the laboratory (and in animals) before being introduced into human medicine. However, evidence from animal experiments, though very helpful, cannot be easily translated to humans, and there comes a moment of truth when an experimental treatment is justified for trial with cancer patients. Such patients are always given a detailed explanation of the reasons for their doctor's opinion that an experimental treatment is justified in their case.

There is an unwritten rule that an unproven experimental therapy is never used on a patient for whom there exists a tried and effective alternative treatment. Experimental therapy is used only when there is a good reason for believing it will be superior to conventional therapy.

Experimental immunotherapy (biological modifiers)

Research on animals and humans has shown a relationship between the body's natural defenses against disease (the immune system) and cancer. For years physicians believed that the immune system was effective only in combating infectious diseases caused by agents such as bacteria and viruses. It is only recently that scientists have learned that the immune system may play a key role in protecting the body against the development of cancer as well as in combating cancer that has already developed. The latter role is not readily apparent, but there is evidence that a competent immune system slows down the rate at which tumors grow and spread.

The immune system consists of lymphocytes (one kind of white blood cells), which act as the body's defense system against foreign organisms such as pollens, bacteria, fungi, cancers, and viruses. One type of lymphocyte, the T cell, is formed originally in the thymus gland, a small lymph gland in the neck near the thyroid gland. T cells are natural killers of foreign cells, including cancer cells.

A second kind of lymphocyte, the B lymphocyte, originates in the bone marrow. The B lymphocyte produces antibodies (gamma globulin) after stimulation from a foreign protein (antigen) and also kills cancer cells.

Another white cell (which, however, does not originate in the lymphatic system) is the monocyte, a large white blood cell that interacts with the T and B lymphocytes and can also kill cancer cells. Unfortunately, sometimes these cells are out of balance, allowing cancer cells to grow. These mechanisms are still being studied to help clarify some of the mysteries.

Immunotherapy attempts to use the body's natural defenses—the T and B lymphocytes and monocytes—to destroy cancer cells. There are documented cases where humans with early and advanced cancer have had complete and partial resolution of tumor after treatment with immunotherapy.

text continued on p. 74

TABLE 2
Chemotherapy drugs: uses and possible side effects

Drug	Route of administration	Disease	Possible side effects
Alkylating agents*			
Chlorambucil (Leukeran)	Oral	Chronic lymphocytic leukemia; lymphomas; breast and ovarian cancer	Nausea, lowered blood counts
Cyclophosphamide (Cytoxan)	Intravenous; oral	Lymphomas, breast or ovary; myeloma, lung; leukemia	Nausea and vomiting, lowered blood counts, hair loss, bloody urine (can be prevented by drinking lots of fluid), chronic lung problems
Nitrogen mustard, HN2 (Mustargen)	Intravenous	Hodgkin's disease; lymphomas; lung, mycosis fungoides; ovarian cancer	Nausea and vomiting, lowered blood counts, hair loss, inflamed veins
Melphalan, Phenylalanine mustard, L–Pam (Alkeran)	Oral	Breast, ovary myeloma; testicular cancer	Mild nausea, lowered blood counts
Busulfan (Myleran)	Oral	Chronic myelogenous leukemia	Nausea, lowered blood counts, chronic lung problems, skin darkening, hair loss, breast enlargement
Triethylenethio-phosphoramide (Thiotepa)	Intravenous; intracavitary to prevent fluid accumulation; local instillation for bladder	Breast, ovarian, and bladder cancer	Nausea and vomiting, lowered blood counts, loss of appetite
Carmustine (BCNU), lomustine (CCNU), semustine (methyl-CCNU)	Oral and intravenous	Brain cancer; melanoma; colon, gastric, lung, pancreas lymphomas; Hodgkin's disease	Nausea and vomiting, lowered blood counts

TABLE 2
Chemotherapy drugs: uses and possible side effects—cont'd

Drug	Route of administration	Disease	Possible side effects
Antimetabolites			
5-Fluorouracil, 5-FU	Intravenous; oral for special reasons	Colon, stomach, breast, pancreas, liver, ovary, bladder, prostate cancers	Nausea and vomiting, diarrhea, mouth sores or ulcers, lowered blood counts, skin darkening (sensitive to sun), hair loss, skin rash, poor muscle coordination, nail changes
Methotrexate (MTX, Amethopterin)	Intravenous; oral; intramuscular; subcutaneous; intra-arterial; intrathecal	Choriocarcinoma; acute leukemia; lymphomas; sarcomas; head and neck, breast, colon, lung, testicular cancers	Nausea and diarrhea, mouth sores, gastrointestinal problems, lowered blood counts
Cytarabine, ara-C, cytosine arabinoside (Cytosar)	Intravenous; intrathecal; subcutaneous	Acute leukemia; lymphomas	Nausea and vomiting, diarrhea, bone marrow depression, mouth sores
6-Mercaptopurine, 6-MP (Purinethol)	Oral	Acute leukemia	Nausea and vomiting, lowered blood counts, mouth sores, skin rash (needs lower dose when used with allopurinol)
Hydroxyurea (Hydrea)	Oral	Head and neck cancer; chronic myelogenous leukemia; kidney cancer	Nausea and vomiting, lowered blood counts
6-Thioguanine, GTG (Thioguanine)	Oral	Acute leukemia	Nausea and vomiting, lowered blood counts, skin rash

continued.

TABLE 2
Chemotherapy drugs: uses and possible side effects — cont'd

Drug	Route of administration	Disease	Possible side effects
Anticancer antibiotics			
Bleomycin (Blenoxane)	Intravenous; intramuscular; subcutaneous; regional arterial infusion	Cancers of head and neck, testicular, cervix, skin; lymphomas; Hodgkin's disease; sarcomas	Nausea and vomiting, skin rash, fever, skin peeling or tenderness, chronic lung problems, mouth sores, hair loss, headache, swelling and pain in joints
Doxorubicin (Adriamycin)	Intravenous	Cancers of breast, bladder, thyroid, lung, ovary; acute leukemia; sarcomas; neuroblastoma; Hodgkin's disease; lymphomas	Nausea and vomiting, red urine, lowered blood counts, total hair loss, mouth sores, liver damage, heart problems (dose related), skin darkening (nails, creases); can reactivate skin reactions from past radiation
Daunorubicin daunomycin, rubidomycin, cerubidine	Intravenous	Acute leukemia	Nausea and vomiting, total hair loss, red urine, lowered blood counts
Dactinomycin actinomycin D (Cosmegen)	Intravenous	Testicular cancer; melanoma; choriocarcinoma; Wilms' tumor; neuroblastoma; rhabdomyosarcoma; Ewing's sarcoma	Nausea and vomiting, swelling of veins, mouth sores, hair loss, lowered blood counts, skin rash
Mithramycin (Mithracin)	Intravenous	Testicular cancer, hypercalcemia	Nausea and vomiting, diarrhea, lowered blood counts (liver and/or kidney damage), mouth sores, loss of appetite

TABLE 2

Chemotherapy drugs: uses and possible side effects—cont'd

Drug	Route of administration	Disease	Possible side effects
Mitomycin, mitomycin-C (Mutamycin)	Intravenous	Gastric, pancreas, colon, breast, head and neck cancers	Nausea and vomiting, lowered blood counts, prolonged anorexia
Streptozocin (Streptozotocin)	Intravenous	Pancreas	Nausea and vomiting, diarrhea, lowered blood sugar, headache, weakness
Plant products-alkaloids			
Vincristine (Oncovin)	Intravenous	Hodgkin's disease; lymphomas, breast; acute leukemias; Wilms' tumor; brain, childhood humors	Nausea; hair loss; constipation; pain in arms, legs, jaw, stomach; numbness or tingling in hands or feet; foot drop, lowered blood counts
Vinblastine (Velban)	Intravenous	Hodgkin's disease, lymphomas; leukemias; testicular and breast cancer	Nausea and vomiting, lowered blood counts, hair loss, mouth sores, loss of reflexes, severe constipation, abdominal pain
Miscellaneous			
Cisplatin, cis-platinum (cis-diamminedichloro-platinum, CDDP) (Platinol)	Intravenous	Testicular, ovarian, head and neck, bladder, prostate, and breast cancers	Severe nausea and vomiting, bone marrow depression, kidney damage, hearing problems (ringing), loss of sensation or dull feeling around arms and legs

continued.

TABLE 2

Chemotherapy drugs: uses and possible side effects—cont'd

Drug	Route of administration	Disease	Possible side effects
Asparaginase (Elspar)	Intravenous; intramuscular	Acute lymphoblastic leukemia; some lymphomas	Nausea, fever, allergic response, abdominal pain, diabetes, liver damage, pancreatitis, mental depression, and blood clotting problems
5-Azacitidine (5-azacytidine)	Intravenous	Acute granulocytic leukemia	Nausea and vomiting, diarrhea, fever, blood count depression, liver damage
Mitotane, o, p'DDD (Lysodren)	Oral	Adrenocortical carcinoma	Nausea and vomiting, diarrhea, mental depression, tremors, visual disturbances, skin rashes, lethargy, drowsiness
Dacarbazine, carboximide (DTIC-Dome imidazole)	Intravenous	Melanoma; lymphomas; Hodgkin's disease; sarcomas	Nausea, vomiting, lowered blood counts, facial flushing, flulike symptoms
Investigational* Hexamethylmelamine	Oral	Lung, ovary, and breast cancer, lymphoma	Nausea and vomiting, bone marrow depression, mental depression
VP16-213 (epipodophyllotoxin)	Intravenous; oral	Lymphomas; monocytic leukemia; lung cancer	Nausea and vomiting, bone marrow depression, hair loss

*Can cause gonadal dysfunction (sterility); long-term use can lead to a slight increase in leukemia.

TABLE 2

Chemotherapy drugs: uses and possible side effects—cont'd

Drug	Route of administration	Disease	Possible side effects
Hormones			
Cortisones Prednisone, dexamethasone, Methylpredniso-lone (Medrol)	Oral	Lymphomas; Hodgkin's disease; breast cancer; acute leukemias; myeloma	Fluid retention (edema), weight gain, increased appetite and sense of well-being; increased blood sugars, high blood pressure, loss of potassium, in-creased risk of infection, skin acne, increased stomach acidity and ulcers, agita-tion or sleepiness
Dexamethasone (Decadron, Hexadrol)	Oral	Brain tumors and metastatic disease in the brain	Fluid retention
DES-Estrogens, diethylstilbestrol, female hor-mones (TACE, Stilphostrol)	Oral	Breast, prostate	Nausea and vomiting, cramps, fluid retention, increased blood calcium, feminization, bleeding (uterine), tender breasts, impotence
Tamoxifen (antiestrogens) (Nolvadex)	Oral	Breast	Nausea (rare vomit-ing), bone pain, vaginal itching, headache, hot flashes
Testosterones (male hormones), (Fluoxymesterone, Halotestin)	Oral	Breast	Nausea and vomiting, hair growth, fluid retention, mascu-linization, jaundice, lowered voice, liver damage

continued.

TABLE 2

Chemotherapy drugs: uses and possible side effects—cont'd

Drug	Route of administration	Disease	Possible side effects
Progesterones, medroxypro- gesterone (Provera-Megase); hydroxyproges- terone caproate (Delalutin)	Intramuscular, oral	Endometrial, kidney, breast, and prostate cancers	Pain on injection, fluid retention, and impotence (rare)

History of immunotherapy. In the early 1900s, Dr. William Bradford Coley at Sloan Kettering Institute observed that some patients with head and neck cancers had tumor control or reduction following streptococcal bacterial infections. He subsequently made a vaccine of mixed bacterial toxins called Coley's toxins (made from streptococcal and staphylococcal bacterial organisms) in the hope of reproducing the results of the cases he had observed. He successfully treated many patients, some of whose tumors disappeared completely.

In 1922, Leon Calmette and Camille Guérin of France developed the Bacillus-Calmette-Guérin (BCG). BCG (the tuberculosis vaccine) or *Coryne- bacterium parvum* (a benign bacterial vaccine), promotes an overall increased activity in the immune system in fighting infections, diseases, and cancer in the early stages. Thus when local melanoma lesions are injected directly with BCG, the results are frequently resolution and control not only of the local tumor that was injected with the BCG but of about one-fifth of the skin tumors located at some distance from the local tumor.

BCG has also been used following surgery for advanced cancer, but the results of treatment of advanced cancers have been less successful than treatment of early cancers. However, there is evidence that patients with certain advanced tumors, such as melanomas, survived longer than expected after treatment with BCG.

BCG and similar therapies have not proved effective when there is cancer involvement of the internal organs such as the gastrointestinal tract, liver, or lungs.

Researchers have traced the natural history of a series of advanced melanomas, kidney, and other tumors. They have discovered that tumor resolution (disappearance of the tumor) occasionally occurs even without therapy, giving credence to the theory of spontaneous remission of cancer. These remissions are believed to be related to the functioning of the immune system, which treats the cancer as a foreign tissue in the same way it would normally reject another person's kidney or heart. Everson and Cole have carefully documented these cases in their book, *The Spontaneous Regression of Cancer* (1966).

In the late 1960s, immunotherapy received a great deal of publicity, generating much expectation and hope. These expectations have not yet been fulfilled, but the hope, in the form of extensive research efforts, continues. These research efforts are now leading to several promising possibilities of treatment through biological modifiers, a new name for immunotherapeutic agents. The biological modifiers currently being studied—transfer factor, interferon, thymosin, and monoclonal antibodies—are described next.

Transfer factor. Transfer factor is a low-molecular-weight dialyzable extract (probably nucleotides) from normal white blood cells (from blood bank donors, patients cured of a similar cancer, or members of the same household who have never had cancer). Transfer factor stimulates the T cells to help correct a deficiency in the immune system.

Many studies of transfer factor are in progress around the country. Our group has been treating people with transfer factor who have invasive melanomas and show no evidence of tumor, but who are nevertheless at a high risk to have a recurrence of their cancer. (High risk is determined by the pathologist based on depth of invasion of the original tumor.) The results of our research look promising, but many more years of research are required.

Transfer factor has been used successfully against diseases that have resisted conventional therapy such as tuberculosis and a fungus called Valley Fever (coccidioidomycosis).

Interferon. Interferon is a group of proteins produced naturally by white blood cells in the body or in the laboratory in response to a viral infection or similar stimulation. It has been used experimentally as a treatment for certain viral diseases such as herpes zoster (shingles), "adult chicken pox." Interferon is being used experimentally against various tumors such as melanomas, breast cancer, lymphomas, and bladder cancer. The preliminary results of these experiments are promising, but they have not yet produced the extensive cures that newspaper articles and other media lead people to expect.

Formerly, synthetic interferon made in the laboratory was less than 1% pure. These early interferons produced many toxic reactions, including fever, hair loss, blood count depression, and rashes. New methods of producing interferon have markedly increased the percentage of purity. Hopefully, these new interferons will produce less toxicity and be more effective against cancer.

Thymosin. Thymosin, another biological modifier, is produced by the thymus gland, the master gland in the body's immune system where T cells originate. Several new types of thymosin are now being made through recombinant-DNA genetic engineering. "Thymosin Fraction 5" has shown promise, when used in conjunction with chemotherapy, for treatment of head and neck cancers and lung carcinoma.

Monoclonal antibodies (hybridomas). Another new experimental technique that is currently creating interest involves some of the newer tools called hybridomas. (A hybridoma is a chimera, a name derived from the Greek beast of mythology who has a lion's head, a goat's body, and a serpent's tail.) In creating monoclonal antibodies, scientists have combined single cells from mice or men that can be programmed to produce specific antibodies that can seek and possibly kill cancer cells and not affect normal cells. These single cells are like B cells and produce specific monoclonal antibodies (a highly specific uniform gamma globulin) programmed to do specific jobs on targets in the body. Hybridomas have a potential for diagnosing as well as for treating cancer. Monoclonal antibody diagnostic kits have recently been approved by the Food and Drug Administration (FDA) to diagnose allergies. A similar process being developed for the diagnosis of cancer will enhance the physician's diagnostic capability.

Monoclonal antibodies are produced as follows: A mouse is injected with a protein (antigen) from a human tumor and the mouse responds by producing antibodies (gamma globulin) against the human tumor. Then the mouse's spleen is removed and cells that can produce the antibodies are separated from the spleen. These activated spleen cells are fused (joined) to tumor cells from a *second* mouse. This fusion results in a new clone of cells—the chimera, which produces monoclonal antibody against a specific antigenic determinant.

By techniques of genetic engineering, the hybrid cells that produce the antibodies can be cloned and are maintained as producing factories in tissue culture. The monoclonal antibody product of these cells is injected into a patient; the antibodies then go directly to the cancer cells. Researchers are studying the possibility of tying cytotoxic chemicals or radioisotopes to the antibodies to enhance their effectiveness against cancer cells. The result would be like a guided missile going to a specific target. When fully developed, this technique will have a remarkable potential in cancer treatment.

Immunotherapy (biological modifiers) is still an unproven form of treatment. When it is effective, it is usually against a small number of cancer cells. Therefore, many of the experiments are set up to prevent recurrence in patients whose cancer has been removed or reduced by surgery or destroyed or reduced by chemotherapy or radiotherapy. The body's ability to develop an immune reaction to a tumor may prove to be the decisive factor in determining which patients are cured of cancer after they have received conventional therapy such as surgery, radiation, or chemotherapy. We must wait for the results of current research before immunotherapy becomes a standard rather than an experimental therapy.

Hyperthermia

Hyperthermia, the use of heat in the treatment of cancer, has been practiced periodically for the last 4000 years. Since 1900, there has been mounting evidence that tumor cells can be killed by heating tumors to 42° to 43° C (108°F) for limited periods of time.

Hyperthermia works because cancer cells are more sensitive to heat than normal cells. Additionally, most tumors have poor circulation (blood supply), which means that they tend to retain heat and cannot eliminate it as well as normal cells.

The heat in a hyperthermia treatment is often delivered by use of a radio-frequency that can heat internally without hurting the skin. Both local tumors and metastatic tumors in most locations in the body (including organs such as the liver) can be treated in this way. After treatment, the dead tumor cells (known as tumor necrosis) are replaced by scar tissue. The use of radiation therapy or chemotherapy concurrently with hyperthermia may enhance the total anticancer therapeutic effect.

Although still considered experimental, hyperthermia may well become a fifth modality of cancer treatment when further improvements in methods of application are combined with appropriate combinations of chemotherapy and/or radiation therapy.

QUACK THERAPIES

Living with cancer creates a state of uncertainty, insecurity, and fear that is at times unendurable. It is not surprising that anxiety can reach a level of panic where a person will be willing to try an unproven method of treatment that has been publicized in the press as a "miracle cure." Resort to one of these therapies occurs among those who are receiving good medical support as well as those who are not. Neither a high level of education nor the ability to reason will deter the desperate patient. A person who has cancer wants a cure. When standard medical therapy cannot *guarantee* a cure, that person may go to any length to obtain a treatment that has not been sanctioned by any reputable doctor, researcher, or government agency. No one wants to die without exhausting every possible means of cure, and a patient is often encouraged by well-meaning friends and family members who have no knowledge of cancer treatment.

Depression and panic can make a patient prey to any speculator who claims to have a cure. Some quack practitioners may sincerely believe their methods are effective; others are just capitalizing on people's misfortune. In any event, quacks with their false cancer cures cost American patients $2–3 billion a year.

The clinical course of cancer is highly variable. As already mentioned, a rare event, such as a remission or cure, can occur without a patient's having received conventional treatment. (Medical literature documents these cases.) However, if this happy event should coincide with or follow treatment by an unproven therapy, the patient will invariably credit that treatment for the improvement. Similarly, a person who achieves a remission while being treated simultaneously by conventional therapy and a quack therapy will tend to believe the quack treatment is responsible for combating the cancer.

Following the appearance of newspaper and magazine articles on miracle cures, physicians are bombarded with questions about these unorthodox methods of treatment. "What about diet? What about megavitamin therapy? What about that new drug that's only available abroad?" Physicians can only reply that in their experience and the experience of other practitioners, these methods have not proved to be of any benefit to cancer patients.

Some of my patients supplement conventional treatment with megadoses of vitamins, Laetrile (a drug derived from apricot pits), coffee enemas, and other unorthodox methods. Although I *neither approve nor condone* the use of these methods, I do not reject such patients for medical therapy, and, if required, I provide them medical literature on the useless treatment. I also tell them about cases of poisoning and even of death from taking Laetrile. But I do not try to argue with them. It is their choice, and I accept the compromise that they take conventional medical therapy.

I have yet to see a single positive result in over 20 years of practice from unorthodox treatment, but my colleagues and I have seen hundreds of patients with progressive advancing cancers who tried a quack therapy first. Sometimes we were able to reverse the process after beginning traditional therapy, but many of these patients lost their chance for cure by opting first for a quack therapy.

Some of these treatments and drugs are available in many parts of the United States in spite of federal and some state laws banning their use. Laetrile is legal in a few states under special circumstances (such as when administered through a university hospital) and is also administered in a clinic in Tijuana, Mexico, as well as in several countries.

In May 1981, researchers from four cancer centers reported the results of the first government-sponsored tests on Laetrile carried out by the National Cancer Institute.* The researchers found the drug to be useless. Patients participating in the test showed no improvement or slowing of the growth of their advanced cancer, and no easing of the symptoms of their disease.

The Pure Food, Drug, and Cosmetic Act, passed by Congress in 1931 and strengthened by the 1962 Kefauver-Harris Amendments, stipulates that a producer of a new drug (or treatment method) must prove that it is not only safe but also effective if it is to be licensed for public use. The act provides for strict controls over investigational and experimental drugs and the sale of prescription drugs. Unless drugs are approved by the FDA, they cannot legally be distributed through interstate commerce. It is a federal crime, reinforced by our postal laws, to advertise or ship such products. Nine states have similar intrastate laws prohibiting distribution and sale of unlicensed drugs and methods, but until more states reinforce the federal legislation, unproved treatments will continue to be promoted and sold. In the states that have not passed their own laws, ways have been found to circumvent the federal ban against false claims in advertising.†

The FDA has published a booklet, *The Big Quack Attack: Medical Devices,* that describes various methods of quackery and directs consumers where to report complaints regarding practitioners of these methods.‡

---

*Paper presented at the American Society of Clinical Oncologists, May 1981. (Dr. Charles Moertel, spokesman for the Mayo Clinic, Rochester, Minnesota.)

†Additional information regarding laetrile and other unproved cancer therapies (Koch, Mucorhicin, Hoxey, Lincoln Staphage, Krebiozin, Bolen test, etc.) that have been banned by the FDA can be obtained from the Food and Drug Administration.

‡The booklet may be obtained from the FDA's Office of Public Affairs, Rockville, Md. 20857, or by calling a local office of the FDA.

8

Steps to recovery: rehabilitation

*Courage, hard work, self-mastery,
and intelligent effort are all
essential to successful life.*

THEODORE ROOSEVELT

Rehabilitation is an important part of total patient care to help a patient
and family toward the goal of recovering and returning to as normal a way of
life as possible. The idea of total patient care is not new, but with the
complexity of today's society and the specialization of modern medicine, it is
very difficult for a physician to give total care.

Cancer, like other chronic diseases, has important psychological and
social as well as medical dimensions. The cancer patient's needs go beyond
basic medical treatment. In the healing arts, an artificial division has often
existed between the mind and body. As medicine has become more specialized, this division between mind and body has tended to be further exaggerated;
in order to heal the whole patient, however, the idea of total patient care must
be shared among members of the medical team.

The medical health care team varies in composition in different areas of the
country because of the nature of local medical facilities and the availability
of personnel. A coordinated medical team usually consists of a physician, an
office staff, and the various members of the hospital team—nurse, licensed
vocational nurse, physical therapist, recreational therapist, dietician, occupational therapist, psychologist, clergy, and medical social worker (sometimes
also the discharge coordinator)—and a home care or hospice team.

When you are an active participant in your medical care and rehabilitation,
you can maintain a sense of control over your disease and your therapy. Only
you can take responsibility for your state of mind, nutritional status, and
physical fitness. The act of taking responsibility is in itself an important factor
in maintaining self-esteem, a feeling of independence, and faith in your ability
to cope. It is a critical part of therapy.

Many resources are available, but it can be difficult for you to take
advantage of them when you are ill. This chapter discusses several ways in
which you can improve your health status. It deals specifically with mental
health, nutrition, exercise, sexuality, and home care services. The principal
participants are you, your family, and your health care team.

79

A patient and family also need advice and information on practical matters such as disability payments and medical insurance, as well as the opportunity to talk with knowledgeable people about the fears and worries related to disease. Not every cancer patient needs or wants to use these professional services. However, each patient should be aware of their availability, encouraged to assess his or her short- and long-term needs with respect to treatment and convalescence, and made to understand that the need does not have to be severe to ask for help.

PSYCHOLOGICAL SUPPORT

It is important to recognize psychological problems early. You can be overwhelmed by the impact of your disease and lose your ability to cope. Once you are able to participate actively, your health care team can help strengthen your will to live by their own positive attitude, by supportive counseling, by projecting realistic goals, and by helping you become involved in an organized program of recovery. To deal with the common problems of alienation, loss of self-esteem, and depression, you will need to call on all your resources. How you eventually do it, only you can decide; there is no right way and no wrong way. I encourage the pursuit of any supportive discipline that appeals to you—from traditional psychiatry to biofeedback, meditation, visualization, and yoga.

I have spoken throughout this book of the fear and loneliness that are triggered by a diagnosis of cancer in any one of its many forms. The word alone is enough to put most people into a state of panic. We confront this wall of fear with our own spiritual and mental reserves and with our ability to express ourselves to others. In so doing, we discover we are neither the first nor the last to suffer from such trauma.

Among the emotions we share is anger. What could be more natural than fury at having your life interrupted—and threatened—by cancer? Anger and profound depression certainly are not going to go away, but their hold on a person can be diluted by confronting and expressing these emotions in a way that will not involve lashing out at loved ones. When we take our anger out on family, friends, or co-workers (all easy targets), we risk alienating the people we most need for support.

There are many other concerns, not the least of them physical. If the effects of the treatment for cancer have resulted in a physical change, a person's self-image can be badly damaged—whether these changes are visible to the public or known only to one's family or spouse. The loss of a limb, a breast, or testicles through surgery, or skin changes from radiation therapy, can be devastating. Adjustment to these changes does not come easily to most people. It is natural to be angry, to grieve, and to mourn when a part of our body is irreparably damaged. But at some point there has to be some acceptance if we are to continue to get something out of life. Acceptance may come sooner or more easily if patients can discuss their feelings with a psychologist, medical social worker, or another patient who has had a similar experience.

Understanding, acceptance, and compromise are necessary to anyone who is undergoing treatment for cancer and learning to live with the emotional turmoil and the sometimes drastic physical changes that can occur. Reaching the stage of compromise may be the key to living with—or without—cancer, because we *all* make compromises every day of our lives.

The difference in making a compromise while fighting for your life is that the stakes are higher than ever before. The learning process can be slow and tortuous. New situations continually arise as you try to deal with the fears of your loved ones, friends, and acquaintances. You must also deal with the often negative attitude of present or future employers, insurance companies, and the general public.

Self-motivation and what you can do for yourself are critical. One of the major themes of this book is that you must become an active partner in the treatment of your illness. You must consider yourself an integral part of the medical team. You should know what is happening in your medical treatment for, with knowledge, your role is assured. In this way, your will to live can be channeled into action.

Even when you are very ill, you have untapped physical and emotional reserves that you can command. If utilized, these reserves will help you to survive yet another day and will become the foundation of your recovery program. When exhausted soldiers march home after a rigorous day, they sometimes begin to march and sing in cadence. They have a revival of mood and spirit and find new energies and strength. So can you, even when exhausted by disease and illness; you too can muster reserve energies.

The problem of work can be a major one for a cancer patient. It isn't until illness deprives us of carrying out our normal responsibilities that we realize how much our self-esteem is related to our productivity and our ability to care for ourselves and others. When cancer patients are unable to return to work or are dependent on family or friends for personal care, household help, and financial aid, they feel like a burden. Just sitting around doing nothing magnifies their problems and often makes them feel worse. That is why it is important to find a way of returning to work in some capacity, whether this be housework, a job, studying, or learning a new skill.

However, returning to one's employment is not always possible. A person's job may be in jeopardy because of prejudice on the part of the employer, who fears disruption of routine or monetary loss from absences for treatment, or who just fears cancer in the abstract. Because of this potential prejudice in the marketplace, a cancer patient may have a hard time finding a job, or—after repeated rejection—may cease looking for work. There is no way to combat such treatment by society except to join the fight for public education about cancer and cancer treatment. The first place to look for a change in attitude may be within ourselves. If we can learn to live with disease—and have a positive attitude—this attitude will affect the thinking of others.

I hope the day will soon come when a potential employer will agree with Darrell Ansbacher (Chap. 16):

I wish I had a chance to talk to a prospective employer about Hodgkin's disease during my interview because I consider it to be one of my greatest achievements. Some people climb the Matterhorn and afterwards they want everyone to know about it and show them slides. In the same way, I'm sorry there's not a place on my resume to show I had Hodgkin's.

It is not always prejudice toward and fear of cancer that prevent cancer patients from being employed. Sometimes they are disabled in a way that prevents them from being able to perform their previous job. One of the greatest needs in our society is for vocational classes and job-retraining programs for those who must change their means of earning a living as a result of illness. Every patient who wants counseling should have recourse to a medical social worker, physical or occupational therapist, and any other professional who can help him or her plan early to match present and potential skills with available jobs.

Work is necessary to our financial as well as our psychological well-being. Illness and a period of unemployment can wipe out years of savings. A cancer patient can discuss with a medical social worker the financial concerns that arise from prolonged hospitalization and convalescence. A medical social worker is equipped to give information on medical insurance and disability benefits; he or she knows of sources of financial aid for home care, transportation to and from therapy, or special medical equipment needed at home.

Cancer patients may have a problem acquiring new medical insurance. Their former health insurance may no longer be available because the company does not want to take the risk of insuring for a disease that does not have a cut-and-dried prognosis. We need new insurance programs designed by people who are willing to assume the risk for cancer patients who are now often denied the benefits they need.

One of the best sources of psychological support for a cancer patient is another person who has had or now has cancer. Who else could be as emphatic or give as practical advice as the person who has experienced it all?

There are several different types of groups organized by and for cancer patients. Reach to Recovery, The International Association of Laryngectomies, I Can Cope and Share and Care are sponsored by the American Cancer Society. The United Ostomy Association and The Leukemia Society of America exist through private support, as does ENCORE (Encouragement, Normalcy, Counseling, Opportunity, Reaching Out, and Energies Revived) and the National YWCA postmastectomy rehabilitation program. These and similar groups and the services they offer are described in Appendix V. They all provide information on physical care, psychological counseling, and other needs.

A typical group of patients who have come together to meet their common needs is called Living with Cancer. Located in New York City, the goal of this group is to break down the feeling of isolation that can engulf a cancer patient. The group provides a network of information by telephone on all aspects of cancer: how to handle expenses; how to apply for disability benefits, Medicaid, insurance, and so on. Lectures are given on nutrition, pain control, up-to-date therapeutic methods, and the psychological problems faced by both patients and their families. Employment problems are also discussed.

Living with Cancer brings patients and their families together to better understand what each is suffering. Cancer information centers similar to this group are badly needed, and new groups are being formed all the time.

NUTRITION

Nutrition should be one of the first considerations in a cancer rehabilitation program. However, it is easy to suffer from progressive malnutrition at such a time because cancer therapy often causes a loss of appetite and taste or otherwise makes it difficult to eat an adequate amount of food. Loss of appetite from depression and anxiety is also very common. Your food can be as important as your medicine.

One problem with malnutrition is that it can evolve slowly and become serious before a person realizes it. A cancer patient may become malnourished almost to the point of starvation, setting up a vicious cycle. Decreased appetite and weight loss result in fatigue and depression; the body is then forced to use its reserves as fuel, leading to further weight loss, weakness, fatigue, and less tolerance to the side effects of radiation therapy or chemotherapy. At the same time, the immune-defense system is less effective, increasing the chances of infection. Malnutrition in general leads to a poorer outlook for survival.

A cancer patient's daily nutritional needs are greater than the normal nutritional requirements. When people are ill or have a fever, their bodies' metabolic requirements are increased by approximately 20 to 25% and additional nutrients are needed just to maintain normal functions such as tissue repair. Good nutrition is also critical to recovery from surgery and to maintenance of the body's tolerance to radiation therapy and chemotherapy. Cure and remission rates also increase with good nutrition. Therefore, every effort must be made at the time of diagnosis or at the initiation of therapy to plan a program to prevent malnutrition. The longer the delay before beginning such a program, the longer the convalescence and the slower the healing process.

Cancer patients should consult their physicians about diet or ask their physicians for a referral to the hospital nutritionist to discuss their dietary needs. They and their families must learn to become involved in ways to improve their nutrition.

At the same time, patients should review their knowledge of the basic food nutrients—proteins, fats, carbohydrates, vitamins, and minerals—and the foods in which they are found. Proteins are needed for growth and repair of body tissue; fats and carbohydrates (starches and sugars) provide energy; and vitamins and minerals are needed to regulate metabolic processes. Because there are more than 50 different nutrients that have been identified as necessary for optimal health, nutritionists often use the Basic Four Plan to provide general guidance to good health. The Basic Four Plan divides nutrients into four groups: protein, milk, vegetable-fruit, and breads-cereals. Minimum daily requirements comprise two servings each from the protein and milk products groups and four servings each from the vegetable-fruit and bread-cereal groups, plus 3 to 4 tablespoons of fats and oils for calories. Multivitamins are added once or twice daily.

With advice from their doctor or a nutritionist, patients can plan a diet that will provide all the necessary additional nutrients. Planning with a professional is also important when a patient is on a low-fat, salt-free, or other special diet.

Early filling is a common problem in cancer patients. This can be counteracted by taking small portions frequently throughout the day. Protein snacks and the use of food supplements in the preparation of food are also helpful, as is the use of convenience foods when one does not wish to cook.

There are ways to combat the many problems that can arise when disease or treatment reduces appetite, makes food unpalatable, or renders eating difficult and painful. Some of these problems are indigestion, loss of appetite, milk intolerance, nausea and vomiting, difficulty in swallowing, bloating, dehydration, diarrhea, dry mouth, heartburn, and esophagitis.

Radiation therapy and chemotherapy sometimes cause alterations in a person's sense of smell and taste. Food in particular can taste slightly bitter, but this problem can be overcome with the addition of sugar, sauces, condiments, or spices.

Several myths concerning cancer and nutrition can lead a cancer patient to adopt an inadequate or inappropriate diet or waste time and money on a quack diet that will not affect the disease course. There is little scientific evidence to support the belief that not eating will "starve" the tumor or that eating adequately will "feed" the tumor.

Many patients ask about the superiority of natural or organic foods over regularly grown foods in the dietary management of cancer. "Natural" is a general term covering all foods that are processed without artificial coloring, preservatives, or any kind of synthetic additives. "Organic" is a more specific term that refers to a method of growing foods in which no chemical fertilizers, pesticides, or herbicides are used.

There is no scientific evidence that natural or organic foods offer any advantage over regular foods so far as nutrient qualities are concerned. Moreover, their greater cost makes them less desirable to people on a budget. Our food supply today is much safer than it used to be when illness from bacterial infestation and spoilage posed a constant threat to infants and older people. There is little evidence that a person who eats regular foods from the supermarket is at any greater risk than a natural foods enthusiast. Concern about the relationship between additives and cancer is based in part on speculation, and the true role of additives is still under investigation. Cancer was in existence long before food additives were invented.

Helpful hints for better nutrition

Whether you are at home or in the hospital, you can make good use of a planned approach to your eating. Your biggest obstacle may be lack of appetite, a common problem of cancer and its treatment. You will probably have to work hard to overcome it, but there are techniques to help you.

In the hospital

- *Consult with the hospital dietician.* When you are in the hospital you have the advantage of being able to consult with the hospital dietician. Have her or him help you plan a balanced daily menu that includes the full range of needed nutrients, particularly proper amounts of protein and calories, and ask her or his advice if you are having any eating problems. The dietician can also help you plan a home nutrition program.
- *Consider adding a high-protein or high-calorie diet supplement to your menu.* Ask the dietician to discuss the various diet supplements with you. She or he may be able to let you taste-test different brands of supplements, and can advise you as to the pros and cons of the various brands.
- *Eat frequent small meals.* Frequent small meals are the best way to ensure that you get enough food, and they can be especially helpful if you have a loss of appetite or difficulty tolerating food.
- *Snack between meals.* The dietician will arrange for you to have snacks, such as high-protein diet supplements, milkshakes, eggnogs, puddings, or sandwiches. If you must interrupt or miss a meal for a test, therapy, or an examination, ask that your food be saved in a warmer, or ask to order another meal when you return to your room.
- *Fill out your daily menu when you are feeling well enough to plan your meals imaginatively.* Have someone help you if necessary. Order food that you like. Consider the protein and calorie values of the food you order, but give thought to its eye appeal and aroma so that it will be as appetizing as possible. Giving variety to your menus will improve your appetite. You may want to save some of your menus to use as examples when you are planning meals at home.
- *Have your family and friends bring your favorite foods.* Favorite foods from home often help your appetite. In some hospitals, families are allowed to use the ward kitchen to prepare special food or to warm up food brought from home.
- *Make your mealtimes pleasant.* Your mealtime atmosphere is important to help you feel like eating. Your family and friends can bring flowers and pictures to brighten your hospital room. Whenever possible, eat with family, friends, or other patients. If you are alone, turn on the radio, television, or music for company. Try to make a mealtime a social time.
- *Avoid stress at mealtimes.* Specific relaxation exercises before meals may be helpful in reducing tension and may improve your appetite.
- *Have an aperitif before meals.* If to your taste, you may find a glass of wine or beer before meals to be relaxing and stimulating to your appetite.
- *Exercise before meals.* You may find that light exercise for 5 to 10 minutes approximately a half hour before meals is helpful in stimulating your appetite. The nurse or physical therapist can show you simple range-of-motion exercises you can do in bed; or, if you can get out of bed, take a walk up and down the hospital corridors.

At home

In addition to the suggestions obviously applicable to both hospital and home (frequent small meals, snacks, possible high-protein supplements, attractive surroundings, exercise, etc.), there are some techniques to have in mind, particularly when you no longer have the hospital facilities and staff available.

- *Plan your daily menu in advance.* Include the proper number of servings from the Basic Four, with particular concern for the necessary amounts of protein and calories. In addition to planning the foods you will eat, it can be helpful to plan the times you will eat.

- *Have help in preparing your meals.* If you are not feeling well, you sometimes won't feel like making the effort to prepare a nutritious diet. A friend or relative may be able to help you by preparing major foods for several days in advance. Home aid in preparing meals is also available in many communities. Also, if you are not feeling well enough to cook, a nutritious diet can be planned using canned, packaged, and frozen foods.

- *Have many portions of food ready to serve.* If you must fix your own meals, or if the person fixing your meals is gone for the day, you may find it easier to fix many small portions of favorite foods and keep them in separate containers ready to serve. It reduces the problem of figuring out what to eat, at a time when your appetite may be poor or you do not feel like cooking. If it is practical for you, a microwave oven is convenient for heating small portions of food quickly.

- *Add extra protein to your diet.* Use fortified milk for drinking and in recipes calling for milk. Use peanut butter, cheese, cottage cheese, and chopped hard-boiled eggs as snacks and devise ways of adding them to recipes.

- *Add extra calories to your diet.* Add cream or butter to soups, cooked cereals, and vegetables. Use gravies, sauces, and sour cream with vegetables, meat, poultry, and fish. Add a high-calorie supplement to your normal recipes.

EXERCISE

Daily exercise can have the same beneficial effect on a person who is ill as it can on the jogger or swimmer. Not only does exercise keep our muscles and tissues in proper condition, but researchers have proved that it helps alleviate depression and even produces a feeling of well-being. It is only the level of exercise that changes for a person who is ill. Following surgery, a person's goal may be just to maintain muscle tone, normal joint motion, and physical strength.

Exercises can be divided into three stages: Stage I, for the bedridden and postsurgery patient, consists of simple range-of-motion exercises that require low energy expenditure. Stage II consists of progressive exercises for sitting and ambulatory patients in the hospital or for outpatients receiving chemotherapy or radiation therapy who do not feel well enough for vigorous exercise. Stage III represents a return to everyday activities such as bicycling, housework, and walking.

Exercise at Stage I is crucial. In acute or chronic illness, when prolonged bed rest is necessary or debility persists, a patient can develop muscular weakness, tissue breakdown, muscle loss, and poor function of vital organs if no attempt is made to exercise. Thus, though rest is needed, total immobility is not desirable. It is detrimental. Simple means of exercise can be arranged for patients in this condition. Muscles in hands and arms can be used by squeezing a rubber ball or lifting a 3-pound Velcro weight. Leg and arm exercises can be carried out whether lying down, sitting, or standing.

Other forms of exercise at this or any stage of convalescence include isotonic and isometric rhythmic, repetitive movements. Massage therapy is also a good means of maintaining circulation and relaxing; it can also reduce the chance of developing bedsores.

In our rehabilitation program, the physician recommends an exercise regimen for a patient, and—with the patient's consent—asks a physical therapist to make a visit. The physical therapist then develops an exercise program tailored to the patient's needs and abilities, often using videotape to demonstrate the exercises. The patient pursues the program at his or her own speed, usually with the assistance of nurses, family members, or friends. The physical therapist returns at regular intervals to check on the patient's progress and to answer questions.

An occupational therapist is often called on to work with patients with special problems such as learning how to function with an artificial limb.

One rule governs the cancer patient and the effect of exercise: the more physical activity, the faster the recovery. Just as an athlete will not achieve proficiency without constant daily training, so the bedridden or convalescing patient will not function at his or her highest potential without daily exercise.

Rules for safe exercising

Some rules for safe and comfortable exercising are necessary to make sure you do not get too tired or hurt yourself.

- Ask your physician if you are ready to exercise. When you are ill or recovering, your physician should determine your limits for you.
- Have someone assist you in doing exercises, for enjoyment and for safety. Having someone there is especially important when you are just beginning to get out of bed, because you may get dizzy when standing up or bending over.
- If you get tired or if your muscles feel sore, *stop* and *rest.*
- *Omit* exercises that seem too difficult; try them again another day when you feel stronger. If you have just had surgery, do not do any exercises using resistance (i.e., those using added weights or elastic stretchers) without checking with your doctor.
- Try to repeat each exercise 3 to 5 times at first. If you feel too tired or weak, do only 1 or 2 repetitions. Gradually increase to 10 to 20 repetitions.
- Try to exercise twice a day, and more often if you feel like it.
- Keep a daily record of your progress.

SEXUALITY

Sexuality in its many aspects can sometimes be affected by a serious illness such as cancer, and by its treatment. By sexuality I mean the feelings we have about ourselves as sexual beings, the ways in which we choose to express these feelings with ourselves and others, and the physical capability each of us has to give and experience sexual pleasure. Sexuality can be expressed in many ways—in how we dress, move, and speak, as well as by kissing, touching, masturbation, and intercourse.

Cancer patients usually have a lowered energy level from their disease and the side effects of therapy. This fatigue, plus changes in body image and anxieties about survival, family, or finances, can place a strain on the expression of sexuality as well as create concerns about sexual desirability. Not surprisingly, people often experience a lowered sexual drive under these circumstances. However, once the immediate crisis has passed, sex again becomes important, although most people have anxiety about resuming sexual activity. The level of resumed sexual activity is usually not greater than that experienced prior to developing cancer, and may be limited by physical changes from surgery, radiotherapy, or chemotherapy. Some people worry about whether they will be able to experience sexual pleasure, whether having sex will hurt them in any way, or whether the fact of their illness is disturbing to their partner, particularly if there have been physical changes as a result of surgery. Their partners may in turn worry about causing harm to their loved one. Some people are even afraid that cancer can be transmitted through sexual intercourse. (There is no basis to this fear.)

Cancer patients who are in a position to start a new sexual relationship can be particularly concerned about the issue of bodily change from surgery. How and when do they talk about these changes, their needs, and their feelings?

Discussing sexual needs and feelings does not come easily to most people. Although some health care personnel are today more aware of the sexual concerns of patients, many patients continue to receive little or no information about sexuality while being treated for, or recovering from, illness. In fact, they may not even be given the opportunity to ask important questions; or perhaps their questions are avoided, making them feel their worries are foolish, unimportant, or inappropriate.

Of course their anxieties are very important and their resolution may be crucial to the continuation or establishment of sexual intimacy. Cancer patients should therefore take the initiative and pose their questions to the person with whom they feel most comfortable, be this their doctor, a medical social worker, nurse, or other qualified staff person. If none of these people has the answers, then patients should ask for a referral to someone who *can* help them—because help is available. Some university centers offer sexual counseling specifically for people with medical illness or physical disability. A doctor or medical social worker should know where to refer patients for such a consultation.

Some sexual problems are physical and cannot be corrected, but sexual satisfaction can still be gained in alternative ways. Impotence following testicular lymph node surgery or from prostatic surgery or radiotherapy requires a specific approach. A penile prosthesis implant may help. Vaginal stenosis (a vagina narrowed by scarring from surgery or radiation) requires another approach. The psychological devastation of a woman who has lost her ovaries or breast from surgery or her hair from chemotherapy are also important body changes requiring special attention.

If a cancer patient was comfortable with and enjoyed his or her sexuality prior to the illness, the chances are excellent that he or she will be able to keep or regain a good sexual self-image despite the changes brought about by cancer. Many people who have cancer or who are the partners of persons with cancer may not experience any change in sexual feelings or behavior. Others may find that increased closeness and communication resulting from the experience of illness enhances their sexuality. Still others may never have considered sexuality to be of great importance in their lives, or may consider it less important now than previously.

A person should not have to give up the comfort and pleasure of intimacy with a loved one just because he or she is in the hospital. Although hospitals and convalescent facilities do not traditionally provide much privacy, many institutions are beginning to recognize this need and now arrange time and space for people to be alone together. In those hospitals where this issue has not yet been addressed, a patient can at least make a *Please knock* or *Do not disturb until* _____ *o'clock* sign and hang it on the door. Some hospitals now provide, on request, an extra cot for overnight visitors. Patients who share a room with another patient might ask their doctor to arrange for private time in another room.

Sexual problems often seem to arise not so much from actual changes in a person's body as from how that person feels about those changes. Both partners may be nervous about initiating sexual activity or communicating feelings, and the waiting game can be mutually misinterpreted as rejection. To think of breaking the silence may be frightening, but I believe that a good move is to make the first move.

The following are some reminders that you, as a patient, might want to keep in mind.

- *Communication is all-important.* The more talking and sharing you can do, the more your awareness of what feels good to you sexually will probably increase. It is rarely easy for anyone to begin talking about sex. You might try initially by sharing with your partner some of the myths or expectations you grew up with about sexuality.
- *Don't let your diagnosis dictate what you can do sexually.* Your sexuality cannot be "diagnosed." You will never know what you are capable of experiencing in terms of sexual pleasure if you don't explore being sexual—new positions, new touches, and above all, new attitudes. You are the sexual expert about yourself; your brain is your best sex organ, and its ability to experience sensation is virtually limitless.
- *You are loved for your total worth, not just for the appearance of your body.* If you were considered loveable or sexually desirable before your

illness, chances are you will be afterward as well. Don't make the mistake of placing so much importance on the way you used to look or feel that you can no longer appreciate your unique worth. Your partner and friends will continue to love and value you as long as you let them. The crisis of illness often brings people who love each other even closer together and enriches their relationships in ways they never expected.

- *You don't have to do it all yourself.* Don't hesitate to seek counseling or information if problems arise. Help is available from a wide range of sources. If you have questions about sexuality or are experiencing some difficulties you wish to discuss further, bring them up with your health care providers or ask them to recommend competent sex counselors or therapists in your area. Other resources that may be available near your home include persons or groups of people who themselves have had cancer and who have had experience in talking about sexual concerns with others.

- *Survival overshadows sexuality.* Remember that stress, depression, worry, and fatigue may temporarily lower your interest in sex. It is normal and natural for someone who loses good health to experience such feelings. When you are ill, just coping with basic everyday decisions may seem like a burden. Taking one day at a time and being patient with yourself is important. Sexual interest and feelings will no doubt return when the immediate crisis of illness has passed.

HOME CARE

Another important phase of rehabilitation is home care for patients and their families. For the majority of patients, the familiar surroundings of home are preferable to a hospital or nursing facility. However, many patients and/or families prolong the period of hospitalization because they fear they will be unable to cope with home care problems. These fears are understandable but they can be overcome. Numerous medical and nonmedical crises can be anticipated and often avoided by training patients and their families in the elements of home care before the patient is discharged from the hospital.

Home care is not for all patients, as it requires a willingness of family and friends to accept the responsibility of providing services on a sustained basis. Often the physical facilities, the equipment, or the availability of the appropriate home helper are not practical.

Therefore, a patient may be better off in a nursing facility. This decision must be made by the attending physician, discharge planners, family, and patient before home care is offered. Not only the patient's physical needs, but also the ability of the patient and family to cope with the psychological stress of the home care situation must be anticipated and carefully assessed. It is often difficult for a patient to endure the indignities that daily dependence on family can bring. The stress of having a chronically ill person at home may be too much for a family already stressed by other circumstances—such as work, their own health and recreation, and other responsibilities.

Patients about to go home from the hospital are often worried about how to deal with pain. If they are being given medication by their nurses and doctors to relieve pain, they often wonder: "Who will give me the medicine at home?" "What if I run out of medicine?" "Suppose I need an injection?" "What if I'm alone and the pain gets worse?"

The first important point to remember is that most pain can be relieved. There are many medications available, and one or more of them will certainly help.

Pain control should begin in the hospital when the physician recommends the type and frequency of medication. The patient and/or family should then keep a record of the effects of the medication. This will help the physician in prescribing future dosages and will prepare the patient and family to be self-reliant in pain control at home. This record-keeping should be continued at home so the patient and family can learn how to use medications more effectively.

Psychological and emotional factors can play a major role in response to pain. Having control over pain helps a patient relax and, as a result, feel less pain and anxiety. Therefore, if injections are necessary, the patient and family can be instructed in the proper techniques by the nurse or the doctor before the patient is discharged from the hospital.

Most patients will require some special equipment or assistive devices not normally found in a home, especially in the bedroom and bathroom. The occupational therapist can assist the patient in learning what equipment is available and how to use it. The hospital discharge planner or medical social worker can also assist the patient in finding out where equipment can be rented or purchased and whether it is covered by insurance.

Maintaining good nutrition is a particular problem for cancer patients because cancer and cancer therapy often cause a loss of appetite or otherwise make it difficult to eat an adequate amount of food.

The hospital dietician can instruct the patient and family in basic nutritional requirements, such as the Basic Four food groups, and explain how to deal with special dietary problems associated with cancer and cancer therapy, such as anorexia, bloating, heartburn, constipation, diarrhea, nausea and vomiting, sore or dry mouth, indigestion, and taste blindness. In many instances special food supplements are required, either with or between meals, to increase daily intake. If nasogastric or jejunal (intestinal) tube feedings are required, appropriate training can be given before discharge. With guidance from the physician, dietician, and the appropriate literature, the patient and family should be able to handle most nutritional problems.

The physical therapist in the hospital can instruct the patient and family in exercises that can be continued at home. Through exercise, patients will feel more confident when they go home and will be less prone to accidents resulting from a weakened condition.

Cancer patients may experience many common problems in body care. The patient and family should be instructed in specific care techniques before the patient's discharge. Patients should be given a practical approach to bowel and bladder care, especially regarding constipation, diarrhea, and incontinence—for example, knowledge of laxatives, how to give an enema, catheter training (indwelling and condom), and dietary management.

Proper skin care helps prevent pressure sores and will make the patient feel generally refreshed. Weight loss and the side effects of radiation or chemotherapy can lower the patient's resistance to infections, so it is important to prevent skin rupture from chafing and bedsores. Patient and family should be instructed by the nurse or physical therapist in the techniques of skin care, such as frequent position changes if the patient is bedbound; the use of an "egg crate" mattress or a foam or sheepskin pad to cushion the patient and provide better air circulation; heat; massage; good hygiene; and the use of talcum and skin lotions.

Patients with colostomies, ileostomies, and ureterostomies will normally be instructed in the care of their ostomies by an enterostomal therapist while they are in the hospital. Support and confidence may also be given to the patient by a visitor from the United Ostomy Association.

One of the fears that patients and families have when going home is what will happen in case of an emergency. The physician can help the patient and family to prepare for an emergency by discussing possible occurrences and procedures for summoning aid and by instructing the family in the appropriate first-aid procedures.

The family needs as much emotional support as the patient. Home care is a tremendous undertaking for family members, who give not only their physical services but also their empathy and compassion. The patient, because of the intensity of the illness, is often able to give little emotional support in return. The family must be helped not to feel guilty for considering their own needs as well as the patient's.

If there is more than one family member, a schedule to rotate responsibilities should be arranged. If one person is the main care giver, he or she must be allotted some free time for physical and mental well-being. A temporary patient stay in a nursing home may sometimes be advisable to allow the family a respite from home care. Psychological counseling or support groups consisting of families of other cancer patients can also provide a needed release of emotions.

RECREATION

Recreation is an important part of living. We all need a break from the routine and stress of daily living. It would seem obvious that recreation is of even greater importance when a person is ill, yet patients often forget about recreation or think it will be too difficult to pursue or somehow inappropriate. It is neither of these things. Many recreational activities can be started while you are still in the hospital, no matter what your limitations, and continued at home.

You may prefer reading or some other solitary pursuit, but there are advantages to giving some time to group participation when you feel well enough. A group offers companionship and the opportunity to discuss your concerns and feelings.

The types of recreation pursued will be as varied and individual as the patients themselves. But whatever you choose for diversion should be just that—fun and a relief from stress. The positive attitude fostered by enjoyment can be critically important for optimum recovery.

HOPE

Hope is an essential part of the will to live. Hope can be maintained as long as there is even a remote chance for survival. It is kindled and nurtured by even minor improvements and is maintained when crises or reversals persist by the positive attitudes of family, friends, and the health support team. Primarily, though, hope will come from within you, if you are willing to do everything you can to improve your health and if you are willing to fight for your life.

Approximately 60% of the people in the United States do not live near major clinical centers; they are treated through their community hospital systems. However, every community has available the rehabilitation resources described in these pages. Cancer patients can obtain a referral to any of these sources of support by asking their doctor, medical social worker, or the personnel at the community hospital or local cancer organizations.

The help is there because the special needs of cancer patients have been recognized both by the professionals in many different fields and by those who themselves have (or have had) cancer. They know they can make a difference in how a person lives with his or her cancer and its treatment.

We always fear the unknown, yet it is amazing how resilient we can be when our day to cope with illness arrives. Most people think they would dissolve in fear and have no courage. But courage is not the lack of fear; it involves learning to live with fear. Participation in a rehabilitation program is part of that learning process.

PART FOUR

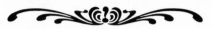

One patient's view of
the doctor-patient relationship

9
Ellen Abbott

I think that doctors can perhaps get some satisfaction, as certainly I as a patient have gotten, in being engaged in the fight. It's us against cancer, and we know we aren't going to win in the end, but, by God, we're going to give it a run for its money. And I find this sort of challenging as a patient.

These are the words of a patient living with a fatal disease, not a dying patient. Ellen Abbott discovered on her forty-third birthday that she had advanced ovarian cancer. From what her family and friends tell me, she had always transmitted a special radiance and joy in living, but she lived the last 3 years of her life with even more enthusiasm than before her illness. The knowledge that she was under a death sentence heightened her zest for life.

At the time of Ellen's treatment I was holding a series of seminars for residents and interns on the problems and concerns of patients faced with terminal cancer. I asked Ellen if she would attend. I felt that the group would benefit from a comparison of her personal experiences with our professional observations, and also that Ellen, with her keen perceptions and analytical mind, could help us to identify and articulate the special problems confronting cancer patients and physicians. Ellen readily agreed to come and became a permanent participant in the seminars.

I also asked Ellen if she would help counsel other cancer patients less well adjusted than she. Soon both physicians and patients were seeking her advice. Implicit in all she said was her belief that life should be lived. She was convinced, as I am, that each person with cancer has the potential to remain productive and to enjoy life during most of his or her illness.

The way Ellen dealt with her own terminal illness is proof that she was able to translate her ideas into action. She was, and will remain, an inspiration to her family and friends, her doctors, and the other patients who had the privilege of knowing her.

I once asked Ellen whether there was anything special she would like to accomplish before she died and she replied that she would like to write a guidebook for other patients, to share with them the positive aspects of her experience with cancer.

I have had a good time of it and I think I could write something that would help others. There are lots of things a patient can do in managing his doctors and family and even his own moods. At the same time a physician has to set the tone in advance for the patient. I'd like to help just some physicians feel, "Gee, I could do this or be that . . ." and also some patients—some in very practical terms and others in a perhaps more philosophical sense—take it easier.

Ellen died before she could write her guidebook, but the following pages contain many of her observations, taken directly from the transcripts of our tape-recorded seminars.

A hundred years ago people grew up on farms. They saw birth and death all the time with the animals. Death was a natural part of life. They saw it as part of the rhythm of life, and one got a larger sense of the seasons, birth, death, life and so on. It's really in the past 50 years in this country and in other industrialized countries that people don't see life and death in the great pattern.

My father was a doctor and so I think that I became realistic at a very young age. I understood that if certain things happened, they were pretty much going to happen. I got this understanding from him, a certain acceptance, so that although like all of us I had never thought I was going to die at all, the minute I heard what had happened to me and how widespread it was, then I knew that nothing was going to change. I don't think you really know if you are going to be afraid or not. I think before I would probably have thought so, but as soon as I knew what was wrong and what was going to happen, I wasn't.

I have no fearful associations with death. I have never thought I was being punished for my sins. I have sinned, I suppose, but I never believed in any sort of cosmic justice or injustice. I never bargained for my life because I didn't think there was anyone who would intervene. I think the universe is neutral. I assume that if you get cancer cells and they spread, the forces of nature are going to go on and you are going to die.

I imagine death as the big sleep. I don't believe in an afterlife; I think it is the end. I know some people despair because of that, but I assume that's the way it is. That's my concept of death and I think that's why I'm not afraid to die—although I want to live as long as I can because I have everything to live for, but that's different from fearing to die.

It helps too that I've always loved life and have no regrets. My father said that he had found that unhappy people were much worse about dying than happy people. They feel they have not lived and they aren't ready to go yet. I don't think that I've lived my life. I thought I'd live to be 90. But I think that the awareness of not having lived while you can must be frustrating to people. An awful lot of people don't live. They don't enjoy life as they go along and then suddenly it's too late.

LIVING

Ellen's early reconciliation with death allowed her more freedom to live. Having made this essential adjustment, she had no fear and was able to redirect her energies. When this psychological process of reconciliation does not occur, the fear of death can immobilize a patient.

The fear of cancer can be equally paralyzing, and Ellen recalled her own exposure to the taboos surrounding that word.

I'm convinced that Roosevelt was right when he said that the only thing we have to fear is fear itself, blind unreasoning fear. By fear I don't mean legitimate fear—I mean, cancer's something to fear, but do you know what I mean? You all know that there is associated with cancer, particularly, this strange aura. Why is it so much worse than other things? I am not being a Pollyanna, but there are other terrible diseases.

There's always been a taboo. A generation ago my own mother—just to give you an idea—a doctor's wife—never used the word cancer, until I got it; and then she spoke it because I always said "cancer." You almost had to whisper, "So-and-so has a malignancy." Now why that's a better word, I don't know. My dad would just say "C.A."

During a meeting of the seminar in which these matters were discussed, an intern remarked that he had seldom seen a doctor successfully handle the problem of death. Ellen was appalled.

I don't think it's as fancy a problem as you all think. People have been dying for thousands of years and managed to carry it off pretty well. It isn't so mysterious and arcane that a good physician, a good human being with respect for another human being, cannot somehow convey both his strength and support.

However, Ellen thought the current wave of books and articles about death might provide a rationale for doctors to avoid meeting their responsibilities to patients. They might be tempted to think that because they were not psychiatrists, they were not qualified to help a patient face death. Still other physicians might take as a personal and professional defeat the eventual loss of two out of three patients. Their tendency might then be to concentrate on patients whom they could cure, absolving themselves of responsibility to their terminal patients with the comforting thought that research will one day provide a cure. In the meantime, many of these patients who were not going to benefit from future research would be walking around half dead, crippled not by cancer but by fear.

Ellen and I therefore felt that physicians should establish realistic goals for the treatment of terminal cancer patients, with victory measured by the number of active years or months gained for each person.

Cancer patients' ability or inability to live fully while undergoing treatment often reflects the way they lived before their cancer was discovered, but Ellen found that a patient-doctor relationship based on candor and trust makes it easier for a patient to concentrate on living.

The physician is the most important person in a terminal patient's life. He may not be the most beloved or valuable, but he has the most telling effect on the kind of life the patient leads. No one—parent, child, husband, lover, or best friend—can take the physician's place. Having had cancer for more than 2 years, I know what a doctor can mean in liberating one to live actively during the remaining time of one's life.

A doctor should recognize that by his own courage and respect for the patient, he can relieve terror. If he shows confidence that he can remain in control of the disease and the pain, it removes an enormous burden from the patient's life. This is the approach my doctors have taken with me. It was never spoken, but they communicated it in their actions and manner. And it has been a wonderful feeling. Instead of seeing each setback and loss of time as a defeat, we turn it around. Each day, week, and month that we pass—particularly if I am free to enjoy life during that time—is a victory.

If I had not trusted my physicians, I would have spent my time wondering, "Where's it going to go next?" or "Is the pain going to be so bad they won't be able to control it?" Instead I told myself, "That's their problem. I have enough to do handling my family and friends and everybody else, doing all the things I want to do." So I put the responsibility on the doctors. Naturally, I tell them my symptoms and cooperate with them. I do everything they tell me, but basically all of the therapy is up to them; I don't have to worry about it.

If a doctor can add to the quality of life of his patient, if he can let the patient live while he's living, there is no greater gift. Even if he could prolong life or save it, I would be willing to say that perhaps the greater gift is this liberating of a life that he is bound to lose ultimately.

When I left the hospital for the first time I asked Dr. John Kerner, my gynecologist, that question I shouldn't have asked, "How long?" That was the only time he ever evaded me, and rightly. Because doctors don't know. He evaded me by saying, "Well, the statistics are quite unreliable, and after all, if you're the 1% ... " And then—it's funny, it was the first time I ever thought consciously about any of this—I said, "Now that I think about it, I don't think I would do anything terribly differently if you said 6 months. I really enjoy life so much the way it is. I would like to go on living pretty much that way." He replied, "I wouldn't put anything off once you start to feel well. The way to live is to live."

THE FIRST MEETINGS BETWEEN PATIENT AND PHYSICIAN

In January 1972, Ellen, my wife, Isadora, and I attended a symposium called Current Concepts in Medical Oncology. One of the speakers was an anthropologist who, like many others there, concentrated on the patient's last days and hours. He suggested that true dying occurred in this final phase of life and that a patient is often abandoned at this most important time. Ellen did not agree with this definition of the "most important time" in the experience of a cancer patient.

I have not gone through the terminal phase yet, but a year ago I believed I was going to die and nearly did. Before the terminal stages, the relationship between patient and physician is formed, and any late efforts to save or correct it are bound to fail. The patient is too consumed by fear and pain to develop a meaningful relationship with anyone at this time.

It is in the earliest meetings, even before the diagnosis, that the tone of the relationship is set. In these encounters, the physician reveals his attitudes toward the disease and the patient. He establishes the foundation of confidence and support on which the patient will later rely. If he shows respect for the patient and his own courage in the face of cancer, he will immediately begin to win the patient's trust. It is important to achieve this before the diagnosis because the physician's manner in presenting the diagnosis and the patient's reaction to it have an enormous effect on the course of the disease.

It happened so quickly that I was completely taken aback and forced to acknowledge what happened. Before the operation I asked my gynecologist to level with me completely. Following surgery, he told me what they had done and what they had not been able to do, and then I knew. I remember I thought, "So." It was resignation. He kept talking, and I cannot recall everything he said, but obviously he was very good in the way he handled me. He was planning radiation therapy. He never pretended that he could save me. He did not say, "You're going to die," but he told me enough so that I knew. Still, he was very positive about therapy. He was not afraid of the disease, and that, along with the respect he showed by being honest, led me to put my confidence in him.

One of the reasons Ellen adjusted so successfully was that Dr. Kerner treated her with sensitivity and respect. Later, while counseling other terminal patients, Ellen often became depressed by stories they told of the unintentional cruelty their primary doctors had shown in telling them about their disease and their prospects for recovery. In many cases the effects of these encounters could not be undone by subsequent supportive efforts of friends, relatives, or physicians.

The nameless, formless fear of cancer and death can be very upsetting to a patient, and this is what is contributed to when a physician is not candid and confident. When the physician is dishonest, the patient thinks, "If my doctor can't tell me, if he can't face it, it must be really terrible. What's the end going to be like?" The patient communicates this fear to his relatives and friends and soon the mood infects everyone. In these circumstances, the patient may refuse to believe anything the doctor tells him and exhaust himself worrying about the progress of the disease.

The physician's demeanor over a good length of time is also important. It isn't just the first interview. It's over and over. It's the whole thing. I think one of the best things that has happened with my doctors is that so often a question is trembling on my lips, and before I can even say it, one of them says, "You realize . . . " or "You know why we're doing so and so . . . " Or sometimes they have anticipated further than that and told me something I would have wanted to know in a day or two.

PAIN

A physician must be flexible and adjust treatment according to changes in a patient's physical and mental condition, because fear of pain and of the future may increase as disease progresses. Ellen Abbott was free from excessive anxiety about pain, but she was realistic about its effects. At one time she suffered a severe relapse from an intestinal obstruction. Unable to eat, she weighed 77 pounds instead of her normal weight of 115, and had to have a tube drain her stomach and intestines. It was then that I first met Ellen, having been called in for consultation and to recommend a new chemotherapeutic regimen. Almost immediately we developed a good doctor-patient relationship, which was further strengthened when she responded to the medical maneuvers. Her partial intestinal obstruction was reversed; she regained 30 pounds and was able to return to active living.

It is not dying but pain that I fear. I am not haunted by it because I do not think my doctor will let me go through unendurable suffering. But pain can be a terribly dehumanizing and degrading experience. You feel like an animal. All you think about is the pain and how to get out of it. There are no higher thoughts, no philosophy, no religion, or anything else. Even your nearest and dearest do not mean much to you. When I felt very sick, the only human thing I did was think about the millions of people in the world who are in agony without a bit of comfort; the napalm and the people in Vietnam without doctors. I thought, "My God, what that must be. Alone, without anyone, lying in a ditch." That hit me. No comfort and nobody to ease them. And here I was with people hovering, offering help and giving help.

I had Demerol when I was so sick last winter, in great pain, and Ernie showed me how to "shoot it" or whatever you do. Sometimes I have terrific pain, but right now, I feel just great. I have narcotics—dolophine, percodan, codeine, and things like that.

But I don't have any temptation to take them except when I really need them, and usually I don't need them. There hasn't been any temptation to abuse drugs.

But at that time (last winter) I really thought I was going to die, although I never completely gave up hope. And it was a slow recovery. I was in bed for 5 to 6 months. Although part of it was very rough, I thought—and this was again partly because of the confidence that had been established with my doctors—that they weren't asking me to go through all that for nothing. I think they probably thought that the chances were very poor of my coming through that crisis, but that on the other hand, if I did, I would have a really good remission, which I have had. I never thought they were saving me just to remain in that state all the time.

At one of the meetings of the seminar an intern asked Ellen whether she would mind discussing her feelings about suicide.

I'd be glad to talk about it. My intellectual feeling is that everybody has a right to his life. I can conceive intellectually of coming to that moment of despair but I'm not yet able to conceive of it emotionally because, as you can see, I'm enjoying myself so much that I want to go on as long as I can.

I'm in the same position you are in. All of you said that when you think about death, it's still a little abstract to you. So although I believe absolutely intellectually that I have the right to take my life when it gets to the point where it's too rough, when the outlay is too great and the pain and the trouble—frankly, emotionally, it's hard to imagine that time.

But if I knew there was never going to be another fairly good remission, where there was going to be any good time, then I would prefer not to have to do it myself. I would say to Ernie or to John, "Let me go." I have that faith in both my doctors.

Ellen panicked only once, when she had a pulmonary embolus, a blood clot in the lungs. She required oxygen and had great difficulty in breathing. There was a tube in her chest to remove collected fluid, and an intravenous tube feeding fluid support and anticoagulants into her vein. At the height of the episode she became panicky. She was cyanotic—ashen colored—gasping for breath as if she were drowning. It was enough to terrify the most resolute person. Her fear lasted less than a day, although her medical crisis continued for 3 days. Later she was remorseful and apologized for not being as noble as she had wanted to be. "It's not the way I want to die," she said. Ellen had repeatedly said she was not afraid of death and had talked to patients about how to maintain their composure. Now she thought she was a failure and felt she had let down her friends, her doctor, and herself. I tried to convince her that her reactions were normal and asked her if she did not feel she had a right to respond like anyone else, but she was not very forgiving of herself.

FAMILY AND FRIENDS

Ellen's high personal standards sometimes led to depression of another kind. She knew that the will to live was important, and she wanted to feel she was making the maximum effort at all times. Occasionally, when she was unable to accomplish as much as she had planned, she would be cheered when I told her that it was her disease, not herself, that was limiting her desire and capacity for achievement. Such depressions were infrequent. Ellen found, on the contrary, that physical activity was all that was reduced. Every other sense and feeling expanded and flourished because of her altered circumstances.

Disease rearranges your values and you cast off things. You do not put up with a lot of stuff in your own self. You reduce the trivia to a minimum. You simplify life, as Thoreau said, when you are under a death warrant.

There is nothing to be afraid of any more when you know you are going to die. It is liberating, very liberating. All the lies are dropped and it cleans up your life. Then everything becomes more poignant, more vivid, the people you love and the people you do not. Relationships become better. You are more aware of the love you feel on both sides, if you know that someone is not going to be there forever. But I also think it's because of the added candor, that you are sharing something together with people who love you.

I always enjoyed life, but I've learned to love it more now. Beauty and music, everything is more poignant. Colors are more vivid. The people I love appear more alive. In a way, my life seems in a rut because I cannot do as much, and I do not feel well part of the time. But it is not a rut, because it is so intense. Everything is heightened, and the awareness is just incredible.

Ellen found that selfishness is essential for survival in the sense that each person has the right to live and die on his or her own terms. She felt it was too complicated to try to protect people, and she was determined to establish an atmosphere of candor in all her relationships.

You have to tell your family and friends. From the beginning I told people what it was. I said it was the big thing, it was cancer. And I don't mean that I didn't act depressed. I said, "I'm going to have all this treatment and everything, but it was pretty bad and they weren't able to get it all." You have to do this, because no one knows how to treat somebody who has cancer. No one will talk about it unless you do. The patient has to set the tone for his surroundings.

Yet one of the surprising reactions was a combination of denial and solicitude. The two things often come together, which is fascinating. I have friends who were as scared of the word as my mother. They wouldn't even say "cancer." They would call it my "disease" or "illness," or "it" or "that." I would very deliberately say, "Well, with cancer ... " a number of times, hoping they would pick it up. Some simply would not say it. Others refused to acknowledge there was anything wrong.

Last year, I had a relapse and went down to 77 pounds. I looked terrible. Some of the people who love me best would visit me and say, "You're looking wonderful." Just patent lies, and yet they would never accept that I really was going to die of it ultimately. And on the other hand they would help me lift packages years after I had surgery. You get weird oversolicitude and second-guessing, such as, "You probably wouldn't want to go because you'd get tired." It's as though you're not a person anymore. But if a patient is tough enough, he can handle it. Over and over you've got to establish the way you're going to handle it and people usually take their cues.

The good thing is, if you're honest, you get past all that and then there is a normal relationship again. Whereas I think if there is a lot of deception, if you're always lying or trying to cover up pain and fatigue, then people think it's worse than it is. If I don't feel good, I don't try to hide it. In fact, you may be full of IVs and terribly sick and everything, but other people will accept it better if you're obviously accepting it in a sense and don't feel destroyed. Then I think they say, "Oh, that's the way it is."

THE PATIENT TREATS HER PHYSICIANS

Doctors are human. We are depressed by patients who are cold and bitter. We are invigorated by patients who are friendly and cooperative. In all my practice Ellen was the epitome of the kind of patient who makes you glad you are a physician. I looked forward to her visits, as did she.

It would be inaccurate to portray Ellen as a patient who did not have recurring medical crises with the usual slow periods of recovery. She also had many episodes of weakness and abdominal swelling and pain from the partial intestinal obstruction. It was her courage, equanimity, and faith in meeting each crisis that made her such a valued patient.

In a subtle way Ellen was effectively giving therapy to the medical team by encouraging us to do our best even though we could not cure her. She felt compassion for us. She would even urge us not to feel discouraged when she was ill from the side effects of a particular therapy, or when her condition worsened. For such patients there even comes a time when they feel sympathy for the doctor because they know their death will be an emotional crisis for the doctor, who is losing a friend. One day during the period of Ellen's pulmonary embolus her mother told a friend, "You know, the thing that's driving Ellen crazy is what it's doing to Ernie."

In essence, Ellen turned something destructive into a positive thing. She used her experience with cancer to help teach some of her physicians how to help terminal patients. During the first meeting of the seminar, Ellen asked the interns there whether they had felt uncomfortable with her or guarded about expressing themselves at the beginning of the evening.

Jim: I think you could probably tell that there was a tremble in my voice when I started expressing some of my ideas, and that was not just because I was having a conversation with someone I'd never known before. It's the fact that you have cancer and you're dying from it.

Ellen: Now, can you tell me, is it easier or harder for you, now that you've talked with me?

Jim: Oh, extremely easier.

Ellen: Isn't it a lot easier to talk, but also to think about it? This isn't why I've done this. That's not why I do it; I do it for my own sake. I'm selfish. But I would still guess it makes it easier, really, on other people, too.

Jim: I was thinking about that while you were talking, when we first came here. And this might be cold, but I was just looking at you as an object, and now I feel so much.

Taylor: As a disease, a disease, not a person!

Jim: And now I see you as a human being. And it's very positive.

Ellen: This is the key . . .

Taylor: Personally, the first thing I was struck by was, "This can't be Ellen. This can't be the one Dr. Rosenbaum was talking about."

Ellen (laughing): She's not sick!

Taylor: She looks beautiful.

When Ellen began to fail, I asked her whether she would like to return to the hospital or remain at home. She replied that she hadn't really thought about it, but that she did not have the horror of hospitals that some people have, and had always had good treatment from the staff at Mt. Zion. However, she said she enjoyed being at home in familiar surroundings, where her family could be comfortable and her friends could visit easily.

As it happened, Ellen died quietly at home. Shortly before she died, she told her mother, "I have no bitterness, no resentment. I don't even hate cancer. You shouldn't grieve for one whose life has been full and happy."

PART FIVE

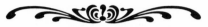

Self-image

Disease is an assault on a person's self-image. A sense of worth is directly related to what we do, how we feel, and how we interact with others, and there are many ways in which having cancer can affect these vital aspects of self. For instance, when cancer patients are unable to work as hard as they did before the illness, or have less energy for family activities than formerly, they may have feelings of shame or guilt. If the disease is terminal, their sense of being defective and somehow to blame for their condition may be intensified.

These destructive feelings do not, however, originate entirely with patients. Healthy people tend, at least subconsciously, to think of someone with a serious disease as lacking in some important way. Such attitudes can result in awkward behavior—avoidance, embarrassment, oversolicitude, a tendency to treat patients as if they were children. None of this escapes patients, who are already feeling sensitive about their condition. To be treated differently now must seem a confirmation of their growing feelings of inadequacy. For these reasons cancer patients, or anyone else with a long-term illness, need an inner certainty of their continuing worth if they are not to fall prey to the attitude of the healthy toward the sick.

Psychological damage can also result from the effects of cancer surgery. A woman whose breast has been removed, and who may even be cured, may have to go through an additional period of anxiety before reaffirming her sexual attractiveness. Surgery that affects the face or neck—areas visible to the public—can also produce self-consciousness and require a period of readjustment. For a person whose livelihood depends on physical perfection—a model or a dancer, for example—the psychological blow of physical impairment can be doubly severe.

Others, accustomed to playing an active role in business and other matters, feel especially humiliated by the loss of autonomy that may accompany progressive disease. When work and accomplishment are a chief source of pleasure and self-definition, slow physical decline can become unbearable.

Most people meet these psychological endurance tests very well, although occasionally a person whose self-esteem was never very high accepts too readily an image of himself or herself as a helpless patient and becomes abandoned to a brooding acceptance of his or her bad luck. Sometimes, conversely, patients will report the emergence of a stronger self-image. They say that before having cancer they often felt hindered in their ability to enjoy themselves, either because of a private fear or neurosis or because of the destructive behavior of someone close to them. The realization that their lives might be cut short made their habitual problems appear trivial and even manageable. I do not mean to imply that these people did not also experience rage, regret, or depression, but the ease with which they began to direct their lives produced a kind of exhilaration, an enhancement of self-esteem.

A cancer patient must struggle against many odds to maintain equanimity. Some people will be awkward in his or her presence because the taboos and fears associated with cancer are not going to vanish overnight. At other times a discouraging medical report will disrupt a patient's calm. Another day one may feel that medical treatment is an endless invasion of his or her sense of dignity and privacy. Each time a person's equilibrium is shattered, it must be slowly regained. Of course, these dynamics become more complicated when cancer is progressive.

Following are the stories of six patients who spoke particularly of the effects of cancer on their self-image, on their way of thinking about themselves and acting in the world.

10

Alice Webster

SPRING 1978

The surgeon assured me before my biopsy that the lump in my breast was only a cyst. Fortunately, I had recently seen a television program on which the results of modified and radical mastectomies were compared, and I made it clear to him that if anything went wrong, he was to perform a modified mastectomy. He said that there were very few surgeons in the San Francisco Bay Area who would perform a modified mastectomy but that if I insisted, he would do one. He said, however, that the problem would not arise since he foresaw no malignancy. I asked him how he could be so sure and he replied, "I can tell by the way the lump feels."

Before going to the hospital, however, I wanted a second opinion and consulted another doctor. He said, "You women are all alike. You all think you have cancer. I don't know what you're upset about. It's nothing but a cyst. We can easily aspirate it, if you wish." Naturally, I responded that my other doctor hadn't made that suggestion. "Other doctor?" he said. "What are you doing here? You should stay with one doctor and take his advice."

I was confused and felt badly that a person should be handled in this way. Nevertheless, I returned to my original surgeon and made arrangements for an overnight stay in the hospital because the biopsy was to be quick and simple. My birthday happened to occur on the same day as the scheduled operation. When I mentioned to the surgeon that I wanted to reschedule the biopsy, he told me that the room was available on that day and that I shouldn't be so concerned. He obviously wasn't. Had I known the end result, I would never have allowed this to happen, for each year the cards and well wishes painfully remind me of that appalling day, and I find myself annually reliving the experience.

My husband had recently lost his teaching job in California and was in New York, where we used to live, looking for a new job. I therefore sent my children, then ages 5 and 2, to the baby-sitter for the night and told her I would pick them up the next afternoon.

When I awoke the next afternoon and found out from a nurse what had happened, I was devastated. I felt that a dirty trick had been played on me, and I felt sorry for my husband because he would have to put up with a woman who had only one breast. Then I realized I could die from it and I thought, "What am I ever going to do? I've got two small children." It was bad. I was afraid and I didn't know what to do. No one was there—not even my husband.

The second day after my mastectomy, my gynecologist, who had originally referred me to the surgeon, came to see me. I asked him if I could hold his hand. He then took my hand and said, "Look, Alice, from now on you're going to be like a gazelle among the lions. The lions get some of the gazelles but not all of them." I felt like there was no chance, no hope. I was surprised at my negative reaction to the doctor's remarks.

Later the same day my surgeon came to my room. He's a doctor who hardly ever makes a mistake, and he didn't seem to be able to handle the situation. I'll never forget the look on his face. He said, "I'm sorry." I felt sorry for him, but I was also angry with him for not telling me there was some chance that it might be malignant.

The surgeon came to see me every day after that, and each time he would look at me and say the same thing, "I'm sorry." One day I asked him, "How long do I have to live? Two years?" "Yes," he replied, "at least two years."

The only professional person who helped me psychologically during my stay in the hospital was a nurse who spent time talking with me. She said, "Don't give up hope. As long as there is a chance, there is hope." I later thanked her for what she did for me because she provided the only glimmer of hope during those first days of shock and grief.

My husband phoned from New York and came out to California for a week. He's very dependent on me and he was upset. A friend told me he cried and said, "How can I live without her?" He's also a perennial optimist who doesn't like to face negative things; nevertheless, he helped me a great deal. He told me he loved me no matter what happened or would happen.

My parents, who were shocked by the news, came to California and helped me after I returned home from the hospital. I also had two friends who helped me immensely by phoning me every day. They let me talk and I just went over and over it. I had other friends, however, who were unable to handle it and who have never phoned or written to me since that time.

On the third day after my mastectomy the surgeon came to change the bandage. He told me I didn't have to look, but I said, "I have to look." And I did. My body had been mutilated. I had to face it. Later, at home, my 2-year-old boy would pull at my blouse to look at my scar. And my 5-year-old daughter was terrified because she thought I was going to die and because she was afraid she might have to endure the same operation when she grew up.

I began radiation treatment as an outpatient shortly after returning home from the hospital. The radiotherapist was a man whose object seemed to be to make women cry, so I said to myself, "I'm not going to cry in front of him." Most doctors hate questions, and unfortunately I would always have several to ask him. His replies were evasive and unhelpful. "It doesn't matter what you eat or what kinds of vitamins you take. You're either going to live or die." Then he'd leave the room.

I had a lot of radiation. My resistance was low and I got the flu, which developed into pneumonia and weakened me. I had always been an energetic person, but at that time I could just manage to get dressed in the morning and then I'd have to sit down for the rest of the day. That was extremely hard for me to handle. A baby-sitter came from 9 until 5, but I had the children alone from 5 until they went to bed. When things happened like my son writing with crayon all over the walls of his bedroom, I didn't even have the strength to deal with it. It was unbelievably frustrating.

At the same time, I was trying to get my feelings together and to face the possibility that I might die. I knew I had to prepare my children for that eventuality. My son was too young to understand the possible implications of my operation. However, my daughter and I were and are extremely close and were able to discuss the matter openly. It was hard for her and for me, but I made her face the fact that I might not be around forever. She would say, "Mommie, I don't want you to die." And I would reply, "I don't want to die either, but we've had 6 good years together and that's what we have to look at." Later I was able to say, "7 good years" and then "8 good years." That has been beautiful—that I have been able to stress the positive.

I took my daughter to the funeral of the grandmother of a friend of hers and explained to her that I wanted her to understand better what a funeral is. It was a lovely experience. People weren't crying. They played the favorite music of the grandmother. When we walked up to the casket, my daughter said, "The body looks just like rubber." And I explained that the spirit isn't there, that it's just the body.

Several months later, as we were driving along in the car, my daughter suddenly said, "Mommie, when you die, I'm going to feel real sad and I'm going to miss you a lot; but I know you're going to be in Heaven, and Heaven must be good." I don't believe in Heaven, and I asked her how she came to that conclusion. She said, "I don't know, but people are too special to have everything end when they die." This came out of the clear blue sky, and I thought, "If she has come that far, that's pretty good." It's hard to believe that good things can come out of this kind of adversity, but my children are stronger. This hasn't destroyed them.

In January 1974, 3 months after my mastectomy, I became upset when I felt a lump in my stomach. I seemed to have all the symptoms of stomach cancer—anemia, slow weight loss, no appetite. All I could think was, "Is this the end?" But when I consulted my doctor, he reassured me that the lump was a piece of cartilage that extended downward from the breastbone. Perfectly normal!

In February another doctor found something "not quite right" in my remaining breast. He qualified his statement by saying he hadn't felt me before, but he told me to see my surgeon as soon as possible and check it out. My heart sank. I was terrified at having to go through it all again. I felt so vulnerable, at the mercy of some unknown monster. However, my surgeon told me it was nothing to be alarmed about. I could have hugged him, and as I left his office, tears rolled uncontrollably down my cheeks.

The turning point in my almost unremitting depression came in April 1974, when I read an article in a San Francisco newspaper about an experimental immunotherapy program that was being set up at the Zellerbach Saroni Tumor Institute at Mount Zion Hospital. It sounded like a chance for life and I hoped it was going to be something to hold onto.

I was very nervous the first time I walked into the Tumor Institute, but everyone was kind and compassionate. They gave me extensive tests. After one of these tests, which involved an injection of radioactive material, one of the doctors told me everything looked normal. I said, "You can't imagine what that means to me."

"I think I can," he replied.

When they told me I was accepted in the program, I was thrilled. I felt it was my one hope. Three donors who had been breast cancer-free for 10 years were the volunteers for me. They donated their blood, which was processed to remove a substance called transfer factor. This was then injected into me in the hope that it would help to build up my immunity against a recurrence. I could hardly wait to get the material in me.

Since that time I have been retested every 6 months for signs of recurrence. So far I have tested negatively and continue to receive transfer factor.

It has now been 4 years since I first walked into the Tumor Institute. During that time I have changed—gradually, but dramatically. The change began the day I decided, "The time I have left, I'm going to use well," and began to rearrange my priorities and look at myself and my life in a more positive way.

I used to have a terrible self-image. I felt every other woman was prettier, more accomplished, and better able to deal with life, so I first had to ask myself, "How much validity is there to these feelings?" Since then I have lost so many hang-ups. A friend who knew me before says I used to keep my personality covered up, that I wore a mask that prevented her from really seeing me. I wore dark clothes, no jewelry, and very little makeup. My husband often told me I dressed like a parochial schoolgirl, and I did! I was very proper, and extremely child-oriented. I lived through my children.

Now my friend sees me as vibrant, fresh, and alive. I feel fulfillment. My family is meaningful to me, but *I'm* meaningful to me now. I'm just as important as other people—and that's a big part of the change. I no longer get inundated with things that don't interest me. I'm learning to say no, whereas before I wondered what people would have thought of me if I said that. And I no longer give a darn what the neighbors think.

Before my mastectomy I went through each day thinking I was immortal. Now I only want to live each day positively. I don't want to waste my energies in negativism. I know where I am because I had to face it. And I can never go back! I'm changing all the time. It's like a renaissance and I love it. I enjoy my husband and children even more than before. I'm very selective with my friends and I enjoy them fully. I like to help them. I enjoy the world around me—nature—and the view from my house.

The house is an example of how I've changed. I have always found it hard to make decisions, but there was my husband looking for a job in New York, wanting to move us back there. I felt it was important to stay in California. I had to make a decision on the house in California in 24 hours, and I was surprised that I was able to do it. Before, I would have followed my husband because that's what I believed was the job of a wife. Now I felt I mattered too. I bought the house, and he is going to get a job out here. Of course, my mother thinks I'm going through menopause, and my husband just sits back and looks at me, wondering at this craziness.

At the time of my surgery, I didn't know I had the option of waiting for a period of time between the biopsy and the mastectomy. I also hadn't heard about the possibility of breast reconstruction, but I'm glad I was at least able to tell the doctor I would only allow him to perform a modified mastectomy. If I had had a radical mastectomy, I would have been doubly devastated. At least I can wear a bathing suit, although the first time I tried to buy one, I almost cried. I felt so conspicuous, and I was afraid to buy one that would reveal too much. I still have to remember not to bend over in my bathing suit, and I have a hard time finding nightgowns that are sexy.

The loss of my breast bothered me all the more because it is an erogenous zone. I wondered how a man could look at me and be turned on. I know a lot of this has to do with my attitude, and I am getting better about it. I attended a sex conference for people who have had cancer surgery, and I'm glad that people are at least acknowledging that there are sexual problems to be worked out for men and women who have cancer.

Nudity in front of the children was another problem. Nudity never concerned me before my mastectomy, but for a long time afterwards it bothered me to be nude in front of my family. Only recently am I able to feel relaxed about it again. Thus though I still have some problems about my body image, when I look in the mirror I think, "That scar saved your life."

This is what I tell women whom I visit for the Reach to Recovery Program,* and it is what I tell audiences whom I lecture on rehabilitation for the American Cancer Society. I do this volunteer work because I feel I can help other women who are undergoing the trauma of a mastectomy. I've been there.

AUTUMN 1978

In retrospect, I realize my husband never wanted to face the fact of my cancer. When they first found the lump, he told me to forget it and it would go away. To this day he tells me that I never had it and that they removed my breast for nothing.

Our marriage went steadily downhill in the last year and a half, so that we are now in divorce proceedings. If I hadn't had cancer, my marriage would probably have held together, but the experience changed me. It made me very strong.

It also changed me by forcing me to look at myself. When you look at

---

*The Reach to Recovery Program of the American Cancer Society consists of a group of women who have had mastectomies and returned to active living. These volunteer women are specially selected and trained to visit new mastectomy patients to show them that they too can return to normal living.

yourself and you don't like what you see, you have to do something about it. Well, you don't *have* to do anything about it. I could have avoided it, but my disease was life-threatening, and I had to face it. I wondered how much time I had left, and I gave a lot of thought to priorities.

Change is so gradual that you hardly know it's happening. At the same time you go through a lot of awfulness when you're facing things, before you get in touch with yourself. Looking back, I don't feel that anything can ever again devastate me the way my cancer experience did. Nothing can be as bad as that, and having survived it, I feel I can survive anything—including my divorce, which is making this a difficult period. However, I know that when it's over I'm going to be in a different place. I'm going to grow with the experience.

I have a feeling of "going forward," and I find myself planning and anticipating the future. But at the same time that I feel the potential of the future, it's also scary and depressing, because being single brings its own problems, such as how to handle meeting men. I'm not the kind of person to get involved right away. That would be too threatening. I have to know the person.

The fact of my mastectomy is not a big problem for me now. My only concern is, when is the right time to tell someone about it? I've decided that this is after you know a person for a while and you can see he has an interest in you, and you are interested in him. You shouldn't wait until you're ready to go to bed. You have to do it at some discreet time beforehand when you know something *could* develop.

It's interesting, looking forward to meeting someone new. It is no longer something I'm going to grab at—I used to feel it was the most important thing in my life. Now, although I feel it would be wonderful, I don't *have* to have it. It's just that I would *like* to have it.

It's as though I have had two second chances—first, with my life; and now with the possibility of a new relationship. So, when my parents feel sorry for me because I'm getting divorced, I tell them, "Don't! What if I didn't have this chance at a new life?"

My new life includes playing tennis, which I began in August. And I've just begun taking skiing lessons. I would never have skied before. I was too afraid. But I don't say no anymore. I want to learn all kinds of things. Even when they don't seem interesting at first, I give them a try. I never used to be that way.

I have been working part-time on a cancer research project, interviewing people, and I'm doing volunteer work with Reach to Recovery, but I no longer want to work exclusively in the field of cancer. For a while, I saw myself only as a cancer patient, until one day a friend said, "Alice, you can spend your life as a cancer patient or as someone who sees herself as sick." She was right. I want to choose to be well and to be in the middle of things.

When I get a job outside the medical world, I will continue to work for Reach to Recovery, however, because I know how important it is to get help when you need it. I not only had a visitor from Reach to Recovery, but I've had counseling twice, and I would have it again if I felt I needed it. I consulted a psychiatric social worker when I had my mastectomy, and a psychologist when my marriage was breaking up. If you get the right person, as I did in both cases, it can be extremely beneficial. If you don't find the right person, you need to look elsewhere until you find someone to whom you can relate.

I still have a lot of fear when it's time for my 6-month tests. It starts when I make the laboratory and doctor appointments, and although it's less and less now, it was really bad for the first 5 years. I was so sure they would find something.

It's terrible beforehand and it's terrible while you're lying there waiting, especially with bone scans, because you lie there for an hour. I have tried to program myself not to think about it. I force myself to think of anything else, and although my mind naturally keeps going back to it, the technique works pretty well. If I have to face it, I will, but until then, I won't think about it unless I have to.

As you proceed from one test to the next, one by one, and they come out negatively, you know that for right now you are completely healthy. It's the greatest feeling in the world.

11
Mort Segal

When Mort Segal was shown the first draft of this chapter, he did not believe that it fully reflected his feelings about his experience with cancer. Because he was a writer, among other things, he began to rewrite the material. Unfortunately, he completed only the first section, entitled "May 16, 1972." Although I urged him many times to continue writing and he often said he wanted to, he never again picked up the manuscript. I believe that if he had tried to complete the chapter, it would have seemed to him that he was completing his life.

MAY 16, 1972

I had a call at home in the evening from an insurance man I know. He urged me to see a client of his, Mort Segal by name. He told me that Segal had just come over to see him that evening to discuss his insurance policies. Segal had learned earlier in the day that he had a malignant cancer, one that "might kill him in 6 to 8 weeks." Segal's doctor had assured him that these weeks would be extremely rewarding in terms of his family and friends. I was told that Segal was "distressed," which was hardly surprising.

Segal was forceful and energetic, very much in command. He was 40 years old, trained as a lawyer, and the managing partner of a national consulting firm specializing in governmental legislative and administrative reforms, governmental reorganization, and the like. It is a field quite outside my experience.

Segal was married and had two young children. He introduced himself as one who had "never been ill" until this "crazy illness" caught up with him. He was annoyed, perhaps even angry, rather as one might feel over having had one's vacation postponed or cut short at the last minute. He appeared determined, at the very outset, to establish a peer relationship with me in regard to the discussion and, even more, the treatment of his disease. He made it clear that he had no intention of merely acquiescing to treatment, as most patients might when consulting their physicians.

Segal made one other point, in very clear and certain terms. He said he would not agree to any treatment unless he was himself satisfied that the likelihood of its success substantially outweighed its physical and psychological inconveniences. "No fishing expeditions," Segal admonished. This point had reference to any of the four cancer therapies: surgery, chemotherapy, radiotherapy, and immunotherapy.

His rationale was that each such treatment intruded on his basic dignity and privacy, surgery more than chemotherapy, chemotherapy more than radiotherapy, and so on. For Segal, this was to be his private "battle." In a way, he almost appeared to relish the contest. Interference from the sidelines, such as by me, was not going to be readily tolerated. Segal said that if it were not for his wife and little children, if he were single and alone, he would not tolerate any interference at all. It was clear that he would be a difficult, headstrong patient.

Having established the rules of our relationship, Segal went on to describe the course of his illness from its beginning. As it happened, its beginning went back nearly a year in time. It wasn't neat, nor did it move in a single direction. But then, these things seldom do.

Segal told me that on June 24 of the previous year, 1971, he quite suddenly had a sharp pain in his right chest. At the time, he was between planes at O'Hare Airport, outside Chicago, on his way back from Washington, D.C., to San Francisco. The pain immobilized him, so that he was unable to board his plane. He assumed he was suffering a heart attack, which he informed me was "pretty much in accord with the way I always thought I would go." His condition attracted some attention among others waiting for planes. Segal said he was embarrassed by the attention, and attempted to diminish the importance of his condition. Nonetheless, he must have looked fairly bad, and finally he allowed himself to be escorted to the airport's first-aid station. His chest pain became progressively more excruciating.

After several hours of waiting at the airport's first-aid station, Segal agreed to go to a nearby hospital. He refused, however, to sit in the wheelchair provided by the attendants who arrived in an ambulance, and refused to ride in the back of the ambulance as well, sitting up front instead. Numerous x-ray films were taken at the hospital. Meanwhile, the excruciating pain slowly subsided. After several demeaning hours of waiting, the physician in charge announced triumphantly that Segal was suffering from constipation. Having missed the last direct flight to San Francisco, he left the hospital by taxi and checked into a nearby hotel. Segal called his wife and merely said that he had missed the last plane. He told her he would catch the first plane out of Chicago the next morning.

On Segal's return to San Francisco, he underwent a number of tests. The pain had completely disappeared during the course of the night in Chicago. This new battery of tests failed to show any problems. It was finally concluded that Segal might have passed a kidney stone. In any case, the incident was consigned to the nether region of medical science, where symptoms wait to be forgotten or recur.

After the June 24 incident, but quite apart from it, Segal decided to take a year's leave of absence from his firm and move to the south of France. His understanding with his partners covered the possibility that he might simply decide to stay there indefinitely. He and his family were due to leave for Paris on October 1. Their house was accordingly rented, the car sold, and furniture readied for storage.

On September 20, however, Segal experienced a second seizure, this time in the midst of an important business meeting. He collapsed and was taken by ambulance to a San Francisco hospital. He arrived with "no perceptible signs of life." An x-ray film revealed total opacity of the right lung. A needle was introduced and pure blood was taken. His perivascular status remained precarious for several hours, but finally stabilized enough to permit exploratory thoracic surgery. During the brief time when Segal regained consciousness before surgery, he expressed distress at his passivity in relation to the physicians and others surrounding him. He said he wasn't accustomed to playing a passive role and found it demeaning, if not emasculating. Before being taken in for surgery, he suggested that the surgeon perform a vasectomy he had long planned but had been equally long in postponing.

Segal spent 9 hours in the operating room. On three different occasions it looked as if he would die. He received 21 pints of blood, and the lower lobe of his right lung was removed. The surgeon also removed a small, exceedingly rare carcinoid-like tumor. The diagnosis was that it was basically benign, although the area ought to be watched. A hospital convalescence of 4 to 6 weeks was anticipated, but Segal managed to have himself released within 7 days. He worked intermittently at his office for several more weeks, and at the end of October boarded a plane for France with his family.

By the end of April 1972, only 6 months after leaving San Francisco, the Segals became thoroughly bored with their leisurely life in France. Accordingly, Segal alone flew back to San Francisco, rented an apartment for his family, who would follow within a month, and went back to work at his old desk in his consulting firm. With some reluctance, he decided that the bucolic life in France could not be his life, and that however much he wanted to be a "family man," close to his wife and children, he could not. He was soon flying around the country, rushing from New York to Honolulu, attending meetings and giving consultations.

During his first month back he discovered that a small lump had developed under the thoracic scar tissue of his right chest wall. His physician diagnosed it as a subcutaneous cyst. Shortly thereafter he had it excised one afternoon in his surgeon's office, under a local anesthetic. The surgeon remarked laconically that the subcutaneous cyst was, in fact, a tumor, and that its development was probably attributable to some cell contamination that remained from the original surgery the previous September.

The biopsy of the tumor, done at another hospital from Segal's original operation, showed that it was not the same type as the original tumor, and that, moreover, it was a rare malignancy—a sarcoma. Further comparison of the slides showed that, in fact, both tumors were the same, which is to say that the original biopsy diagnosis had been incorrect. Segal was informed that he had a highly malignant, rare tumor of the blood vessel lining, called hemangiopericytoma. His hemangiopericytoma proved to be the ninth such tumor, in that presentation, known anywhere in the world. It was at that point that

Segal's surgeon informed him that the tumor "might kill" him "in 6 to 8 weeks." That evening Segal called his insurance man, who in turn called me.

LATE OCTOBER 1972

Segal refused all treatment for the 4 months following his diagnosis, preferring to enjoy the short time he was told remained to him. During that time and from then on, my role in his case was that of a consulting physician, working closely with Dr. Herman A. Schwartz, head of oncology at Kaiser Hospital, which was a participant in Segal's health-insurance plan. I explained to Segal that the surgeon's figure was based on an estimate and that the outcome of any one case could not be determined by average statistics, especially when they were based on a sample of only eight other cases. Each case, whether cardiac or cancer, must be considered individually. Segal's reply was always, "If I'm going to die, I want to do it my way."

However, when Segal found he was still alive in mid-October, he became interested in consultations about chemotherapy. (His tumor was not operable for cure at that time, and it was not considered primarily radiosensitive.) He told me that during the 6 weeks following his prognosis he had leaped from bed each morning ready to do battle with death and that each evening he had had the satisfaction of having won. When the 6 weeks passed and he was still functioning and well, he felt even more exhilarated, believing that by an act of will he had succeeded in defeating cancer and death.

Although Segal had never been ill himself, he knew what prolonged disease could do to a person's resolve to die with dignity and grace. His father had contracted Parkinson's disease 15 years before and at the time was adamant about wishing to live only as long as he could take care of himself. His decline was imperceptibly slow, and as the years passed and his debility increased, he abandoned his resolve. Although totally incapacitated, he clung to life. This experience left an indelible impression on Segal and was certainly an important reason for his reluctance to accept treatment.

Another reason, certainly, was that illness is humiliating because a person has to depend on the decisions of others for treatment of a disease he or she does not completely understand. A doctor tells a patient that certain physical manifestations have been detected and that a particular treatment may be effective in restoring health. The patient must then trust the physician. Segal was not used to being in this relationship to someone else. He saw his life in terms of his own will.

Basically I really like the kind of person I've made myself become, and that's what it's all about—whether my will prevails over my doctors', whether I will control the course of my illness and its effects on me. I can do that in a variety of ways, one of which is the decision whether to take treatment or not. It is my intention to die with dignity, not to waste away. I'm not going to go down the tube slowly. The trick is to figure out when that may happen and to act before you lose the option.

We had many sessions, with questions and more questions. Segal played the role of defense attorney and was also his own client. I reminded him of the adage that lawyers who conduct their own defense have fools for clients. I could reason with Segal, but I always felt I was losing, and I was surprised to find I had finally won his agreement to try to fight his cancer. Presumably he had come to see me because he had decided to take therapy, but he needed to have these arguments first, partly to let me know he was not "turning himself over to me." To assuage his last vestiges of doubt, I sent him to the M. D. Anderson Hospital in Houston for consultation. The concurrence of those doctors with a plan for chemotherapy made Segal receptive to treatment, although he always managed to add another "condition." When he yielded on one issue, he wanted compromise on another.

With the understanding that we didn't know how such a rare tumor would respond to drugs, Dr. Schwartz instituted a four-drug chemotherapy program, to be administered by the physicians at Kaiser Hospital.

LATE NOVEMBER 1972

Segal received injections 5 mornings a week every 3 weeks and suffered side effects of nausea, vomiting, hair loss, and fatigue. But once he had made the decision to try the program, his determination to see it through prevailed.

The dosage in his daily injections was reduced but the vomiting continued, causing physical discomfort as well as embarrassment. The nausea began just as Segal arrived at work after his morning injection, and it came in unpredictable waves. If he got an attack while in a meeting or on the telephone, he had to excuse himself and rush to the bathroom, where he would vomit for several minutes. These attacks were usually dry heaves and the sound reverberated through the office. He began keeping a bowl in his office, eliminating the dash to the bathroom. Although Segal described these maneuvers with his customary humor, the procedure obviously offended his sense of privacy. We changed the chemotherapy schedule, and his physicians began to administer injections in the evening so he could work uninterrupted during the day.

Chemotherapy also disrupted Segal's travel schedule. He was so uncomfortable during the 5 days he received injections that he stayed close to home and then tried to squeeze 3 weeks of travel into 2. The vomiting and fatigue reduced his efficiency to such an extent that he often worked all night at the office, returning home around 5:00 AM for a few hours of sleep before returning to the office. He was determined to maintain his former level of productivity, which in the past had involved working 80 to 90 hours a week and traveling almost a quarter of a million miles a year.

DECEMBER 18, 1972

X-ray films showed changes in Segal's lungs; his disease had returned, which meant that we had to consider surgery. A resection could possibly have reduced the size of the tumor, making it easier to control the residual tumor with chemotherapy and perhaps immunotherapy.

But Segal was against surgery. He recalled with some chagrin that after his first operation he accidentally saw his medical folder, which contained the comment "Shows considerable anxiety about dying." Questioned by Segal, his physician told him, "You were very anxious about dying before the operation; you asked if you were going to die." Segal then asked me whether this had been intellectual curiosity or fear. "Fear. Not weeping, but real fear," I said. This surprised Segal, for fear had no place in his self-image. "My concept of dignity is not to weep when I am dying." The incident had other ramifications—an intrusion on privacy, the humiliation of dependence on the decisions of others, a feeling of anxiety such as some people feel when another person is driving the car.

Segal was determined not to let false hope interfere with his reason, creating the paradox that his emotions in the form of his desire for independence were leading him to make unsound decisions. He refused to yield to my medical experience.

I felt somewhat ambiguous on that point, however, because I believe a patient should participate as much as possible in decisions concerning his treatment. But Segal's need for authority outweighed his knowledge, a fact that caused him some conflict.

This is the first time that I've been in a position where, technically, someone knows significantly more than I do. I have to believe you aren't trumping up enthusiasm to talk me into one more treatment.

The members of the Tumor Board at Segal's hospital were to recommend whether surgery should be performed. Segal remained opposed to an operation but held hours of discussions with his wife, close friends, and doctors. I feel that patients often obtain better medical results when they encourage their physicians to act positively, so I was pleased when Segal eventually acquiesced to surgery.

LATE JANUARY 1973

On the day Segal was scheduled to enter the hospital, the members of the Tumor Board decided his tumor was too advanced to be treated surgically. Segal's wife, Janet, describes this decision as an enormous letdown for Segal, after he had prepared himself psychologically for the operation. "It was the most painful period for Mort. He kept doing, saying, laughing, joking, directing, inspiring, enraging, but he knew he wasn't going to win the war he cared most about."

EARLY MARCH 1973

We continued with a program of chemotherapy, but Segal resented the loss of time involved in going for treatment and the interruption in his travel schedule, although he now dismissed the side effects as "inconvenient." I asked him if having cancer had made him change the way he lives.

I don't put things off now, but I never did. I never worried about quitting a job or dropping everything and going off to live in France. Janet and I haven't let ourselves be constrained by finances or the children. People ask me why I don't take a vacation or do something I've always wanted to do. I've always done what I wanted, and what I want to do now is work. My regret in dying isn't for the things I haven't done but for the time I won't have to do more. By rights I should have another 15 or 20 good years, and now they're gone. You know, I used to kid myself that I never got to spend time with my family because I had to work so hard, but after the 6 months in France I realized that I work all the time because I like it. If you feel good about yourself, if you are doing what you want to do, you don't change your life just because you're sick.

JUNE 22, 1973

The tumor in Segal's right chest grew steadily and appeared to be invading his liver. We decided to discontinue chemotherapy because there had been no improvement after six sequences of drugs; and despite Segal's light dismissal of the side effects as little more than annoying, they were in fact severe and humiliating. Segal never complained and yet he had become so sensitized that he would vomit at the sight of the syringe in anticipation of the side effects to follow.

We started an experimental immunotherapy program in hopes of inhibiting tumor growth. We were dubious about whether this would do much good, which meant that we had to reconsider surgery. Segal agreed to surgery more readily this time; months of nausea had convinced him that it might be less of an imposition on his freedom than chemotherapy had been. Also, in Segal's case there was a progression of the tumor. We asked the consultants in Houston to review his case.

JULY 9, 1973

The physicians in Houston recommended a surgeon at UCLA and Segal flew to Los Angeles to consult with him. They talked at length about the quality of life and the doctor told him that if the operation was a success, he might expect to have from 18 to 24 months of good life ahead of him. The doctor then showed him a graph based on the doubling growth rate of his tumor and assured him that without an operation he would be dead in 5.2 months. He also said that if they were unable to remove the total tumor, if the operation were a failure, Segal would not have long to live.

Although this doctor is a leading surgeon with extensive medical knowledge, he was playing prophet when he produced a figure like 5.2 months. Growth rates change; the nourishment to the tumor changes; and the body's immune system may affect these as well as other factors. Predictions have some validity, but no matter how much one knows about tumor growth rates, they provide incomplete data when the total situation of a patient is considered.

Segal didn't waver in his determination to die rather than become an invalid, so the operation became his only major option.

JULY 23, 1973

Segal and Janet came to my office to review all the points in favor of the operation before going to Los Angeles. Segal was satisfied that he and the surgeon had the same goals in mind, but I think Janet wanted to hear the arguments for herself. She was upset. I think she felt that her husband's case had not been properly handled and that he should have had the operation in January. Possibly his chances would have been better then. In any case, they now faced three possibilities. As Segal put it,

I might die on the operating table, in which case everything is settled. They might make the resection and I'll get another 2 years, maybe more. Or they'll see that they can't resect and just close me up again. The last eventuality will be the hardest to live with, so I'm preparing myself for that. Besides, there's no choice now. I'm hurt and I'm tired. Without the surgery I'm going to be bedridden. Then I'll be dead.

JULY 30, 1973

The operation was performed and the tumor was not resectable. It appeared to be invading the liver and was highly friable. An attempted resection could have led to fragmentation, causing rapid spread of the malignancy.

My wife and I flew to Los Angeles the next day to be with Mort and Janet. When we entered the room, Mort was alert and cheerful, but when Janet and Isadora left his expression changed. He said, "Ernie, that was the last try. You begin to hope and that breaks you. All a man has at the end is his dignity."

We talked for a long time, and he told me about an experience he had had on a recent trip to Point Barrow, in Alaska.

I've seen any number of pictures of the tundra and the Arctic wastes, but until I was up there I had not visualized how frightening, how truly frightening it is to be up there. The size is beyond conception. It isn't like the photographs, with borders. It's without borders. It's without words. I chartered a small plane and flew across the North Slope for hundreds of miles. There is nothing—no life, no polar bears, just snow. You can walk for 1800 miles over the pole and down into Siberia. There is just nothing out there. I thought of the foolishness—or the incredible bravery—of the men in 1903 who started out across the ice cover, risking death. I've been close to death, but it's one thing to be there all of a sudden and not to whimper, and it's another to march across a plain resolutely, knowing that when you get there, you drop off. And it's another yet to know that you are marching across the plain to the edge, but kind of blindfolded so that you get to see only occasionally. Treatment is that experience. It's marching across a plain resolutely, sometimes blindfolded, which is when you are receiving treatment or are in a remission or whatever; but sometimes just seeing that you are getting closer. Suddenly the blindfold comes off and you are really close and it comes as a surprise. That is why people become freaked by their experience with treatment. And that's how people break. It's the uncertainty. There are lots of people who could march there with certainty and with dignity. But there will be a breakthrough on the horizon, which is now so close, and it will suddenly be extended—perhaps to infinity. How many times can people take that? I don't think I can take it, and I consider myself a very strong person.

MID-AUGUST 1973

Segal had phenomenal recuperative powers. After the exploratory lapa-rotomy (abdominal surgery), he was eating the following day and flew home 3 days later. That evening, 5 days after surgery, he attended a fund-raising party for the Friends of Cancer Immunology (FOCI) in San Francisco, brought several of his friends, and spent 4 hours helping to raise funds for cancer research. I am sure he was exhausted afterward, but that was his style—to maintain a high standard of performance.

I visited Segal at home late one afternoon. He had tried to keep up his active pace—a day each in New York, Washington, Denver, and New Orleans; but he was forced to take a day off because he was feeling so weak. He said:

I'm becoming a kvetch, Ernie. But it's hard to do otherwise. I hope that Janet doesn't remember me as one. It's shocking to think that one has 9 years of marriage, and a partnership, and that the last week is what people will remember you for. Of course I don't believe that, but I think the last week is an important week. I want Janet to remember me as I am today, not as I might be, should I become a weakly weeping kvetch. I don't want my children to remember me that way, either. I don't want to be that way. I demand it of myself. And I'll not let anyone deny it to me.

I told you that when I went to Los Angeles I had prepared for the eventuality that the tumor would be inoperable. It was the only possibility I thought about because I knew it would be the most difficult to manage. If I'd gone down there hoping, I'd have been destroyed. Afterwards, I was upset but not devastated; and I was mostly upset because Janet was, and because I was going to have a lot of pain and discomfort for a couple of weeks when I might have been well. If you don't have much time, a couple of weeks is valuable.

Segal talked again about the treachery involved in hoping (which it is clear that he did, despite himself), and of how people do not have the resources to repeat very often the process of gaining, and then losing, hope. He also spoke of the horror that chemotherapy had been for him.

It's an indescribably awful experience. It's like going every morning and having an injection of stomach flu. You do it every morning, and you do it yourself. It isn't like, "If I'd only worn boots, I wouldn't have caught stomach flu." You're going out to be whipped every day. You think people get depressed or are cowards because they're not willing to take it. But, goddammit, it takes away from you. When I think of the things I've gone through, I'm appalled. I don't know where I found the resources. I've got to be satisfied that I can still live with quality. I think treatment risks doing a great disservice to people who want not to be bothered anymore. But that isn't the same as folding up with no hope and going into a catatonic state, waiting to die. That's obviously one kind of reaction. But there are a whole bunch of people who just don't want to futz around anymore. They want to do their thing and then they want to drop dead. But treatment does terrible things. I could talk about the injections and get sick—actually throw up thinking about them—even though I haven't had them lately. A cerebral person like me doesn't want to be tied to a bodily function that affects his mind. The point is that you really change, Ernie.

The results of Segal's treatment were only fair, because chemotherapy merely slowed down the growth of his tumor. But his side effects were out of proportion to the strength of the drug. Sometimes anxiety or the anticipation of bad results from a previous experience can increase toxicity; and although Segal appeared calm on all occasions, he was undoubtedly conditioned by his prior toxic experiences. Conversely, a patient who approaches therapy with a positive attitude often has less toxicity.

After the operation in Los Angeles I had been worried about Segal's becoming despondent and had recommended that he talk with a psychiatrist.

You think I'm depressed. You're wrong. I'm not depressed, let me assure you. I talked to my friends since you suggested I get psychiatric help. They don't think I've changed at all. And I don't think so. You're projecting. I am not voicing a more positive or negative view than I otherwise would. Except as things become more negative, you demand more positivism. You respond to negative impulses with greater positive adrenalin. I don't respond more or less to negative impulses. I persevere. And that's an important difference between us. You are far more genuine than I am, and I admire you for it, but I don't think either of us would trade places.

Nevertheless, Segal was always aware of what pain and time could do to him. He kept open the option of suicide at the appropriate moment. I asked him if he thought he could do it.

I spent a lot of time thinking about that. I don't doubt my ability to do it, but it's a continuous battle between you and me to decide whose will is going to prevail. I have to guard against hoping too much. You might talk me into one treatment after another until I lose perspective. I fear I'll be worn down through a process of attrition, which will involve on the one hand my physical illness but the result of which will be that my perceptions and my rationality will be impaired or distracted. Then I'll become like everyone else after a while—hanging on. The most rational, the most powerful, the most independent among us are subject to being worn down, the only difference being that some of us act at this point while some of us wait too long.

I don't think you would consciously wait too long to let me go, but your threshold is different than mine. And you don't know what it's like. It's like what Negroes call the Black Experience. You can't know what it's like to be black unless you really are a black. And it's not even enough to be black. You have to be black in a special situation.

I tried to reassure him by saying, "I've promised you won't suffer and that I'm not going to keep you alive when there's no hope."

But we have different senses of hope. I'm not going for a 5% chance. Maybe you would. I want to be sure it's the decision I'd make.

I didn't doubt that Segal could kill himself, yet this rarely happens among cancer patients. A person's capacity to endure seems to grow as the need arises.

MID-SEPTEMBER 1973

After the operation in July, Segal refused all further treatment, although the tumor grew steadily. Most days he worked an average of 16 hours, but one day in September he returned early from a business trip because of a new pain in his back and chest. His spirits were low. He said, "Dying slowly is like psyching yourself to be executed tomorrow morning at dawn and learning at dawn that it's going to be put off for another day, and that goes on day after day. And it breaks the spirit."

Nevertheless, he agreed to have angiograms in preparation for the possibility of introducing chemotherapy directly into the arterial system that feeds the tumor. He also agreed to radiation treatments that might relieve his pain by shrinking the tumor.

NOVEMBER 27, 1973

The angiograms showed that the tumor was pressing against Segal's liver but had not yet invaded it; they also revealed the growth of a second tumor behind his heart. We gave him radiation for the second tumor, but another method of dealing with such a tumor would have been to insert a tube in the aorta, the major artery in the body, and to apply chemotherapy directly to the tumor. This would have meant carrying around a pump with a chemotherapy reservoir and making frequent visits to the hospital. Segal's philosophy and self-image did not include that kind of dependence on tubes, and he vetoed the idea.

Radiation provided sufficient pain relief to enable Segal to work, even though his treatment schedule was sometimes upset by business trips. However, I think that the best medicine is not always the best medical care. It is more important that a patient have freedom to live and work.

Segal had by this time survived almost 5 of the 5.2 months predicted by his Los Angeles surgeon.

JANUARY 5, 1974

I asked Segal how he felt about the reprieve he was receiving through the radiation treatments.

It doesn't seem like a reprieve to me. It just means I'll live a little longer. I wasn't looking for a reprieve. I was looking for energy and achievement. A reprieve doesn't provide that.

I wanted to leave behind me a kind of statement. I thought I had plenty of time, but more achievement will be denied me. One achieves and makes statements on different levels. One of the statements we obviously make is our children and how they grow up, the chain of immortality they represent. That will be denied me. And even if they remember me, it doesn't matter. I won't have had the impact on Rebecca and Josh that the next 10 to 15 years would have meant. They will not be my statement.

Another statement is made in our work and what we accomplish in the marketplace of ideas, money, business, or whatever. When I walk down Montgomery Street, I think, "Some of these people will accomplish things. I won't." I have every reason to believe I would have achieved more in my work, but I've run out of time.

A third statement, which I think I have achieved, is that indefinable quality of being a good person. There are a lot of people who love me because I am really a pretty decent and interesting guy. That is important to me, the achievement of love.

I've run out of time because I've run out of energy. I'm in a holding action. It takes everything I have just to keep moving. It's difficult to maintain one's grace. If this year were a repeat of last year, I don't believe I'd go through it. It's no longer cancer and me. Each new treatment has removed me from the privacy of my own dealings with cancer. To you and the other doctors I'm just a tool. It's a war of attrition with constantly more troops. It's not my war anymore.

Although Segal said he was worn down psychologically, he still strove for excellence and precision in his work and was, I am told, a catalyst in fostering these qualities in his associates.

MID-FEBRUARY 1974

After neurological consultation for progressive back pain, Segal entered the hospital for a myelogram. The diagnosis was recurrent tumor invading the sciatic nerve, so radiotherapy was reinstituted and provided some relief from pain. But when the radiotherapy was only partly completed, he decided to go home and receive the treatments as an outpatient. He never would stay in a hospital a minute longer than necessary.

In addition to giving Segal radiotherapy for pain relief, we tried to teach him how to give himself pain shots, but he was not sufficiently interested to become proficient. Even when his pain was severe, he would sometimes postpone receiving a shot as a test of strength.

LATE FEBRUARY 1974

When a person has cancer and life can no longer be measured in quantity, quality becomes the objective. Segal achieved this quality before he had cancer, but he continued throughout treatment to make the most of each day. During the last 2 weeks of February he became too weak to go to the office and spent most of his time in a rented hospital bed in a sunny corner of his living room. He enjoyed being at home with his family and would invite his friends over for cocktails, sometimes holding meetings or advising friends and colleagues.

He continued to go to the hospital for radiotherapy treatment, but as the pain increased, he became more of an invalid. Going to the bathroom, three rooms away, was a chore. He almost required pain medicine for the trip. The back pain increased; the muscle spasms became intense, wracking his entire body. I remember being called by Segal, who was almost in tears, at 5:00 one morning to come over and give him a shot. He received his evening shots from a psychiatrist neighbor, and with those, the pills, and the muscle relaxers, he made one day at a time.

Finally the trips to the hospital for radiotherapy became too difficult and treatment was discontinued.

Segal might possibly have gained some extra weeks or months of life from another round of chemotherapy, but he did not want any more treatments. He was tired. In 1 year he had had 5 months of intensive chemotherapy, surgery, radiation therapy, and immunotherapy—the whole breadth of medical treatment for cancer. But he did say that the past year and a half had been worth it because he had the chance to enjoy his family and to watch the personality of his small son develop.

MARCH 9, 1974

I stopped at Segal's home and found him sitting up in bed, bright-eyed, talking excitedly on the telephone. When he hung up, he looked around the room at Janet and me and appeared immensely pleased about something. He had recently revised the charter for a large eastern city, and the call had been from the chairman of a Senate committee, informing him of legislative approval and congratulating him on the excellence of his work. (Segal had worked so hard and so well that few of his business associates ever knew he had cancer.)

Isadora and I decided to have a luncheon to celebrate Segal's success. The weather was unusually nice, and Janet and Mort invited several of their friends. We sat around eating and drinking wine, discussing the president's problems and other topics. It was one of those memorable days, and Segal was at his best.

During the next 3 days Segal's debility increased, however. He would lapse into a partial coma and then reawaken to capture additional moments with Janet and his children, his mother, and his friends. He said he appreciated more and more during those weeks having those he loved constantly with him. And although he did not want help, he needed it and accepted it graciously.

MARCH 13, 1974

Janet was with him, and his mother and children were near, when Segal lapsed into a coma and died, at home, on the morning of March 13.

He succeeded until the last several weeks in not allowing cancer to interfere with his way of life. Even then, while physically spent from pain and the sedation of pain-relieving drugs, he managed to finish two important projects. He also kept his sense of humor.

Segal also maintained his self-respect and autonomy in his relationship with me, refusing to suffer many of the humiliations and indignities of a person who would sell his soul for a few more pills or days of life. It is impossible for the self-image of a man like Segal not to suffer from dying slowly; but Segal did not break in the end, as he had feared. He met his challenge with courage and accomplished what he most wanted, to live and die with style and dignity.

12

Joan Stansfield

*I think perhaps self-awareness, self-concern, and self-love without egomania are
things we should all be able to reach without first running into a brick wall. It shouldn't
take a fatal diagnosis to make us look at things squarely and deal with them straight on,
or stop lying to ourselves. But I'm afraid for most of us it does. I think I've straightened
myself out in the areas where I was deluding myself. In fact, I discovered while I was
in the hospital that I'm a stronger person than I might have anticipated. I am just a bit
gutsier than I thought, and I'm delighted to know that.*

Joan lived in San Francisco on a steep hill lined with vividly and variously
colored Victorian houses, but the apartment she shared with her three children was somewhat small for their needs. Mornings were hectic, with Joan
rushing to her job downtown. Mike, 18 years old and a senior in high school,
usually had an early morning class, so it fell to 20-year-old Derek to take his
sister, Cathy, who was 5 years old, to the day-care center on his way to classes
at City College.

A frequent visitor at the apartment was Joan's ex-husband, Jack, who lived
several streets away, and a ringing telephone often signaled a frantic call from
Joan's mother, who lived alone across town. Joan would have been living with
Jack if he had not had a drinking problem, and she might have lived with her
mother if she had not been a smothering, overconcerned parent. As it was,
Joan's emotional endurance was often severely tested as she sought to maintain an equilibrium in these relationships.

The consequence of her husband's problem was that Joan had worked
for years to provide steady financial support for her children. At 42 she
still had all these responsibilities, and, in addition, her daily routine was
affected by cancer and cancer therapy. She worried about the future in terms
of her responsibilities because she knew she would probably die of the
disease.

Joan is the most reliable and eloquent witness to her own experience with
cancer, and I hope her story, assembled from tape-recorded conversations,
will give some idea of the kinds of difficulties a cancer patient with family
burdens may encounter. More than that, in Joan we see a person faced with
terminal cancer who discovered untapped resources of strength and flexibility
and who as a result refused to let cancer claim more than the necessary
portion of her time and energy.

I waited quite a while before consulting a physician because 4½ years ago I had a similar irritation that forced me to stop nursing my daughter, Cathy. When the inflammation reappeared, it was much easier to assume it was a recurrence of that problem rather than something more serious. However, a time came when I knew. I knew because I had no pain, and I was aware that a malignant growth is often characterized by an absence of pain. I simply had a feeling of great sickness; and when I finally did have pain, my breast cancer had metastasized.

Since the diagnosis, the changes in my attitude have been subtle. I'm not even sure it's good for me to discuss them because I think one can analyze almost anything out of existence. But I remember that I wasn't particularly content with my life. I had problems with my mother and my ex-husband and I was certain that illness would be more than I could handle. When I realized I was going into the hospital, I wanted to give up altogether. Yet I'm a fairly cheerful person and, given a choice, I prefer to look on the better side of a situation. So after surgery, when I was able to assess my position, I decided, "All right, I have cancer. I will live with it. I won't necessarily die of it."

I think my father had something to do with that decision. We were very close, although I don't remember a great deal about him except that he loved gardening, hiking, and camping. When we went walking together on Sundays, he always made a walking stick for me. And my friends adored him because he was one of those fathers who would squat down to their level when he spoke to them.

He contracted Hodgkin's disease when I was 5 years old, and it must have been pretty advanced at the time of diagnosis because he collapsed and couldn't speak. I have always been in the habit of thinking that he died of cancer, but you know how little flash cards settle themselves down in the back of your brain? Well, last week I flashed on the thought that my father did not die of cancer. Although he had been given a year to live, he actually lived for 7 years altogether after receiving radiation therapy. He died eventually of coronary thrombosis. So I suddenly thought, "My father did not die of cancer; I do not have to die of cancer. That's a point to concentrate on."

Another quite different influence in my past that has helped me was a certain fatalism acquired from my Scots Presbyterian upbringing. Although intellectually I now reject much of what I was taught, I still respond emotionally to the concept of God's will. What will be will be. I knew that when breast cancer metastasizes, it may go to the lungs, then to the rib cage or to the bone marrow, which is pretty bad and pretty ugly. Nevertheless, if you're going to have cancer, what a great time to have it! This is a real breakthrough period in cancer research, and if I don't make it until they find a cure, that's my problem.

I think I'm pretty good at not lying to myself. Maybe I'm too good at recognizing reality, but while I was in the hospital deciding to live with cancer, I learned about priorities. There are a great many concerns which have gone way down on my list. My mother, for one. She's a weeper and a sufferer; the violins are going all the time. After my operation she demanded of the doctor, "How long will it be?" He, thinking she meant how long would I be away from work, said "Six weeks." While I was coming out of the anesthesia, I could hear her on the telephone beside my bed informing everyone we knew that "Joan has 6 weeks to live."

In our relationship I am the mother and she is the child, although she rationalizes her dependence as "Joan needs me." It has been that way since my father died when I was 12 and she began acting out saving him by dragging me off to all kinds of clinics. About every 6 months I had to have a complete physical examination. She was sure there was something terribly wrong with me and that she would save me. I see this now; I wasn't aware of it at the time except that I knew I wasn't ill. But by the time I was 16, just graduating from high school, I think I must have been quite close to a breakdown just from being hassled by this widow who was going through her own changes, a sort of prolonged menopause. A very wise friend took me to her gynecologist and I was given a series of B_1 treatments which really helped me.

My mother is a hysteric personality and that kind of person usually creates a very inhibited child, which I was. What I needed was a sense of her confidence in me, but she could not give that; it's so easy to control people when you make them feel inept.

Now she is partly senile and lives in a past of 40 years ago. When she first moved to San Francisco, I would go with her every Sunday to a nearby Congregational Church where the congregation is composed largely of retired people her own age. They made overtures of friendship, which she rejected because of her need to live her life through me. Now she is lonely, but some people can be lonely anywhere. She feels left out, the self-sacrificing mother, the only one who can help, so the boys and I humor her and try to make her feel better. However, when I'm around her, I'm constantly reminded of how ill I am. She phones me every morning and says, "You poor thing." I am the cross she has to bear and she is helping me. Oh, is she helping me! With help like that, I don't even need cancer.

The other family problem which has descended in my list of priorities is my ex-husband's alcoholism. We separated for the second time 6 months after Cathy was born because I didn't want to go through that again with her. In the early years of our marriage I know I did all the wrong things, but then we both had therapy and I realized I was playing doormat and a lot of other roles, because alcoholism is a great game. Yet it is almost impossible not to become involved, to remain objective while someone stomps around and breaks up the furniture.

But we try to be objective, and the boys have a good feeling for Jack. They accept their father for what he is and for what he is able to give. He taught them both music; he worked with them in scouting; and even before that we were into camping, hiking, climbing, and all that. So they are able to be grateful, to recognize and enjoy the good qualities and just swing with him when he is unable to function.

Although I cannot live with Jack, I still have strong feelings of respect and admiration for his positive qualities, and I trust him more than anybody I know, which is why I was able to let him help me last year when I was in the hospital. He is fantastic in a crisis situation. He moved in with the children, gave financial aid, moral support, and all kinds of things. Day-to-day is his problem, accepting responsibility on a continuing basis. It's all such a colossal bore because alcoholics are so extremely predictable.

He now recognizes his drinking as something he must deal with; and although this is a problem that affects me deeply, it is one from which I must withdraw. I cannot help him.

With the change in priorities, it's me first, then Cathy, and then the boys, because they are old enough to be on their own. Yet I've learned more from them than from anyone else; I'm pleased to have known them and to be their mother.

Cathy was unplanned, and this whole situation seems especially unfair to her. I feel I owe her a little bit more. But feeling sorry for her when she does not understand why we feel sorry for her is the most destructive thing I can think of. The boys know my cancer is terminal, but Cathy knows only as much as she can understand. She sees the television spots of the American Cancer Society on television and announces, "You have that too," as though it were a status symbol. She doesn't know it's fatal, but she knows it is something serious and that everyone is trying to find out about it.

Actually we don't talk very much about cancer; life goes on pretty normally, and the domestic chores get done. The boys get their own breakfasts and Derek takes Cathy to the day-care center, where I pick her up in the late afternoon. She and I go to the supermarket after that, although I often feel weak in my legs by then and have to lean on the shopping cart for support. We all help with cooking dinner and doing dishes, but extra projects such as covering the chair in the living room just don't get done. My principal problem is fatigue. I find it very frustrating that I doze off as I sit down to read in the evening.

Otherwise, cancer has not altered my life in any major way. I miss backpacking and other physical activity, but I can live with that. I can also live with this nap of red fuzz on my head and this wig which doesn't resemble my own hair—and even the prosthetic device that gives me a bust line.

The only thing I find debilitating is dealing with people who make unfair emotional demands. Then I begin to get a physical reaction—sweat and a sense of weakness. I actually sweat and that's a nuisance with this wig, because it gets damp and then when I go outside it gets cold. I kind of resent that, but I hope it doesn't show because it's no one's fault; yet I think that is when I am aware of my illness, when someone makes a demand that I don't feel I can fulfill or that I choose not to fulfill. When the demand is really unreasonable, my reaction is that I don't have time for that kind of nonsense. Fardels I can bear, fools I won't.

I have always tried to live one day at a time, but I think I'm better at it now. My job is fairly stressful—a hassle, really. As supervisor of telephone representatives in the customer service department of a major health plan, I build case loads for 20 employees and handle the inquiries and complaints they are unable to deal with. Although I enjoy the people I work with, and dealing with the public, the organization itself has been invaded by systems engineers and efficiency experts who do not understand the concept of service, in which quality should be valued over quantity. I try to handle all this well without going overboard, but I'm a thorough person and don't like to leave things hanging. So I try to conserve—not so much physical energy as coping and imaginative energy—my resources that are most affected by my disease and my therapy.

Chemotherapy began the day I left the hospital in 1972. My liver was enlarged and invaded by cancer and I had early signs of jaundice. That first drug reversed the entire process and I became normal, but after 5 months I reached toxicity. The side effects were severe. I was dropping things and having memory lapses, so I kept, at my oncologist's request, a record of my symptoms over a period of 12 days:

Wednesday,	March 15	Heavy gas pains, no stool. Took laxative.
Thursday,	March 16	Diarrhea. Stay home. Sleep.
Friday,	March 17	Work half day. Ill; no stool. Laxative.
Saturday,	March 18	Sleep until 2:00 PM. Perk up in the evening.
Sunday,	March 19	Sleep most of the day.
Monday,	March 20	Stay home in bed.
Tuesday,	March 21	Pain, ill. Work half day.
Wednesday,	March 22	Heavy gas pains; no stool. Laxative.
Thursday,	March 23	Diarrhea all day. Stay home. Try to sleep.
Friday,	March 24	Work all day.Sleep from 7:30 PM Friday to 11:00 AM Saturday.
Saturday,	March 25	Grocery shop at very slow tempo. Drag through day. Perk up in evening.
Sunday,	March 26	Slept nearly all day. Washed out. Some diarrhea. Splitting headache.
Incidentals:		Mouth sores in corner, spreading inside. Slow healing of minor scrapes. Greatly lowered pain threshold. Memory failure. Heartburn. Gas.

At that point my therapy was changed to another drug. The first one had done its job; the second maintained my remission. Two weeks after the changeover, I felt alert, my memory improved, and I was much more cheerful. I had been constantly aware of illness on the first drug but now I thought of myself as a well person who gets tired easily or who has pain sometimes. Unless I run into the weepers, I forget I have cancer.

Speaking of weepers, yesterday a difficult customer was directed to me for special handling. He wanted reimbursement for a flight he had taken to Tijuana for Laetrile treatment, but such coverage was not included in his contract. I needed some information from him but he was too angry and self-pitying to cooperate. Finally he blurted out, "Listen, lady, I've got terminal cancer." So I replied, "Isn't that a coincidence! So have I." Needless to say, he began to cooperate and even invited me to join a group of cancer patients that meets regularly and issues a newspaper on the latest drugs. I can understand going that route, but I choose not to.

Today I had an appointment for chemotherapy review, so after lunch I took a bus to the office of my oncologist. Of my three doctors—internist, surgeon, and oncologist— he is the one on whom I am most dependent right now. It's interesting, though. Neither he nor either of the other two ever said, "Why didn't you come to us sooner?" They just analyzed the situation and did their best once I got there.

The first time I met my oncologist, Dr. Rosenbaum, I was still in the hospital. I liked him immediately. He was very matter-of-fact, very low key. I just liked him, liked his face. You can't explain reactions like that, but I'm quite sure that if I hadn't liked him, I wouldn't be responding in quite the same way to chemotherapy. And when I do have discomfort, I am better able to tolerate it because of the confidence I have in him.

I'm even pleased by the atmosphere in his waiting room. There is little chitchat among the patients, no gloomy comparisons of symptoms. This isn't the result of any directive from him. I think people behave the way they do because that's the way they are with him. It's a very subtle thing, as are all aspects of one's attitude toward living with cancer.

The first thing I do during an office visit is give my blood to Sophie, my personal vampire; then, since the wait may be a half hour or more, I lie on the examining table and take a nap.

The interval between office visits has varied from 1 to 3 weeks, but I'm a little uncomfortable with the 3-week span. It isn't anything terribly inspiring that he says to me or that I ask him. It's just seeing him and "How are you?" and "You look great!" And he usually teases me about the wig. But I know he is frightfully busy and I always worry that I'm taking up too much time and asking too many questions. Therefore, I either write down the questions or get them firmly in mind so I can ask them quickly and absorb the answers, because those answers are terribly important to me.

When Dr. Rosenbaum was on vacation, I didn't get nervous, but I did cross streets very carefully. I didn't make any waves anywhere because I didn't have him to run to. Anybody could have helped, I suppose, but I felt a responsibility to behave myself.

I think if I had to define an effective physician, I would say one who sees and treats in each patient more than the physiological aspects of his problem. When Dr. Rosenbaum is planning a treatment program for me, I know he takes into consideration my various responsibilities and sources of tension and concern. For example, he changed my chemotherapy so I could continue working and keep my home together, and he has helped me arrange that my cousin become Cathy's legal guardian when I die.

We talked today about whether or not I should apply for Aid to the Totally Disabled.* Cancer that is neither cured nor controlled is considered ample qualification for receiving help, and I asked Dr. Rosenbaum whether he would consider it ethically feasible to recommend me. He said he wanted me to understand he was pleased with my progress but at the same time would be willing to give the authorities the necessary medical information. The question is complex, however, and I'm not really good at making heavy decisions. I have a tendency to look at both sides very carefully and to conclude that either way will work. I guess I don't have a strong enough ego to say, "*That's* what I'm going to do." Although I have good disability coverage in my health plan, that would not go into effect until 6 months after I stop working. Social Security Disability benefits require a wait of 5 months. I have always worked to provide a steady, predictable income for my family and I have a responsibility to feed my children. Because of these financial considerations, I will have to weigh the pros and cons carefully. On the other hand, if I'm going to go on disability eventually, why not do it now when I'm functioning fairly well? I'm good at self-starting and could accomplish a lot without the discipline of an 8:00 to 4:30 routine.

Yet I have never been a well enough organized person to have a life goal. I think living a useful life is more important to me, and that again is why the decision about disability is so important. Can I be more useful to Cathy and the boys if I go on disability and am available, doing things I consider important, or is it better to go on in one's little rut? I think you can overdramatize this a bit. One simply needs to make a choice. I could walk out the door right now, get hit by a truck, and not have done all my great life-dream things.

I mentioned disability to my mother, very casually, as a possibility only, because I didn't want her to freak out again and think I had only 2 weeks to live. Her immediate reaction was, "Of course you won't be able to make it financially, so I'll move in," at which point I decided, "Forget disability for the time being."

I don't know what course my illness will take. I have told Dr. Rosenbaum I have very strong feelings about the slow and dirty aspects of dying with cancer. Although I have no religious or other strong feelings about suicide, I am constrained by a nonsuicide clause in my insurance policy. I definitely believe in euthanasia, yet if I were a physician I don't know whether I'd be capable of making a professional decision. I just know what my own personal emotional feelings are, and I can't bear the thought of putting my family through what I've seen so many families go through. It's all so pointless. It's all so stupid. It's an ego trip too. I don't want to be remembered as that stinking body lying on the bed for days and days, turning into a complaining, demanding thing. Because that's the kind of memory that sticks.

I remember when I was a child being taken to visit a maiden aunt who was sick. It was summertime in a small town in an old house, and she was dying in an upstairs room of cancer of the intestines. She only had a sheet over her because of the heat but the sheet was draped over a wooden frame so it wouldn't touch the bones which were protruding through her skin. The weight of the sheet would have been agony for her.

---

*As of January 1974 a person can apply for Supplemental Security Income for the Aged, Blind, and Disabled. It is advisable, when possible, to apply for this aid and for Social Security Disability 3 to 6 months in advance of the need. People who think they may qualify for such help, now or in the future, should ask their local Social Security office for further information.

I remember the stench and I remember the revulsion. And I think of her when I think of getting to the slow and dirty stage.

I have no fear, just an attitude about not rotting, and a desire to protect my children from things that are unnecessarily unpleasant. But there is no point in thinking about that now. I'm not there and can't predict what kind of strength I'll have for coping if that time comes. I will have to do it day by day, as I do now.

"Now" is not so different from yesterday. I don't think I perceive color, sound, all the senses, more deeply, but I do relish them more. Sunsets I have always enjoyed, but now I really wallow in a good sunset. But I don't think, "This may be my last sunset." I can't play that role. This may be an overreaction to my mother and her "Sarah Bernhardt is alive and well" routine, but it is also an attempt to be honest in my emotional reactions instead of overdramatizing them. One is so Hollywood-oriented. People with final diagnoses always do beautiful romantic things like going off to Mexico. I am just aware that I take more time to enjoy things, like walking on a raw day in San Francisco with a cold wind in my face.

I have mentioned that one must often treat the family as well as the patient. This was true of Joan's mother, for whom I could not help feeling sympathy. Elderly, arthritic, and nearly blind, she wanted to give comfort to her only child. And she was fearful of her own lonely future. During episodes when Joan was hospitalized, I felt her mother needed comfort and compassion and I tried to reassure her of her usefulness to Joan. At the same time Joan needed some respite from her mother's constant attendance, some moments of peace in which to recover.

As with all patients, Joan's life circumstances—the need to support her family and maintain a household—helped me to determine the type of treatment she should receive. She could not continue to take a drug that knocked her off her feet for several hours a day. She also needed my steady interest and concern; and I think my availability and our short, frank conversations provided this for her, as well as the hope of achieving stability in her disease, which she did for many months.

In a sense Joan required less emotional support from me than Mort Segal. Where he needed encouragement to continue treatment, Joan simply wanted advice and reassurance. Thus my role differs with each patient, although it is not something I think about ahead of time. Patients tend to cast me in the roles they require, and I try to respond appropriately as their needs become evident. Like them, I meet one situation at a time, one day at a time.

13

Elisabeth Lee

I've never been one of those women who runs around buying lots of clothes and having her hair done. I'm neither young nor the world's most beautiful woman, but I liked my body and wanted to have all the pieces. I'll never quite accept the loss of my breasts.

What happened to me is a little different from what happens to most women who develop breast cancer. Fifteen years ago I had a biopsy for cysts in my breasts. The test results were negative, but after that the doctors watched me closely. Other cysts developed and disappeared. Then 2 years ago, in April 1973, my gynecologist ordered a xeromammogram because I had a new cyst in each breast. Nothing showed up in the test results. Nevertheless, after further consultation the doctors agreed that I shouldn't take any chances and that biopsies of the cysts should be performed.

I agreed to have the biopsies but I was in an utter panic. This is the first part of the emotional crisis for a woman in whom cancer of the breast is suspected. She continuously wonders whether she'll emerge from the operation with both breasts, one breast, or no breasts. Moreover, I was, and still am, very frightened of the effects of anesthesia.

To my great relief, when I awoke from the operation I still had both breasts. The lumps had been benign.

Then a month later, when I went to see my surgeon for a checkup of the biopsy incisions, he told me that although the cysts had been benign, the cells around one of the cysts were beginning to change. He wanted to remove that breast. He said he hadn't told me before because he wanted to be certain beforehand. He wanted additional consultative opinions on the biopsies. However, I wish I had known he was thinking about it because I would have had time to prepare myself. I'm the kind of person who would rather know. I need time. I think I could accept almost anything if I just had time to think it through carefully.

The first thing I did was telephone my husband, who was on a business trip. He became more upset than I did because he knew I was upset. He's a very concerned and sensitive man.

I couldn't believe it was happening to me. I was terrified. I had been born late in my parents' life and was consequently exposed to some fairly Victorian attitudes, one of which was my mother's belief that the removal of a breast is the worst thing that can happen to a woman. I now know it isn't the worst thing, but I thought it was at the time and told the doctor how I felt. He said most women feel the same way, that they'd rather he took out inches or feet of intestine than go near a breast.

What made my case unusual was that the cells in question showed only local and early changes. They were becoming malignant, but there was a 65% chance that the tumor might never progress. Such early detection is rare, and I felt that I had an option to do nothing. However, my surgeon didn't agree. He said it was the ideal time to operate, and that it would be suicide not to have it done as soon as possible. He felt that when a person has a 30 to 35% chance of getting cancer, and a nearly 100% chance of prevention and cure by surgery, there should be no question as to the course to follow. He gave me 2 weeks to think it over, and I told him that during that interval I wanted to talk to other doctors. I explained that it wasn't a lack of faith in him. I just didn't want to have any regrets. I wanted to be positive that it really had to be done. What if someone along the line had made a mistake? He wasn't offended.

I consulted several doctors, one of whom was a close friend. This doctor also sympathized with my need for certainty and arranged a consultation with Dr. Rosenbaum, who recommended that I have both breasts removed at the same time. He said that my breast tumor was uncommon and that because of its particular pathology there was approximately a 25% chance that the same process was occurring in the other breast.

I also consulted other women who had had mastectomies, but I was very careful whom I chose. I sought out women who seemed to have common sense, because some people become very emotional and tend to say such things as "You must do this" and "You mustn't do that." One friend who had had a radical mastectomy several months earlier said simply, "It's not the kind of thing you want. It's the kind of thing you accept and live with."

There were many considerations. I have three children, who were then 11, 13, and 15. I wondered what would happen to them if I didn't have the operation and I died. And if I did have the operation, how would that affect my relationship with my husband? Would he still want to go to bed with me? Could I let him go to bed with me? The doctors assured me that a marriage that is solid doesn't suffer from the removal of one breast or two breasts, but I wasn't so sure. I told my husband that if I lost my breast I'd never again go to bed with him. He said, "That's rubbish. I love you and it makes no difference to me." I still couldn't believe it wouldn't change our relationship. We discussed the fact that losing a breast is equivalent to a man's losing his testicles. Telling him all my apprehensions was a great relief.

As the results came in from the doctors I consulted, I became more and more convinced that the operation was necessary. Their opinions were unanimous. Nevertheless, I needed that period of time for reflection.

There was one other doctor who helped me. He said he had had a patient who was faced with a decision similar to mine. She told the doctor she would think it over and talk to her husband about it. Then she phoned him a week later and announced that she would prefer to die with her body intact. The doctor persisted and suggested she think it over, but she never called back. She died.

I decided to have one breast removed. I think that if I had had another week to decide, or if I had been able to talk to just one woman who had had both breasts removed at the same time, I might have chosen to have a double mastectomy.

My husband was very supportive. I know that some husbands aren't, and that would be the end as far as I'm concerned. We decided not to tell our 11-year-old the full details because we felt he was too young, but we told the older two. They were very frightened, especially our 13-year-old boy. When Dr. Rosenbaum was told about their reactions, he invited the four of us to his office and explained everything to the children. He treated them as adults, presenting my case exactly as it had developed and explaining the rationale for surgery. He told them where they could obtain reading material, if they wanted to, and encouraged them to ask questions. After an hour of discussion, they accepted it very well, which was an enormous relief to me. If a mother knows her children aren't upset, it helps her to get through her ordeal.

Fortunately, my mother lives with us, so there was someone available to take care of the children. The temporary absence of a mother must be a tremendous burden in families where no extra help is available. Of course, relatives and friends do step in, but I think these are problems that doctors don't always have time to consider.

The night before the operation my surgeon visited me and talked with my husband and me. He was very kind. My husband had previously asked him and Dr. Rosenbaum whether it might not be possible to remove only the inside of the breast and leave the shell and the nipple. We had heard of cases where this was done and silicone implanted later. This was therefore considered in the plan, although the surgeon warned us that if anything more was found during the operation, it would be necessary to perform a radical mastectomy.

The possibility that they might leave the shell was a great help to me psychologically. But I also seemed to have lived through certain emotions. When I went to the hospital for the biopsy 6 weeks earlier, I had been very frightened, and when the possibility of the mastectomy was first mentioned, I was in an utter panic, a quiet panic but an all-engulfing one. Now I was reasonably calm. Since that time I have talked to others and am convinced that most people go through similar sequences of emotion.

It proved possible to keep the shell of my breast, although I began to wonder whether they'd really found all the troublesome cells. I thought, "Perhaps they missed a couple. Maybe I'm going to die of breast cancer anyway and needn't have gone through all this." Then I pushed all that to the back of my mind and put my faith in the doctors, and in God.

Suddenly it was time to go home and begin my real adjustment. I discussed my feelings openly with my family, the doctors, and a few close friends, but I knew it would be hard for me if many people knew; and it's amazing how you can do all this without anyone's finding out. I suppose I didn't want people to know because I'm a perfectionist and this made me less than perfect. Some people want everyone to know. I feel that what happens to my body is a private matter.

Through some oversight, I was never given any information about prosthetic devices, although I now know the American Cancer Society's Reach to Recovery Program* provides all kinds of valuable information, not only about the different textures of prosthetic devices and where to buy them, but about special bathing suits, other sport clothes, and nightgowns for women who've had mastectomies. So there I was, on my way out to dinner one evening, and flat on one side. First I tried cotton, then Kleenex. All of us pushed it around to see how it looked. The children knew it was serious but they joked about it too, and that was something that really helped me.

The next day I phoned some stores and found I could buy devices that ranged from $1 to $70. I settled on the $1 item. I was lucky to have enough tissue left to keep my bra from riding up, because not being able to keep a bra in place can be a real problem for a woman, psychologically and practically. A suction device that really works is quite expensive. However, a plastic surgeon told me that even when women must have the entire breast removed, he can still put a little something there to provide some bulk.

I have painful memories too. I thought I'd never take a bath again. I just didn't want to look at myself. I used to run around the house with no clothes on and my children would come in and talk to me while I was taking a bath. Now I locked the bathroom door. I wouldn't even let my husband see me without clothes, and I still make love with my nightgown on. I felt my husband didn't deserve all this. After all, in

*See Chapter 25.

our culture foreplay usually begins with the breast, and I felt, "Why does he have to have someone who's mutilated when there are other women in the world?" I'm a somewhat insecure person, and this brought out many of my insecurities.

I told Dr. Rosenbaum how I felt, and we had a long, frank talk about the realities of my situation, my marriage, and my attitude toward my body and sexual relations. He suggested I see a psychiatrist, and I did speak to one several times. He helped me a great deal, although I still find it hard to relate to my husband in bed as well as I did before. I know it's my fault and that it's all in my head, but it's still difficult.

Luckily, I didn't have a lot of time to worry after the operation. I'm in a position where I can be very helpful to my husband in his work. I've always been involved in doing things for him and the children. One of them was graduating from junior high school and another was preparing to go away for the summer, so fortunately I was busier than usual.

The summer passed quickly, and on the advice of Dr. Rosenbaum, but with the surgeon's reluctant approval, I entered the hospital in October 1973 to have my other breast removed. Just before the operation I again began to have second thoughts. Dr. Rosenbaum visited me, and after a supportive talk I mustered the courage to remain for the second surgery. As suspected, the results of the operation showed multiple areas of early cancer in the other breast.

It is now March 1975 and I still have not had the silicone implants. The surgeon wanted me to wait 6 months after the removal of the second breast. He said it was for reasons of infection, but I think he wanted to be sure nothing recurred, which was fine with me because that was one of my first concerns regarding implants. If something occurs under the implant, how will they find it? I also wonder whether it's wise to put foreign substances in your body, although Dr. Rosenbaum tells me the silicone is actually inside a plastic bag. It's like a Baggie with the proper shape, so there are no strange substances seeping into your system.

There is another problem. They tell me that because of the way they had to perform the operations on my breasts, one side may not look as good as the other after the implants are made. They may have to do that side twice. At least it can be done under local anesthetic, which removes one of my greatest fears.

I'm still considering the possibility of reconstruction, although my condition doesn't bother me the way it once did. Dr. Rosenbaum feels that if I can reduce the amount of disfigurement it's worth my having the implants. He has told me that I won't be the same as before, but he thinks I might get some emotional satisfaction from having them. As far as the shells are concerned, I have no feeling in one side, but some feeling is beginning to return to the skin and nipple on the other side. That may be unusual, as I was told not to expect any feeling. I think surgeons prefer to be cautious in predicting the results of an operation because each case is so different.

On the plus side, I know I have every chance for a complete cure because my cancer was caught before it really got started. If I'd waited 5 or 10 years, it might have been a different story. I'm grateful it's over and that there were doctors who were wise enough to pursue an elusive problem and find out what the trouble was. I'm thankful it was operative because there are many people who can't have surgery or who have a cancer in an area where early detection is difficult.

I was lucky in many other ways. I had a loving, supportive husband and children who needed me. It would have been harder if I had been 21 years old and had never had children. It would have been harder if my children had already grown up and gone away. I didn't have to worry about expense, which was more than it might have been because I had the separate operations. Even though we have good insurance, there's a great deal that's not covered. I also had enough money to consult a psychiatrist. This is a luxury when the main problem is medical, but it's just as important.

If I have undergone any other psychological changes than the ones I've described, I think I've developed a greater feeling of responsibility for others. When doctors have given their skill to save you, you feel it is incumbent upon you to do something with your life. When you look back over the years, the most important thing will be what you've done to help people. Although I'm still involved with my family's activities, I try to find more time to help other people. I especially want to help women who are faced with the alternatives I was faced with. I would first urge them to overcome their fear of going to the doctor; and I would urge them not to postpone surgery, if it is recommended. They will experience the same stages of fear, disbelief, and acceptance that I did. They will be devastated at first, but they will find that as they cope successfully with each stage of fright and denial, they will slowly build the emotional strength that will see them through their ordeal. After a while the feelings of devastation and nakedness will be eased. And they will be grateful, as I am, to be alive.

ELISABETH LEE – WINTER 1981

I telephoned Elisabeth Lee one day in February and asked her if she would be willing to be interviewed for a second edition of *Living with Cancer,* to talk about her feelings about cancer now that time has passed. She readily volunteered and we met at her home.

ER: Your life is back together again. You're active and working. What has happened since your surgery and recovery in 1974?

EL: In the last 5 years I think I have forgotten in many ways about what happened to me. Although I have my regular checkups, I don't think about it because I don't think you can continue to let the fear of cancer overwhelm you. You have to go forward. I have gone back to work. The children have grown up and are in college, and my husband and I are alone for the most part.

I think that what helped me the most was my husband, because he is a very accepting man, and this cancer and my operations have never been of any concern to him. I can visualize many marriages that have difficulties under the same circumstances.

I'm thinking now of going into full-time work, and one of my concerns is that they might ask me something about my health. My response will be, "My health is excellent." And it is.

ER: As far as we're concerned, you're cured.

EL: I think that one's psychological attitude is very important. If I feel I'm not cured, I might not be cured. I think what happens to you emotionally sometimes triggers off cancer. I've read, for example, that when someone suffers a sudden shock, they are more apt to have cancer. Is that correct?

ER: We all have cancer within our bodies. The evidence shows that in the first year of bereavement there is a higher incidence of cancer. The cancer that is already there somehow becomes more prominent, probably because the body, which normally has control over its tissues, loses that control under stress. For example, under stress of shock, you will have more adrenalin and cortisone and hormonal changes that can affect tissue growth. So there is something happening—but the cancer is in the person already. We have trillions of cells, and when an occasional cell is malignant, it usually doesn't grow because the body controls it.

EL: And I believe it's important to keep up your body's health defenses by exercising and eating properly.

I sometimes wonder—I did have cancer of the thyroid in 1966-1967, and I wonder whether this will happen again. It's happened twice now. I don't think of the breast operation as having been for cancer. (That's one way of rationalizing.) But I wonder whether something might happen again in the next few years. But, then, I don't wonder very often because there is no point in it. If it happens, it happens, and then I'll come to you and you'll take care of me.

ER: I think you may have a right to say—in your rare case—that you never had cancer of the breast. It's the kind of thing you see in the cervix, where you do Pap smears all the time, and then you see cells changing and you do something about it. In a breast you can't do a type of Pap smear. There is no nipple test and no secretion test. But your mammograms showed carcinoma in situ in several areas of both breasts. The risk was there, and I'm glad we performed the surgery. I think it did two things for you. You have avoided the high risk of breast cancer and you have peace of mind instead of being terrified every day of your life.

EL: There is no doubt that I did the right thing. In fact, I have read recently that this kind of surgery is done with people *before* they develop carcinoma in situ, and I think that's not a bad idea because they can have the implants right away. It saves a great deal of worry and concern over many years. If I were doing it again, I would do exactly that because surgery is different today than it was 10 or 15 years ago.

ER: Surgery is improving every year. Tell me your thoughts about implants. You've seen two different plastic surgeons, if I'm correct. About 5 years ago, you were really considering an implant because you thought it would help you feel more comfortable about your body.

EL: I have talked to Dr. M and Dr. V about the possibility of implants. Dr. M is opposed to it, Dr. V is going to work on Dr. M because he thinks he is being a trifle conservative. Dr. M thinks something could develop underneath the breast implant, but I keep telling him that no one could tell anything the last time until they did the surgery. By having the implants, I can check to see if everything is nice and clean. He tells me not to worry, that everything is probably fine, and I think it would be foolish to go against his recommendations at this point. If I decide to do it later on, Dr. V will be happy to do it. In fact, I am talking to him about a face lift. It sounds ridiculous but I thought it might be fun.

ER: How has your life changed now that you're out of that phase of 5 or 6 years ago? Are you enjoying life more? Are your fears different?

EL: I still have some concerns; also, my father had cancer of the colon, so my history is not the greatest. I think people inherit a tendency to cancer, so I check carefully about all these various possibilities and then I forget about them until 3 or 4 months have passed and it's time to be tested again. I feel it is more important to enjoy life. As you grow older, how much time is left? No matter what you have gone through, as you grow older you feel you should enjoy more and give more—simultaneously. Fortunately, my husband's and my relationship with our children is a close one and my relationship with my husband is a good one too.

Women at certain ages tend to get anxious about what they're going to do. I have been involved with helping women get back to work in a women's reentry program. And what I would really like to do is get a smashing job helping reentry women; then, when I have been successful, I'd like to tell people what you can do even if you have had health problems. I would like to be an example to women. I want to help middle-aged and older women have confidence that they can do something. As long as you feel you can do something, you can. Much of it is psychological. Also, many women feel they are not women anymore after they have had operations like mine, but they are just as much women as they were before.

ER: You're much more convincing now than you were 6 years ago!

EL: I think I realize that the loss of my breasts doesn't make any difference. Most people don't know it's happened. And my family has faith in me. It takes a while to accept it, but there are so many people out there who cannot be helped. It would be foolish to sit around and weep and moan. I am very grateful after all you have done for me and for my life.

ER: You have done a lot for yourself. Don't you think your attitude helped a tremendous amount? You can put faith in a doctor but then you have to go and do it yourself. You have to go to the hospital, walk in the door, and have the operation.

EL: I think you have to take what comes down the pike (and I am glad to say my children have learned this from my experience). You can't run away from it. You face it; you solve it; and you go on to the next problem. And in between you have a great many pleasures. I think that for a woman who is alone and has these problems, it must be very difficult. If my husband were to die, then I think I might have problems. I have been discussing this with a friend who has had radical mastectomies on both sides. What if you are single and dating? Do you stop going out with someone? Do you tell him about this? I told my friend, "I cannot imagine anyone marrying me with this problem." She said, "If the man wouldn't marry you with this problem, he isn't worth marrying," which is an interesting answer.

ER: She's right. Still, people are so afraid of the disease, afraid it's contagious—which is ridiculous—but that's what makes people different.

EL: Right. And today I told a friend about what had happened. It has been very hard for me to discuss my mastectomies with anybody whom I didn't tell originally; and I didn't tell very many people. The doctors and family knew and one or two close friends. This friend is a woman whom I met since that time. We have become very good friends, and it has taken me 3 years to get around to mentioning this to her. Now that is interesting—that I wouldn't discuss it. I wouldn't discuss it with many people because I'm a very private person. I don't discuss how many times I go to bed with my husband a week or anything of that nature. There are certain things that are private.

ER: Don't you think that having survived some traumatic years, you have matured to a higher level of handling your problems?

EL: That's something that should happen as you go along, although it doesn't happen to everyone. I wish I had been this mature some years ago because it is the only way to survive.

ER: Do you think that, knowing Dr. M's recommendations, if you had a choice and the surgeons were willing, you would have your breast reconstruction done now?

EL: Yes.

ER: Why are you so positive now when you weren't positive 2 years ago?

EL: Because it is the only way I can get anybody to do a biopsy. That may be one of the reasons, although it sounds ludicrous.

ER: Are you still worried?

EL: There is an increasing amount of tissue in my right side.

ER: There has to be some.

EL: The other side does not have that tissue and that is one of my reasons. Furthermore, I would just like to do it. One of my prime problems is getting the proper kind of prosthetic device for bathing suits. They don't make any more of the kind I've always used—and I don't feel like spending several hundred dollars on them . . . Foam rubber does not work with bathing suits.

ER: What else has changed in the last few years?

EL: I have developed a greater feeling of self-confidence—just in general. I think that a feeling of self-confidence and self-worth help you to accept any problem you may have. When I look around at most of the people I know, I conclude that they are not accomplishing much. They are doing things like playing bridge—unlike your wife, who is doing something worthwhile. And I think I have also done a great deal that is worthwhile, so I have more feeling about my worth. My husband and I love each other, we respect and love our children, and they reciprocate our feeling, and I have helped many people who were not able to help themselves.

ER: If you had an opportunity to give some advice to other women, what would it be?

EL: My advice would be, first of all, to be sure they have their breasts checked regularly—either by a physician or by themselves. It's very important. If they find they have a problem, they should take whatever steps are necessary surgically, or with any other kind of treatment. But I think they should get several opinions before proceeding. You have to be sure in your own mind, and if you follow one person's advice without seeking another opinion, you might think later on, "I shouldn't have done it that way." You have to be perfectly positive concerning the route you choose to follow. Then you follow it and you accept it.

ER: How would you respond if you had a recurrence? A person like you who has faced cancer in themselves or their family often shows a better ability to cope with recurrence because they have acquired coping mechanisms. They've had to fight their way through all the battles and they've achieved a level of knowledge that they can do it.

EL: I am not sure how I would respond to a recurrence. My experience does enable me to face other crises much more calmly and with much more fortitude. You face one thing that is not good, and you go on to the next. I am not sure it helps that much if you face cancer and you are not cured. Then I am not sure what happens. I was in a very fortunate position. Let's say someone has had a mastectomy; she has a recurrence in the other breast; then she has chemotherapy; and then she starts losing weight. At that point it is very difficult to face anything. I would be frightened, I think.

You must remember I have had both thyroid and breast cancer. I really feel good about myself. I feel I have faced something and accepted it. I have had the best possible care.

ER: Also, you have a maturity now that you didn't have 5 years ago.

EL: Wouldn't I have had that anyway without all this happening?

ER: Probably you would have it but not with the same quality. I always feel it's a shame that people have to go through great trauma to mature to the level where they can cope with life's problems.

EL: I think that's what life is all about.

14

Louise Milner

"How could this happen to me?"

"It didn't happen to you, Mr. Milner. It happened to your wife," replied the surgeon. He had just performed a radical mastectomy on Louise Milner, aged 28. When Louise discovered the lump in her right breast a few weeks earlier, she had asked her husband how he would feel if she were to lose her breast. His quick reply stunned her: "I couldn't bear it. I can't stand cripples."

Today, 5 years later, Louise sits opposite me at my desk and moves carefully in her chair to find a comfortable position. Her right arm is swollen and half paralyzed from nerve damage. Skin metastases cover her chest, shoulders, and neck. Less than one lung is functional. She talks about her life before cancer and sighs, "I'll never get over losing my breast."

The eldest of three daughters of Russian immigrants, Louise was already a beauty in her teens. She received modeling offers, was envied and adored for her long blond hair, lovely face, and exquisite figure. She enjoyed a close family life but felt her parents were overprotective and wanted to be independent of them. Because "nice Russian girls" did not leave home and get their own apartments, marriage appeared to be the logical means of escape; and when Louise met David Milner, he seemed to have the proper credentials: tall, blond, a "Greek god," and an engineer. But after 1 year of marriage Louise, 6 months pregnant, fled to Los Angeles and got a divorce. David had spent most of his evenings gambling, often lying about where he had been, and he was hostile to the idea of having a child.

After her daughter, Sandra, was born, Louise began to model and dance professionally and to learn the techniques of staging fashion shows. During the next 2 years her career flourished and she was offered numerous jobs in the Nevada gambling resorts. It was while dancing in one of these clubs that she met, and married 3 months later, Gil Smithfield, a general practitioner from the area. Louise became his office manager, acting as receptionist, bookkeeper, and part time nurse in addition to continuing her career of modeling and arranging fashion shows at the local clubs. She also ran a ballet school and a charm school. Life would have been ideal except that this time her husband's addiction was other women. Louise was distraught much of the time, and a sense of inadequacy began to grow. "I even tried to model myself after each of his new lovers," she remarked. She tried to please at the same time that she felt she was being used; and she was therefore angry with herself and with Gil. A particularly notorious affair with a visiting celebrity precipitated a suicide attempt by Louise and resulted in plans for divorce.

Louise's first husband, David, read a vague account of these happenings in a gossip column, guessed that Louise was involved, and immediately wrote her to offer his support. They began corresponding. David expressed regret for his past behavior, spoke of his longing to be with his daughter, and reminisced tenderly about his love for Louise. Louise says she cared too much for Gil to feel she could stay away from him if she were alone. She needed someone—so, hurt and lonely, she divorced Gil and remarried David. The marriage seemed to be working until Louise discovered the lump in her breast.

It is not unusual to hear a beautiful woman complain that she sometimes does not feel loved for her true self. This was how Louise felt when David became impotent after her mastectomy. A day came when he moved out of the house, telling her he couldn't make love to "someone like that." David's view of Louise became her view of herself. She felt that she made people uncomfortable, that she was flawed, no longer desirable, and there followed a series of experiences that confirmed these facts for her.

Actually it had begun in the hospital. Doctors and nurses would glance into Louise's room and then hurry away, avoiding eye contact. She would call out to them, "Please come in. It's all right." Yet they quickly made excuses to leave.

One evening a resident, having perceived Louise's ostracism, went to her room and, with the best of intentions, told her she might cry if she wished. Louise informed him she was not ready to cry, but he urged her again. He was compassionate, but his analysis of Louise's emotional state was inaccurate; and he appeared confused when she failed to react according to his preconception of her.

Out of the hospital Louise observed the same tentative behavior in many friends and relatives. One friend would not visit her after the mastectomy for fear she would "catch" cancer. There were, of course, positive experiences too, kindness and concern from unexpected quarters. Nevertheless, Louise was generally demoralized and forlorn when she entered her surgeon's waiting room for a follow-up visit. In the waiting room was one other patient, a woman with only half a face. Louise became terrified, thinking, "My God! Am I going to die looking like that?" and burst into tears as she entered the surgeon's inner office. When she explained why she was upset, he berated her, "You baby! You don't have that kind of cancer." Louise did not know what kind of cancer she had, only that she needed reassurance. Then the surgeon told her to raise her arm as high as she could, and when Louise failed to raise it higher than her shoulder, he again became impatient. "It's got to be higher!" Louise said she was trying; he told her she was not. She wept some more and promised herself that by the next visit she would raise her arm high enough to strangle him.

When, by the next appointment, Louise was able to raise her arm and told him how angry he had made her, he crowed, "But you see? It worked! Your arm is up where it should be." Louise was not impressed. She felt he could have achieved the same result with a gentler approach.

Several weeks later Louise sat in another waiting room at a local hospital, where she had gone for a cobalt treatment. She passed the time chatting with a patient who, on hearing the purpose of Louise's visit, related lurid tales of the effect cobalt had on her girlfriend's father's best friend. The friend had lost 60 pounds; his hair had fallen out; and he had had frequent blood transfusions. Louise was horrified at the time, but fortunately she found that she gained 15 pounds, kept her hair, and needed no transfusions. She is now very definite about the adverse effect such tales may have on an inexperienced patient: "If I met someone who was going to have chemotherapy, I would not mention the possibility of nausea because that might produce a worse reaction than he might otherwise experience."

Louise also feels strongly that medical technicians ought to be allowed to discuss the results of tests with patients. There is usually a lapse of hours or days before a patient learns the results of the latest test from the doctor. It would be better, Louise thinks, to hear a white lie, a word of encouragement from the technicians, to reduce worry in that interval. "Worry is what makes you unable to sleep or eat, and much of the time it's responsible for depression. People are more frightened by the silence of those technicians than they would be if they'd just say everything is fine. No wonder people give up."

After her second divorce from David, Louise moved, with Sandra, into her parents' home in San Francisco. Her parents did everything they could to make Louise feel comfortable and welcome, but what she really wanted was a man to tell her she was still a desirable woman. Although the operation had revealed that her cancer had metastasized, Louise was in relatively good health, and she wanted to enjoy life. Again, however, the reactions of others did nothing to restore her confidence. She recalls an evening when her mother happened to be in her room while she was undressing. Louise had removed the prosthesis that fitted into her bra and replaced her breast, and her mother said, "Turn around, honey, so I can see your incision." But when Louise turned around, her mother gasped, "Oh, my poor baby," and burst into tears.

Nevertheless, during a visit to Los Angeles Louise summoned the courage to telephone a man she had dated between her marriages to David and Gil, a man who had kept in touch with her through the years and always assured her of unflagging devotion. They had lunch several times but Louise did not tell him about her operation or her cancer. Then one evening on his sailboat, as he was telling her of his affection and of his admiration for her beauty, Louise interrupted him. "Before you go any further, I want you to know that I have cancer and that I've had a breast removed." Louise reports that he catapulted to the other side of the boat, hitting his head on the boom, and stared at her. She told him to take her home, and she never heard from him again.

Back in San Francisco, Louise accepted invitations from time to time from men she found attractive. She was fearful of repeating the experience of Los Angeles, yet in different ways she did repeat it, over and over. She would go out with someone once or twice and then defensively blurt out her news. Protestations would follow that this "made no difference," but that was usually the end of the relationship. Louise now acknowledges that although she occasionally met with insensitivity, she was also insensitive in her bluntness, and she courted rejection in order to avoid future emotional pain. Her increased vulnerability only sharpened her defenses and reinforced her self-rejection and her loneliness.

Then Louise met Alex. His wife had died of cancer, and he was familiar with the disease. The word did not paralyze him. Louise says, "He was kind and serious, and we were compatible, a good couple. And I was very happy."

Two years passed in this way, until Louise suffered a recurrence of her disease. She spent a month in the hospital recovering from an oophorectomy and exploratory surgery, and during all that time she did not hear from Alex. Finally she phoned him. He announced he was getting married to someone else; he loved her, would always remember her, but he could not go through with her what he had gone through with his wife. Louise said later, "He really hadn't minded about the mastectomy; he was afraid of the cancer that was still in my body."

Louise did not date again. "It hurt my feelings too much. I couldn't take another rejection." She withdrew into the safer world of family and friends. But even at home there were problems. Her family was loving and devoted, but Louise felt they too were angry with her for being ill. She would try to allot the same time and energy to their activities that she had before, but when she became exhausted trying to please them, she was full of resentment.

During this time, the fourth year after Louise's mastectomy, cancer spread to her liver and lungs. Chemotherapy was begun and her initial response was good, with excellent control of the cancer; but after several months she was often nauseated and suffered from attacks of anxiety that developed into long periods of depression. She felt that she was a burden to her family and a bad mother to Sandra. "Do you have any idea how useless I am and how painful it is for me to live?" she asked several times. I tried to make Louise understand how important she was to Sandra and that the grandparents could never take her place, but her mood did not improve. Then I reduced and altered the chemotherapy, and although her mental anguish decreased, the disease itself began to progress slowly. Suddenly, in a moment of desperation, Louise cast her hopes in another direction.

Telling me she was going to Hawaii for a vacation, Louise flew to Tijuana for Laetrile treatment, even though she was familiar with the controversy over Laetrile's therapeutic value. Mort Segal spoke of the loss of hope that erodes the spirit; for Louise, too, the apparent failure of chemotherapy to stem the growth of her cancer destroyed her faith in conventional medicine.

In Tijuana Louise stayed in a hotel that offers a special menu for cancer patients who have come for Laetrile treatments. At the clinic itself, she recalls, there were six doctors, plus nurses and other staff; but in the waiting room there were never fewer than 75 people. For 2 months Louise visited this clinic and received Laetrile orally and by injection, but the doctors made no attempt to monitor her physical response. Specifically, no x-ray films were taken of her chest; and her disease continued to progress.

Although Louise experienced no improvement, she struggled to maintain a semblance of enthusiasm as an encouragement to the patients who had become her friends. They came to her when their own spirits were low, and Louise sadly recalls, "All those people around me were dying."

By the time Louise decided to return to San Francisco, she was critically ill. Almost the moment she came into my office she blurted out the truth about her absence. She was embarrassed and hoped she hadn't offended me by seeking other help, but I could understand what motivated her and I don't believe in worrying about the past. I put Louise in the hospital, where an x-ray examination revealed that her right lung had collapsed into a cancerous mass and her chest cavity was filled with fluid. I then summoned a thoracic surgeon, who placed a drainage tube in her chest and removed five quarts of liquid. The right lung had atrophied and would never function again; the left lung was being invaded by cancer. She had progressive disease on her skin all across her chest, and more liver involvement. If an x-ray film had been taken of her chest while she was in Tijuana, it might have been possible to save part of her right lung.

I immediately began a new course of intensive chemotherapy. Louise's hair did fall out this time and she again had side effects, but the rapid progression of the cancer was halted.

The experience in Tijuana had made Louise fearful of dying. She felt constantly short of breath and did not feel secure unless she was close to an oxygen tank. Several times she was hospitalized because she couldn't breathe, but these episodes were in reality anxiety attacks. One day she confided in me, "I think I'm going to die." I replied, "I don't think so. Why do you?" Then, to reassure her that I would always relieve her pain, I promised her, "I won't let you suffer." The reversals in her health and the length of her illness had predisposed Louise to misinterpretations; she thought my statement meant that she was indeed about to die, and she went home and spoke to no one for several days. Fortunately, the misunderstanding was cleared up in a subsequent telephone conversation, and Louise's spirits improved.

By and large, however, the months following Louise's return from Mexico were the most psychologically debilitating since her mastectomy. The progression of her malignancy had caused her to lose hope, and she again contemplated suicide. I could only hope that her fear of death and the strong prohibition against suicide in her Russian Orthodox background would deter her from resorting to such a measure. But a patient's state of mind is often his or her most destructive symptom, and I was therefore afraid that Louise might die soon anyway if her mood did not change. The effect that patients' emotions have on their physical status is one reason statistics are not reliable. They simply cannot predict how a given individual will respond to a particular treatment for a particular type of cancer.

I explained to Louise that she had been taking a drug that might have caused some of her depression and anxiety and that we would stop using it. I also gave her an antidepressant. We talked again about how much Sandra needed her and how, if Louise could live well with cancer, this could be a legacy for Sandra. The downward trend of Louise's spirits was finally reversed—largely,

I think, because I acted contrary to my medical preference by withdrawing chemotherapy and using hormonal therapy instead. This ran the risk of more rapid physical deterioration, but freedom from the drug's side effects gave Louise energy to meet her emotional needs. She said one day, "You don't know how much your telling me to 'cheer up, don't give up' is like food to me. When you tell me I have a future, I know you're not just saying it to pacify me. And that, to me, is more than anyone could do. It cheers me up for weeks."

Since her mastectomy, Louise had avoided most of her former associates in the fashion and design world. She did not want them to see her in her present condition, and she felt she had nothing to offer them anymore. "I had to do something else," she recalls. And she did. With her right hand almost nonfunctional, she trained herself to work with her left. At first she could neither thread a needle nor write. Hemming a dress took hours. But gradually she became proficient and began to take pleasure in sewing and other crafts. She designed dresses and bathing suits with high necks and loose flowing sleeves for women who had had mastectomies. She made sand candles and macramé chokers, earrings, and nets for hanging plants. She painted in oils and began an organic vegetable garden in the backyard. With her creative energy thus channeled, Louise began to feel useful; she was delighted when her efforts gave enjoyment to others. At the same time she began to find more pleasure in reading and to study psychic phenomena and reincarnation. She does Alpha mind control and healing meditation every morning and evening and says that Alpha has changed her way of thinking about herself. "I used to demand perfection of myself and my friends. Now I am easier about everything. I also suddenly realized I didn't care what people thought of me, that I was a pretty nice person and shouldn't have been so hard on myself. Before, I always felt I wasn't doing enough. Now I know I did more than the average, and I've found I like myself. In Alpha you simply program yourself for positive thinking and action."

Thus by the spring of 1973 Louise's condition had stabilized and she was relatively content. Sometimes during her office visits she would share with me her complaints about her family and tell me their criticisms of her. I would remind her that when a person is ill over a long period of time, ordinary aggravations can be magnified to proportions that stun both patient and family.

Louise's experiences seemed to parallel Ellen's to the extent that many people either ignored her illness or were oversolicitous. This was illustrated during and after a family vacation at their summer cabin. Louise said, "They seemed to forget I was sick and would urge me to go to the beach one minute and take a hike the next. I would explain that I couldn't be in the sun for very long and they would offer to bring an umbrella. If I refused, they would say I was no fun anymore, so of course I did all the things they wanted." Within 2 weeks she was rushed back to San Francisco by ambulance, barely able to breathe. It would be difficult as well as futile to assign blame. Louise knew she should not overexercise. At the same time it is easy to imagine a collective will on the part of sisters, nieces, and nephews to relive the carefree years and try to forget Louise's cancer.

In the hospital Louise was given sedatives, oxygen, and narcotics for her pain, and she slowly recovered. However, her self-pity at having cancer and a relapse, and her anger at herself for not being able to say no were projected onto her family and friends. I felt that because she had such anger, it should be vented, and I urged her to telephone the people with whom she was most angry and to explain her feelings and the reasons for them. Louise did this, and it helped. Speaking out about her feelings has become one of the means with which she now deals with cancer. Her family, finding it hard to take at times, calls her the "Queen Bee," and Louise readily admits that she is sometimes demanding, quarrelsome, and impatient. But this is at least an honest reaction, and an open one. She is not harboring any emotionally exhausting secret animosities.

At the same time that Louise was accusing people of indifference and insensitivity, she was furious with her mother for being overprotective and solicitous. "The first night I was in the hospital after that vacation, my mother came over with chicken soup and enough apples, bananas, and peaches to fill the drawer beside my bed. She made me call the commissary and order ice cream, cookies, and milk and wouldn't leave until they were delivered. The next night, when my IV tube was hurting, I pulled it out and she screamed at me. The house doctor came and said the tube had pulled clear of the vein, that the fluid was making my tissues swell and I had been right to pull it out. Then all day long, just as I was dozing off, she would telephone me. She phoned me eight times in one morning."

It is not difficult to understand a frantic mother who equates every drop of IV and mouthful of food with an improvement in health. I suggested to Louise that she gently ask her mother not to telephone so frequently, but Louise insisted this would hurt her mother's feelings. I therefore spoke to her father, who explained that Louise's mother was always hoping for a miracle and that fussing over Louise was just her way of trying to make one happen. I told him there were no miracles, that Louise needed good care and rest. After that Louise's mother retreated to some extent, and I hoped she understood that my meddling was done in the interest of her daughter's health. Even if Louise had been exaggerating, I felt that my first responsibility was to meet her needs and to let her know I would support her.

Besides her mother's calls, in her first 2 days in the hospital Louise received 25 calls from relatives and friends asking, "How are you?" Barely able to breathe, operating at 40% of normal lung capacity, Louise labored to reply to such questions. "People should ask something you can answer 'yes' or 'no' to, or they should just offer their sympathy and ask if there's anything they can do. What if I replied that I was getting blood transfusions, and that I was nauseated and in pain with a 105 fever?" The phone calls were irritating, but they provided reassurance that people cared, and they also became a means through which she could vent anger at her disease. She did not have the phone turned off.

Talking over these episodes with Louise reminded me of the day she came into my office and I asked her how she was feeling. She smiled and said,

"Marvelous," and we continued with the examination. That evening I told Isadora, who had also talked with Louise that day, how pleased I was that she felt so well and was in such good spirits. My wife shook her head and replied, "Louise just said that to make you feel good. She told me she deliberately dressed up and made herself look good so you'd be pleased."

I needed to be reminded how much we doctors encourage deceptions like Louise's, in and out of hospital. Too often patients feel they must tell their doctors, family, and friends what they want to hear. Gaiety and good sportsmanship are rewarded; complaining or frankness is shunned. It should be possible to say, "Thanks, I feel lousy," without having people disapprove or turn away.

Louise has managed her life very wisely since the family vacation and its aftermath. Naturally, her condition and her moods vacillate, but she has learned what to expect from herself and others; she has learned, as Ellen hoped cancer patients would learn, that she can have a lot to do with her own and other people's attitudes toward her cancer.

For instance, Louise was aware that, despite all the open grieving by her parents and relatives, Sandra had not cried for months and that she was having one bad cold after another. Louise took Sandra aside and told her that any time she wanted to cry it would be all right, that as long as Louise knew she was not physically ill, she would ask no questions. Sandra looked surprised, closed the door to her room, and cried for 2 days. She stopped getting colds and began to bring friends home from school for the first time in a year.

At first Louise was worried that her appearance might frighten or embarrass Sandra's teenage girl friends, but instead she found them relaxed, refreshingly open, and easy to talk to. Louise showed them her wigless head and told them to call her "chrome dome." On successive visits, they measured the growth of her hair. They asked her what it was like to be dying and whether she was afraid, and they expressed their fears for themselves and their parents. At other times they simply shared their everyday problems about school and boyfriends. Their candor delighted Louise, and she came to consider these relationships among her most valuable.

Sandra, who has just turned 15, spends hours asking Louise about Louise's own childhood. Louise has observed the traditional jealousy between some of her friends and their teenage daughters, and she feels this has been circumvented in her relationship with Sandra, partly because of her cancer.

In December 1973 Louise went to a Christmas party at the company where she had been a designer and a model. She had not visited her former coworkers for 5 years, and they were thrilled when she accepted their invitation. The owner of the firm gave her a long two-piece royal blue outfit with a matching fur collar and hat, which she wore to my office just before the New Year. Her hair had grown back. She was stunning. No one would have guessed she had cancer. Before rushing off to a New Year's Eve party, she let me take her picture.

Since that time, Louise has created a way of life around the often terrible limitations imposed by her disease. She is still on hormonal therapy, and her fears about pain have been mitigated by access to pain-relieving shots, which I taught her to administer to herself. "I know the pain will go away when I want it to. And it's funny how that cuts the pain down. If you have to worry about how to control pain, it seems aggravated. But, more than that, I know you won't let me suffer with half my face gone. I was always afraid of being a vegetable, of being doped up and not knowing for months what was going on. I don't know how you'll do it, but I know you won't let that happen. And that gives me security."

Louise, sitting across from me at my desk, has brought several of her latest paintings to show me. She is pleased that I like them and remarks, "I remember your saying, 'Louise, you must fill each day and live each day.' I never really knew what you meant because as each day came along I would think, 'Tomorrow I'm going to do this, and next week I'm going to do that.' I was always planning what I was going to do tomorrow but never doing anything today. Now I fill every day so full, unless it's a day when I'm not feeling well, that I sometimes don't get to all my projects. Do you realize it's been 5 years since I began receiving medical treatment? And next week I'm going to Hawaii for a vacation." Louise smiles and adds, "I'm really going to Hawaii this time."

15

John Peterson

John Peterson was referred to me in the spring of 1971, a year after undergoing surgery and radiotherapy for melanoma. An alert, youthful-looking man of 50, he began in a direct manner to describe his experience with cancer. I sensed a feeling of sadness and discouragement, and as his tale unfolded, I understood why.

On his return from a vacation with his family in the summer of 1969, John noticed a lump on the side of his neck. It was hard, and approximately half the size of a Ping-Pong ball. It did not hurt, but it was unusual; and he could not avoid being aware of it as he shaved each morning. Although anything relating to doctors and medicine had always triggered strong anxiety in John, he did in this case consult his family doctor, who assured him the strange lump was a common occurrence, a cyst. He declined to treat it, saying it would go away of its own accord, and asked John to return in a couple of weeks for routine observation. John returned in 2 weeks, and a month after that, but always received the same advice.

The cyst failed to disappear as predicted, and John naturally began to wonder whether the diagnosis had been accurate. Because the doctor was also his friend and had consistently reassured him, John was reluctant to bother him again. But when his friend became ill for a short time the following January, John took the opportunity to consult another doctor in the same office. This doctor was equally certain the lump was a cyst, but suggested they go ahead and check it out by removing it surgically. He then referred John to a surgeon at the local hospital. After meticulously probing the spot, the surgeon announced, "Yes, we might as well remove it. These cysts can get nasty."

John did not look forward to the prospect of being unconscious and letting another person cut into his body. Moreover, he remembered a minor operation he had undergone as a small boy. The anesthetic wore off before the operation was finished, leaving John frightened and distrustful. However, he was now an adult, and he was pleased with the approach of the two doctors. Accordingly, he arranged to take a day or two of vacation from his job as assistant manager of a nearby lumberyard. The time would be well spent if the troublesome cyst could be removed. He entered the hospital on a Tuesday afternoon in January 1970 to prepare for minor surgery the following morning.

It was almost dark outside the hospital window when John awoke from the anesthetic on Wednesday afternoon. He tried to turn his head to survey his surroundings, but movement was painful and difficult. He touched his neck where the cyst had been. The bandaging seemed excessive, and the soreness surprised him, but he assumed this to be routine. Nevertheless, as a precaution he groped for the call button and told the nurse on duty he would like to talk with the surgeon as soon as it was convenient, half apologizing that he merely wanted reassurance that everything was all right.

A dinner tray was placed before John. He found it difficult to bend his head downward and consequently had to lift his plate to eye level to see what was on it. He picked at his food until his wife, Sue, arrived. She too was surprised at the degree of soreness and apparent extensiveness of the operation. At John's request she asked the nurses whether the surgeon would be coming by that evening. They told her they had left a message with his answering service and would probably hear from him shortly, although Sue guessed they were having trouble locating him. In any event, Sue and John were confident that he would appear before John's release on Thursday morning.

But the following morning the surgeon neither appeared nor telephone instructions for John's dismissal from the hospital. As a result, each time a footstep or a voice echoed in the corridor, John glanced expectantly toward the door. His uneasiness grew as he repeated to himself the comforting litany, "It was just a cyst. Nothing could have gone wrong. The surgeon's a very busy man."

The nurse who brought John's breakfast and medication assured him that the tenderness in his neck was normal, but when he asked where the surgeon was or whether the operation had gone well, she suddenly appeared ignorant of his case. John's anxiety sharpened. As each hour passed, it became increasingly difficult to convince himself he was a victim of oversight or neglect. He could see that the nurses were sympathetic as well as nervously evasive; and when Sue joined him for dinner that evening, she also appeared anxious.

By dawn on Friday John realized he dreaded the surgeon's visit. The day before, passing footsteps had made him start in hope. Now he was relieved when they continued down the corridor. He lay still and waited.

He must have dozed off. A doctor he did not recognize was standing beside his bed. "Mr. Peterson, I'm the surgeon who assisted at your operation. Your surgeon had to leave town for several days and therefore asked me to speak to you. I'm going to be very frank with you, Mr. Peterson. You have incurable cancer. It's melanoma."

John had never heard of melanoma, and said so, whereupon the assistant surgeon told him, "A biopsy of the cyst reveals that you have a vicious type of malignancy, one with a highly unpredictable growth pattern. We're planning a more extensive operation next week, but I must warn you that just when you think you've got it all, it pops up in another area." Sometime during this recitation, John realized that his surgeon must have suspected he had cancer and failed to warn him. He began to cry, but the effort caused pain around his incision. Hesitantly he asked the doctor to tell Sue the diagnosis so she would receive a clear explanation of his disease and his prospects.

The second phase of the operation was performed a week after John was told he had melanoma. This surgery was more radical than the first and involved the removal of surrounding muscles.

John remained in the hospital another 10 days and rested at home for a week before returning to work, his neck still in bandages. His family and friends were astonished at how quickly he got back on his feet. Radiation treatment was planned as a preventive measure to destroy any cancer cells the surgery might have missed, but such treatment cannot be given until a surgical wound has healed. In spite of his determined recovery, John's incision was particularly slow in healing, so it wasn't until 6 weeks after the second surgery that he began weekly trips for treatment to a radiotherapist in San Francisco. The therapy lasted 3 months, and on the days he made the 2-hour round trip he still managed to work at least half a day.

On the importance of work in his life John once told me, "Work is all I know. I grew up during the Depression and my family was poor. I've worked since I was old enough to pull a grocery cart. I worked during vacations, after school, and on weekends. I even worked during the gym period at school. Consequently I never learned to play and never participated in sports like other children. Now, all these years later, I'm not content if I'm not working."

But John had other pleasures besides work. They may even have been accentuated by his cancer experience and the unpredictability of a recurrence. Sue is certain that the possibility of his melanoma's returning was always at the back of his mind, but she remembers that he was cheerful and tried hard to live each day. Looking back at this period of their lives, she recalls that they made more trips and in some ways enjoyed themselves more than in the years before cancer disrupted their lives. This was also partly due to their circumstances, the increased freedom of having their two older children on their own and the two younger ones almost ready for college. They spent much of their time improving their home inside and out, painting, rebuilding, and gardening. "We're both orderly people. We like things to be nice," John explained. The few hours when they weren't working at their jobs or on their home, they listened to their stereo, with the added pleasure of knowing their older son was studying to be a concert pianist.

In December 1970 Sue and John observed their thirtieth wedding anniversary and planned to celebrate by taking a long-hoped-for trip to Italy in the spring. Regrettably, the worst occurred in February 1971, when a new lump appeared near the site of the original tumor, only a year after the diagnosis of melanoma. Sue canceled their reservations and John reentered the hospital for tests.

The surgeon who had performed the first operation had moved to another city, but the former assistant surgeon was available. He performed a biopsy and removed the tumor. He then told John he might have to lose his right arm, although later he changed his mind, saying that since the cancer had probably spread to other areas, removal of his arm would only cause extra pain and discomfort. "If I were you," he said, "I'd go home and forget about treatment. Your cancer has spread too far. Chemotherapy will only make you miserable during your remaining life. I've seen cases like this before."

John did go home, but he needed to take action against the surgeon's harsh pronouncement. That need brought John back to San Francisco to consult his radiotherapist, who referred him to me.

From the day of our first meeting and our talk about his background, his present life and work, and his discouraging encounters with two physicians, I knew my first goal must be to try to inspire hope. Thus I talked about control of his disease, about the possibility that the growth of his tumor might be slowed down or arrested. I told him how chemotherapy and experimental immunotherapy had led to improvement in many cases of melanoma; but I could not, of course, make any promises of cure. "I can only tell you what realistic results we can hope for. You can't quit until you've tried," I urged. John nodded, but because of all he had been told, faith in treatment would come only with success. For the moment his sadness prevailed over all my reasoning.

John consented to a program of experimental immunotherapy in the spring of 1971. He subsequently experienced periodic brief episodes of high fever, flulike symptoms, and a rash as a consequence of BCG immunotherapy, but the tumors in his neck were significantly reduced in size. Several months later frequent nausea took away his appetite; he tired easily and lost weight. Yet despite these discomforts tumor growth was controlled for over a year. John's desire to fight was sustained because he was able to work full time. This was evidence that he was not going to deteriorate as rapidly as had been predicted, evidence that in turn reinforced his courage to continue.

In the summer of 1972 John, Sue, and their two younger children made a trip to Canada. Just after their return, we discovered John's tumors had begun to grow again. Concurrently he began to dread the side effects of the drugs; and as his anxiety increased, he began to have attacks of nausea before treatment. In addition, he had pain in his right shoulder and numbness in his fingertips.

A month later, in September 1972, we discovered that John's disease had progressed to his lungs and liver. This meant that immunotherapy had ceased to forestall tumor progression, so we initiated a program that combined immunotherapy with chemotherapy. Unfortunately, the addition of the chemotherapy produced a stronger reaction of nausea than before, with the result that, in anticipation of his injections, John often vomited before reaching my office. But the chemotherapy also achieved a remission for several months.

Treatments were scheduled at 2- to 3-week intervals, and the accompanying nausea, which always humiliated John, lasted 2 days. A greater humiliation was experienced the following spring when his cancer once again advanced and the side effects from a new chemotherapeutic program forced him to cut his workday from 8 to 5 hours. The forces of physical decline, side effects from treatment, and severe depression and anxiety merged and began to shatter his self-image.

John now left the office at 3:00 each afternoon. Tired rather than sleepy, he lay on his bed, often too weak to get up yet too nervous for sleep, trying to remember ever having been in bed at 4:00 in the afternoon. He felt defeated and ashamed. Angry with himself, he was easily annoyed with others. Unhappy at being, as he saw it, a burden rather than a sustaining force, he became less communicative. The days were long and monotonous.

One day during an office visit Sue, John, and I talked about the additional time John now spent at home, and I asked him if he had any hobbies or interests.

He replied, "All I've ever done is sleep, eat, and work. I have no hobbies. I don't read. Television bores me. I don't play cards. I do enjoy listening to the stereo, but you can't do that all the time. I want to work in the garden or go backpacking with my younger son, but I'm no longer able to do those things. And I see all kinds of things to do around the house, such as washing the windows, but I have no strength for that either. Consequently I'm depressed and everyone irritates me — Sue, the children. I no longer have any patience."

"How do your children react to your illness?" I ventured.

"I think they take it as a matter of course. Sometimes I even wonder if they're concerned about it. They don't help at home. They don't even clean up their rooms. The children of today are wrapped up in themselves. They've been spoiled.

"I wanted our children to have the education I didn't have," John continued. "I held down three jobs at one point. I worked at night so they could have all the extras, but the result is that they've never learned to do things. They aren't lazy — they're hard workers — but they've never known want. They've never known what it was to give every extra penny they earned for the support of the household."

Here Sue intervened. "It's difficult for John to put himself in the children's place, to understand that they see the world from a different perspective than he does. They're good children, but times have changed.

"John's mother became very ill when we were first married. As a matter of course John spent his summer vacation with her and took care of her while she was down and out."

"In this day and age it just isn't there," John sighed.

I met the Peterson children a few weeks later. We discussed the progression of their father's cancer, and his prognosis. They said they would do anything to relieve his anxiety and lessen his pain, that they felt helpless in the face of medical failure and advancing disease. Coupled with their frustration was the emotional fatigue of witnessing suffering that changes little from day to day. When disease is acute, or illness sudden, medical change in a patient may be rapid and dramatic. With a chronic illness such as John's, a patient's suffering may begin to be taken for granted by those around him.

John's children needed the distraction of school, friends, and sports. They also understood their father's need for encouragement and sympathy. I have often witnessed this particular conflict of needs, the solution to which lies in mutual understanding. To deal with impending loss, those close to a patient need to pursue their everyday activities, to establish and maintain an ongoing life. At the same time the help they give their loved one can be mutually rewarding. The patient receives emotional support while the family members fulfill their need to show their love.

During the late spring and early summer of 1973, John was given several combinations of chemotherapy, with little success. Each failure to achieve another remission led to a further decrease in physical stamina and deeper depression. His shame at not doing his share of the work consumed him, and as a consequence he withdrew even more into himself.

One day he said, "I used to help Sue, but now I come home at night and I'm unable to do anything."

"He used to do a lot," Sue confirmed.

"Since the kids don't always pitch in, Sue's stuck fixing dinner, getting it on the table, and doing the dishes. Then she has to correct papers for her second-grade class, which means she doesn't get to bed until after midnight."

I wondered whether it would be possible for them to spend more time together, but Sue responded, "We spend lots of time together, but we could spend better time. John is lonely, and I'm lonely. And we shouldn't be. We should be closer than ever before. But we don't talk together."

"It's just that I get very depressed by my illness," John said. "I sometimes feel my family would be better off if I were gone and it were over with. They wouldn't be burdened with me any longer—particularly Sue."

"We don't feel that way," Sue said firmly.

John persisted. "But I feel that way."

"So he withdraws into himself and doesn't communicate."

"I realize I keep too much to myself."

"We used to talk freely. There was a warmth."

"I think we still do."

"Much less."

I broke the ensuing silence. "John, do you feel that by talking about it, you just add to their burden?"

"It's not that. I don't like to talk about my illness. I look ill. I feel ill. There's all this sickness in the house. Why in the world should I carry on? What's there to be gained? I'm not enjoying life."

Sue interrupted, "Dr. Rosenbaum thinks this extended time should be lived. Your attitude can help you to live it."

John turned toward us. "But what if you're not capable of living it?"

Toward the end of July John had another remission from his cancer as a result of taking BCG and chemotherapy. His neck masses were again reduced in size, although he felt sick and weak intermittently. Then in August the flulike symptoms from the BCG recurred. Yet however much John was suffering physically, I was still convinced that depression was playing a role in depriving him of any possibility of enjoyment. John agreed. One afternoon toward the end of August he commented, "The last couple of months have been the worst I've ever put in. I feel so weak all the time. I'm beginning to wonder whether it's cancer or nerves."

"Which do you think it is?" I asked.

"It could be nerves. We went to San Francisco to the Ice Follies on Sunday. I wasn't going to go, but I did, and I felt better. I forgot myself and found I had more strength than I realized.

"It's the normal day's routine that gets to me. I get up tired. I go to bed tired. I come home tired. I work 5 hours a day, from 8 to 11 in the morning—and I find I can barely make it till 11—when I come home and have some pudding and half-and-half to settle my stomach. I rest before having a bite of lunch, although I don't eat much. Then I go back to work at 1:00 and by 3 I'm ready to come home again. At that time I have a 7-Up float and sleep until 6. When dinner's over, I go back to bed, usually around 8:00. And it's the same routine day in and day out.

"That's why I'm continually wondering whether I'm doing the right thing taking chemotherapy. As you know, my last surgeon told me, 'You'll just be sick continually and it won't do you one bit of good.' Well, I am sick a good deal of the time, and I'm of no use at home or in the office, even though my employers are kind enough to pay me. I freely admit I've thought of suicide many times. But at least I should probably stop chemotherapy and let nature take its course."

"Yet you agree that chemotherapy isn't causing all your problems," I reminded him.

"I don't think the actual process of chemotherapy is doing it. I think it's the fear of it, and the anticipation, and not knowing what's going to happen. I need to have everything cut and dried ahead of me. Yesterday I went out and bought a funeral plot. I plan ahead."

"So there it is. He's planning for death," Sue blurted out.

But I could not agree. "Most of us just ignore the fact that someday we're going to die. I think you were right to make those arrangements. It takes a lot of courage not to leave it to someone else. But now you've taken care of that, and from now on I think that concentrating too much on death in the unpredictable future can defeat you in the present. Is there any way you can think of to approach the present differently, to try to counteract some of the depression?"

"I don't know how to counteract it."

"It's a vicious circle," Sue added.

"How do you feel about living in the present, Sue?" I asked.

"Well, I feel that if he only has 6 months, I'd rather live those 6 months. I'm in it as much as he is because we're living together. And yet I can't expect him to go beyond his physical capabilities. But within those capabilities we should do things together and enjoy the time we have."

"It would be nice if you could get away for weekends," I suggested.

"We were going to go away this weekend, but John panicked and we had to cancel."

John explained, "I didn't think I could eat out in restaurants for 2 or 3 days."

I did not think John should "let nature take its course," but I could appreciate his desire for some respite from chemotherapy. Lately he had suffered the side effects without experiencing the benefits of treatment. We discussed the matter at length and agreed to eliminate chemotherapy treatments for the month of September.

"All we'll do is take some x-rays and carefully watch your case," I said. "It'll give you a rest and a chance to regain your equilibrium. We haven't kidded each other, John. You're in trouble."

John looked out the window. "That's something that's always bothered me. Am I going to make it this year? Am I going to make it next year?"

"I hope you're going to make it this year. Your troubles may well stabilize. Next year is a question mark. I hope to get you through this year in halfway decent shape."

"Like I am today?"

"Yes. I also hope you'll get those reservations back and have a nice weekend. Even if you can't enjoy your meals, you can still relax and walk in the woods."

"You're right. I always worry about something before it happens. I'm high-strung."

"That's true," Sue affirmed. "Even before cancer, he was this type of person."

I said, "Cancer just magnifies your problems—the ones you've had all your life. They become accentuated under stress."

Sue and John got their reservations back and then had to cancel again. Despair and cancer had effectively incapacitated John and he now began to deteriorate rapidly. His neck nodules grew, his liver became enlarged, and his pain was persistent. Even then he continued to work several hours a day. He was anxious to complete the year's work for financial reasons. "At the end of December I get a commission on the year's sales, and our sales were good this year. Money is important to me. After all, that's what I'm working for. We use everything we have on two incomes."

In mid-September John and I discussed his medical alternatives. They were limited. He had been through all the major chemotherapeutic regimens, and unless a new one was developed, any further treatment would only be detrimental. However, there was one possibility. "There is a new drug you might try," I told him, "although it's not specifically for melanoma. It's simple and nontoxic, so if you get sick, it won't be the drug. All you have to do is take three capsules a day at home."

John began taking the new drug in early October, but other problems intervened. Intense pain in a lesion in his hip brought him to the hospital in the middle of the month. I told him we would try to relieve the pain with local radiation. "Melanoma is an odd thing. It can be sensitive or insensitive to radiation. You can't tell ahead of time. But you're in a pain pattern right now and our job is to get you some relief or to break the pattern altogether. Sometimes I've knocked people out for a whole day with complete sedation and analgesia and broken the pattern."

"How long will I be out of work?" was John's natural response.

"If we have success with radiation, you should get pain relief between 7 and 21 days, but you may be too fatigued to return to work immediately. Our job now is to get you through this acute phase."

We talked some more about medication and other details, but before leaving his room, I asked, "John, during the intervals these last weeks and months when you had some relief from pain and nausea, did you experience any happiness at all, or has it been one struggle day after day?"

The sadness in his eyes reminded me of that first day in my office. "It's been one struggle day after day. There have been no good days, really—not in the last 2 months."

I was regretful. "What bothers me is, we've made all these moves to give you a better quality of life. But there is no way to prophesy the results of treatment. One can only treat, wait, and hope. And we still hope to knock down your present pain so that you can be comfortable."

By the end of October John was despondent. The radiation was not completely effective in reducing his pain, which meant that he was partly dependent on narcotics. Surgery was not a possibility; the available regimens of chemotherapy and immunotherapy had been exhausted. X-ray films showed that the nodules in his lungs had grown and that his melanoma had spread to his brain.

Sue and the children were traveling 2 hours each day to visit John, as were other close relatives and friends. At that time our only medical option was to keep John comfortably sedated, so we agreed with his family that it would be best to return him to his hometown hospital. However, before making the transfer, John asked, "Is it going to come slowly, or is it going to come quickly? The only thing I worry about and fear is going out slowly with all this pain and mental anguish for myself and my family. If I suffer, my family suffers."

I reassured him he would not suffer, adding, "I've talked to the doctors who will be in charge at your local hospital and they're very capable. Also, you know I'll always be available for consultation."

John died 2 weeks later, in his hometown hospital, with as much pain relief and comfort as his doctors could administer.

When I look back at John's experience with cancer, my admiration for him increases. His case is an example of the frustrations that can arise for both patient and physician. Here was a man whose character was shaped by a youth of poverty, of early and endless work, who in adulthood was to find his deepest satisfactions in hard work. It was the means by which he expressed love and achieved self-esteem. When his disease progressed and therapy failed, I wanted to give him hope, but I could not combat his feeling of worthlessness when he was unable to work.

John suffered many of the worst potential problems that may arise for a cancer patient—the failure of early detection, the insensitivity of two of his doctors, his predisposition against treatment, and medical failure after the achievement of initial control through immunotherapy and chemotherapy. If chemotherapy had been more successful for a longer period, perhaps John's attitude toward therapy would have been more positive. Yet in retrospect I would still advocate therapy for John because one never knows who may respond, or when. I continue to give new patients the advice I gave John that first day in my office, "You can't quit until you've tried."

And John did try. Sue recently told me, "In September of 1972, when John was informed that his melanoma had spread to his liver and lungs, it was the first time he knew he couldn't lick it. He gathered us together in the living room and explained that all he could gain was time. Even then, although he later had moments of being morose because of the inconvenience, side effects, and eventually the futility, of treatment, he never really lost heart until the last few weeks of his life." Further, when I asked Sue to assess the value of treatment, she said, "It was worth it for John and it was worth it for his family. We had him 4 years. We might have had him for only 2."

PART SIX

The family

A family faced with the life-threatening illness of one of its members has the dual problem of trying to control its own fear and anxiety while giving encouragement and support to the patient. This is just the first of many dichotomies that can arise between inner feelings and outward behavior. It can produce a situation in which members of the family and friends spend their time wondering how to ease the emotional suffering of the patient while the patient is busy worrying about the despair of the loved ones. Each of them is searching for the most tactful way to deal with the other. In this search they may consider trying a candid approach but reject that option as potentially devastating. I am convinced, however, that a deliberate policy of candor and openness will create an atmosphere that is beneficial to all concerned.

Living with Cancer is based on my belief that candor creates confidence and trust between a doctor and the patient and his or her family. Candor between patients and their families can achieve similar results by removing the burden of secrecy and opening the door for the alleviation of apprehensions. Candor is not easily achieved. Some people are not in the habit of speaking of their deepest concerns. Even those who have established a close relationship may become fainthearted in the presence of cancer and the threat of death. To achieve openness and to maintain it under stress is part of the challenge of living with cancer.

As a doctor I think I can be a catalyst in helping a family establish open communication about cancer and the terrors it evokes. In the early chapters of this book I described how I try to initiate a relationship based on candor by holding frank discussions with each patient and family about the particular medical problem and its implications for their future. I emphasize the importance of asking questions and discussing problems as they arise, to forestall a more serious anxiety state. Having been brought together in this way and having experienced the relief that open discussion can bring, they will, I hope, continue to relate to each other candidly about their cancer problems after they leave my office.

If they do continue such discussions in the privacy of their home, they will reap the benefits I mentioned. They need not lead a double life, hiding their real feelings while trying to guess what the other is thinking. Hearing what the other is experiencing can never be as devastating as what the imagination can conjure. Fears and frustrations can be talked about as they arise and not left to fester until they become too frightening to mention, or until a habit of withholding evolves into irretrievable isolation. The confrontation of each other's fears therefore becomes a means of keeping those fears under control. This will allow the relationship to operate in a new realm, where despair can sometimes be minimized or set aside, and enjoyment and pleasure can resume their rightful place.

Candor between patients and their families and friends includes a recognition of each other's needs as well as fears. A family needs to give, to feel it is doing something practical to hasten the patient's recovery, whether that patient is at home or in the hospital.

The separation caused by hospitalization is particularly traumatic; it can cause extreme emotional distress to the members of a family. They leave the hospital each evening and worry whether their loved one will ever again lead a normal life, or whether he or she will even leave the hospital. Feeling impotent, they need to give of themselves. Fortunately, there are many practical services a patient's family can perform for him or her while the patient is in the hospital—services such as feeding, walking, turning, massaging. These, along with the offer of special foods, a favorite pillow, or a comforting hand, become the routine of the daily hospital visit, giving solace to family and patient alike.

When a person is critically ill, it is not unusual for at least one family member to be in attendance around the clock. This may involve sleeping in a chair beside the patient's bed or arriving early in the morning. To obtain up-to-date information on the patient's condition, relatives may rearrange their schedules so as to be present when the doctor makes rounds or a particularly helpful nurse is on duty.

When a person is at home, functioning well, there are still many opportunities to give emotional support through practical means. One need only consider the trials cancer patients must sometimes undergo. They may be anxious about a visit to the doctor, wondering whether a new problem will be discovered or a new treatment recommended. They may not have transportation to and from the doctor's office, or may be dreading the side effects from the day's treatment. A spouse, parent, or friend can offer a ride or accompaniment on the bus. If family members are working and unable to be with the patient during the day, there is still the evening, when the side effects of therapy may have to be endured. Patient and family benefit from any means by which love and encouragement can be expressed.

To be realistic, however, not every family is able to be open, loving, or intelligently supportive, before or after a crisis. Even people who feel they have a stable relationship may find it severely threatened by the pressures of long-term illness. Latent problems may emerge. Formerly controlled anger or guilt may surface in sudden attack or recrimination, indifferent or oversolicitous behavior. Just the exhaustion and frustration of constant worry and care may break the most loyal supporter.

Lengthy illness can also break the most courageous of patients. When a person has fought long and hard against cancer, lost and regained hope many times, and then realizes the battle is not to be won, he or she may at times experience rage and depression that will seek as their target the nearest available person—spouse, child, parent, or the nurse on duty. This anger is usually manifested as irritation over trivial matters that in normal times would not even concern the patient. The person under attack needs to understand that this is not a rejection but a cry of anguish.

In addition to anger and depression, a patient must also endure the endless boredom of being ill, as well as the fear of being a burden when special attention is really wanted and needed. Ironically, the people from whom the patient wants this attention may be suffering from the same tedium or from feelings of inadequacy and guilt for being unable to relieve his or her suffering. They may not be able to cope with the reality in which the patient is imprisoned. The result may be a gradual diminishment of attention and care by the family and increased bitterness and fear of isolation in the patient.

No one should be blamed for the way he or she responds to the crisis of a long-term illness or the threat of change and loss. Some people and some relationships grow stronger; some waver and hold together; others collapse. I believe that those who strive toward the ideal of candor and sharing in their relationships can not only hold together but also experience new depths of love, respect, and understanding.

I have often thought it is a shame that some people have to develop a fatal disease before they realize the value of life and love, family and friends. I am not implying that just because a person has cancer a light will shine or bells ring out, or that he or she will become clairvoyant. This heightened appreciation may simply evolve from the common effort of patient, family, friends, and doctor to find solutions to the medical and emotional problems that cancer can bring. It is the successful interaction of these people that contributes to mutual understanding and strengthens love. It is these experiences that give life its worth and dignity.

Following are the stories of several patients, each of whom is unique—in himself or herself, in type of cancer and medical outlook, in the availability and willingness of family and friends to provide support, and in the degree of candor all allow to exist.

16

Darrell Ansbacher

SEPTEMBER 1973

"When Darrell feels bad, we feel bad. We let our empathy flow to him and hope that it gives him strength. Every single one of his problems is our problem, and because we share, it becomes easier to bear all around."

Mr. Ansbacher smiled at Darrell, the younger of his two sons, who was about to complete a course of radiotherapy for Hodgkin's disease. The disease had been discovered the previous June when Darrell, aged 18, home for the summer from his freshman year in college, had consulted his family physician about a swelling in his groin. Darrell had been confident that a shot of penicillin would dispense with the problem. However, a negative examination and blood tests alerted his physician to other possibilities and he arranged for a biopsy the following day.

It was now a warm evening in September, when summer comes to San Francisco. I had stopped at the Ansbacher home to chat with Darrell and his parents about their experiences during the past 3 months.

"Has Darrell's illness brought you closer together as a family?" I asked.

"People say a crisis brings a family together, but that hasn't been the case in our family," Mr. Ansbacher replied. "We've always been close. Our children have always felt they could come to us, and vice versa. Moreover, I remember when all this happened, Darrell was with his friend Roger, and Roger came out of the house and said, 'You know, Darrell is worried about you.' That's the kind of relationship we have in this family."

We then discussed the period of the diagnosis.

"I was very fortunate," said Darrell. "I know that some people can have Hodgkin's for years and not know it. A doctor who was less concerned and less skillful than our family physician might not have observed the symptoms and recommended that I have the proper tests and a biopsy.

"However, even though I was undergoing all those tests, I don't think I was really aware that it might be something serious until you told me I had a malignancy in my lymph nodes but that the possibility of leukemia had been eliminated."

Mr. Ansbacher added, "When we were told a malignancy was diagnosed, the blow was incredible. Then, as the results came in and we discovered it was

167

Hodgkin's, and we were told what the prospects were at that stage of the game, all of a sudden I was happy with Hodgkin's. You're grateful for small favors."

His wife nodded in agreement. "The first relief was that there was a chance for a complete cure, so we were free to concentrate on the next step, which we felt had to be carried out as quickly and efficiently as possible. I think as parents our biggest comfort was our involvement in getting things done fast and well."

Events did move swiftly for the Ansbachers. In the days following Darrell's visit to his family doctor, he had a bone-marrow examination, a biopsy of the swelling in his groin, x-ray examinations of the chest, a lymphangiogram, and an intravenous pyelogram, as part of the preliminary staging of the amount of disease. When the approximate degree of Hodgkin's disease had been determined, Darrell and his parents were referred for consultation and further explanation to Dr. Henry Kaplan, a leading authority on Hodgkin's disease at Stanford University Medical School. I alerted them to the probability that he would recommend exploratory abdominal surgery, a procedure that is now almost routine in determining more precisely the extent of spread of the disease. In such exploratory surgery a biopsy of the liver and lymph nodes is performed, and the spleen removed. After early childhood, the spleen, essentially a large lymph node, is considered expendable — it has served its function of providing the body with an immune defense system (lymphocytes) while the body is developing its own system of antibodies. Thus it can be removed and examined without interfering with any natural functions. If the spleen is unaffected by Hodgkin's disease, it is almost certain that the liver is unaffected; if the spleen shows evidence of disease, then there may be liver involvement.

"I was very apprehensive about how the details were going to be conveyed to us by Dr. Kaplan," Mr. Ansbacher recalled. "Was he going to ask my wife and me to come into his office while Darrell waited outside, or would he take Darrell into his office and leave us outside? He did neither of those things. He invited us all into his office, saying, 'I'm going to tell each one of you the same thing at the same time. Nobody is going to be kept in the dark about anything.' Then he laid it on the line very bluntly, without any reservations, telling Darrell, 'You may as well forget about the next year of your life because it's going to be a very difficult year.' However, he also confirmed your reassuring statements that in Darrell's case there was an 80 to 90% chance for a complete cure.

"Of course since that conversation we've found the system of sharing information has worked so well that we've made a pledge to each other to continue it."

In the 10 days following the original biopsy, Darrell underwent 3 days of tests at Mount Zion Hospital, visited Dr. Kaplan and was tested at Stanford, and entered Mount Zion on July 4 in preparation for exploratory surgery the next day.

Darrell said, "There was a party the night before I was admitted to the hospital. It was a strange experience going to this party, knowing that the next day I was admitting myself to the hospital. I was actually letting myself in for it. Nevertheless, since it was to be done, I was lucky not to have to wait to be admitted until after the holiday."

"I think a doctor should keep in mind that waiting a week, or even over a weekend, for an operation may seem normal to him, but may be an excruciating interval for a patient and his family," Mrs. Ansbacher added.

In the exploratory surgery on July 5 Darrell's spleen and appendix were removed, his lymph nodes resected, and bone marrow and liver biopsies taken. The results were pretty much as we had suspected—slight spleen and lymph node involvement and a good chance for complete cure. However, a cure could not be effected without complete nodal radiation and a course of complementary chemotherapy.

Of the lengthy process of cure, Mr. Ansbacher commented, "We have decided to take each day as it comes. That's the only way we ourselves can cope, and we hope our attitude flows to Darrell so he can cope with it too."

"How much have these last weeks of traveling to Stanford for radiation disrupted your lives?" I inquired.

"First of all, we don't think in terms of our lives being disrupted. My wife and I have never considered that anything our children required was a sacrifice. The word 'sacrifice' never entered our vocabulary because we never thought it or felt it. What has disrupted our lives, though, is the sorrow of seeing a child agonizing and losing weight.

"We take turns driving Darrell to Stanford. My wife goes twice a week. I go once. And Richard, my older son, goes once. But we never forget that Darrell has to go 4 days in a row. Our only goal is to make him feel better. But when I went today, I came away feeling better for having gone. When I don't go, I don't feel so good. I also went into the radiation room with him once, just to see. I felt that way I could empathize even more with him. They explained how the various lead shields are made, how thick they are, and how Darrell was being prepared for the treatment. They gave me a feeling it was being done right—not that I'd know if it weren't. But I'd seen it. I felt better. And I think the family needs to be made to feel better too. It's a heavy burden for us."

"We've had other help, too," said his wife thoughtfully. "Do you remember the social worker who was in the radiation area the first day?" Turning to me, she explained, "She sat down and spoke briefly to all of us, telling us what was going to happen; and then when Darrell was having his treatment, she told us what the various unpleasant effects might be, such as nausea, weight loss, fatigue, diarrhea, and the loss of his hair in patches. She said there are no two patients alike. That's terribly important to know.

"We also talked about the relief to a patient of having advance knowledge of his side effects. If and when they occur, he needn't worry that something new and terrible is happening. But the social worker then said that most people tend not to ask questions, that they come into the hospital with no idea of what's wrong and don't appear very interested in finding out.

"However, I don't think it's a lack of interest," Mrs. Ansbacher continued. "Sometimes people feel that if they ask a question, the doctor will think they are questioning his medical expertise."

"I have a good example of a patient being uninformed," said Darrell. "Yesterday I was sitting in the waiting room and I heard an elderly man on the other side of the door say something like, 'I don't understand why you have to take my blood to find out how I am. You're radiating me. I had pain in my right leg and you took out my left kidney.' Then he jokingly added, 'I'm glad I didn't have a pain in my foot or you would have cut my head off.'

"When he came out I explained to him why they took his blood. I told him how the blood count gives an indication as to how efficiently the body is functioning in spite of the radiation and how imperative it is that the body maintain a certain blood count. The man obviously had cancer and didn't know it. He even had a kidney removed without being told why."

"People are also overawed by doctors and don't want to bother them," Mr. Ansbacher commented. "Yet a question that may sound silly to a doctor isn't silly to his patient. It's terribly important that I be able to ask about anything that concerns me without being ridiculed. Nothing has happened to Darrell since June 21 for which we didn't seek out an explanation."

One thing that happened to Darrell was a daily bout with nausea following his radiation treatment. I asked him if the nausea had eased up lately, and I was also curious to know what he actually experienced each day as he went into the radiation room.

"First of all," Darrell began, "it's a very odd sensation to know that all I have to do not to be sick on any given day is to skip my radiation treatment. I have to keep reminding myself that it's for my own good.

"The routine helps me. I get up at 6:30 each day that I'm scheduled for treatment, and I'm there for the first appointment at 8:00. I usually have to wait a few minutes in a room with other people, most of whom are worse off than I am, with no hair on their heads, beady eyes, and some burn marks on their bodies. When my turn comes, I go into a room, take off my clothes, and put on a robe. Then I enter the radiation room. I have the same room and the same technicians each time, which is really important to me because it reinforces the routine. The room, which is underground, is about four times larger than a regular x-ray room, and it's oval-shaped, with thick cement walls. The only furniture, aside from the x-ray table, consists of three work tables laden with huge lead blocks. Each patient has a set of lead blocks that is prepared specifically to his measurements and that delineates the areas to be radiated. When you lie on the x-ray table, a mesh screen apparatus constructed like a breakfast tray is placed over you, and your particular lead block is placed on top of that. Your body is marked, so the blocks are replaced accurately each time. When the technician who has set up the screen and the block leaves the room, she goes to a window about 8 by 4 in. and pushes a button that slides the heavy door into place. The door is inside the wall: that is, when it has slid into place, nothing is visible but a flat cement wall.

"By this time you've removed your robe, of course, so there you are, naked. It's like a waiting room for—somewhere.

"There's also an odor of lead, and a high-pitched noise for as long as you're being radiated. For me it's a minute and a half, so each time I hold a countdown and think that this is one less time I'll have to be there.

"And that's it. We travel 2 hours each day for 1½ minutes of treatment. Although I usually do the driving on the way down, whoever has come with me that day drives back, because the nausea begins almost immediately.

"I do everything I can to establish and maintain routine to make it easier on myself. We park in the same place each day and walk to the cafeteria, where I have a Pepsi-Cola and a doughnut. I find that helps when the nausea comes. Although I vomited after the first few treatments, I now find I can think my way out of it. I'm home by 9:30 and lie on my bed with a container next to me, just in case. Then I generally goof off, watching game shows and doing puzzles until I feel better later in the day.

"The reason I try to reinforce the routine is to establish a rhythm that will make the end of treatment seem to come more quickly. It's like climbing a steep hill in San Francisco. If you keep your eye on the cracks in the cement instead of on the top of the hill, you'll seem to reach your goal in less time.

"However, to answer the rest of your question, the nausea really hasn't abated. But as you know, I've always had a weak stomach, so none of us is too worried about the meaning of the nausea. As a matter of fact, my mother is apt to urge me to go to a summer school class or to visit a friend."

"True," laughed his father. "I'm much more apt to say, 'If you don't feel well, just lie around.' I've been overprotective with both our boys in that respect. When I see Darrell with an upset stomach, I haven't the heart to urge him to do something to occupy his mind, as the doctors have recommended."

Mrs. Ansbacher observed, "Yet Darrell knows that when he goes out and is active mentally, when he doesn't have the opportunity to think about himself quite as much, he feels good when he comes home. We've all had that experience. So you just wonder how far the mind involves itself with the body."

Darrell knew. "The power of the mind to ignore the body is just incredible. Sometimes it even works adversely. I can be feeling bad but go out and be active anyway, and then later find myself wishing I hadn't."

"I think Darrell's age raises a question here," said his mother. "How much do you insist that he do, and how much do you let him make up his own mind? He's been away at college and had a year of independence. He's at a cross-road. We know we have valuable experience that might be of help, but how do we get it across without sounding like a parent-child relationship? Of course, some decisions were never in our hands. If the doctors say you have to have your spleen removed, or radiation therapy, or chemotherapy, these are just not decisions. We don't tell Darrell he's got to go through these things. He's old enough to know that's what he has to do and that if we could avoid it, we would. All we can do is act on these doctors' decisions in concert with one another and share whatever comes."

Darrell offered eloquent testimony of his parents' handling of the issue of independence. "My brother and I were always given opportunities to exercise independence. We've never felt we were being overprotected for more than an hour or so. It's never been one of those 'They'll never let me do anything' kind of things. Yet I've had friends whose parents went one step too far in cutting the cord—where the kids had to leave the house. Other kids just stayed away for 3 or 4 days at a time as opposed to going home. And when they finally did leave, it was the greatest thing in their lives. I've never had that experience, nor has Richard.

"But I think that whether you're dependent on your parents or not, when you're sick, you go to them. I was like that when I was 8. I'm like that at 18. And I'll probably be like that when I'm 28. If I get anything that exceeds the flu, I'll call home."

"I've often told Darrell how concerned I am about people who are alone, without family or friends. That must be really crushing. How increasingly debilitating that must be when a situation is already serious," his father said.

"There are some psychologists who say a person won't get better unless he knows it's important to someone that he does get better," said Darrell. "As far as getting better goes, one thing we've never really talked about is that by having treatment I'm interrupting my life for a year instead of losing it in 5 or 10 years. It means there's no alternative to treatment, but it also means I haven't been concerned with death."

"But we can empathize much more now with people who are really faced with an end," said Mrs. Ansbacher.

And her husband quickly confirmed this feeling. "Obviously since this has happened to us, I feel much closer to other families with problems."

I told Mr. Ansbacher I had been curious to know how his family crisis had affected his relationships with his friends.

"Many people in the last 3 months have told me, 'We have good thoughts for you. Our prayers are with you.' I know these people aren't going to go home and pray for Darrell Ansbacher; I don't take them literally. But these words have been a tremendous comfort to us all. I really think that people's good thoughts for you can help."

"There is something very Jewish about our situation," Darrell said. "It's the sense of strength from the community, the strength of people coming together. Our family is in a position where we've had that kind of help and comfort, mostly from fellow Jews, members of our congregation. The cards, telephone calls, gifts, and things like that have really helped."

His mother elaborated on the beliefs that underlay that strength. "It isn't a holier-than-thou attitude. It isn't a matter of belief in God per se. It's a sense of the life force. I feel man has been put on Earth with a marvelous brain to think with. When I go to services I don't necessarily pray to God. I go there to be in an atmosphere where I marvel at Creation with all its faults and to find where I fit into it.

"Cancer is where nature has gone wrong, but I still know there are scientists with brains who can think up cures. That fits in too. I have a very comfortable attitude toward life. Whatever will be will be. I'll fight for what I have to, but I have a calm attitude about when my time will come, or my husband's time will come. I have this attitude because of our religious background. I feel I have something to hold on to."

Darrell returned to college 1 month late, at the end of October, upon completion of his radiation treatments. He had only 6 weeks in Los Angeles, free of all therapy, before coming back to San Francisco at the end of the fall quarter, in time to begin his first 28-day cycle of a 6-month course of chemotherapy. The cycle consisted of an intravenous shot on the first and the eighth days of the cycle, in addition to pills taken orally on the first 14 days. The fifteenth through twenty-eighth days were free of medication.

Darrell and I talked in my office the day after he had received his first shot of the second cycle. He planned to return to Los Angeles the next day and to commute to San Francisco on the days he was to receive his shots. I first asked him how being a month late at college had worked out for him.

"I had put a huge amount of emphasis on getting back to school at the beginning of the quarter. I'm not sure why. It wasn't that necessary, although part of it was that I had made plans with several people. I did get out of time with a lot of people but that was more because I was taking eight units and they were taking full loads. I couldn't keep up with them."

I then commented on the tremendous role his parents had played in helping him through his operation and his radiation treatments, and asked, "How did they react when you returned to school?"

"When I first left, they were both a little timid about it. They weren't sure it was the right thing to do. But now they see that I thrive in Los Angeles, so even though their first response is, 'Let's keep him at home where we can protect him,' they're happy to have me be there.

"I think a lot of my problem has been psychological, my nerves. This is probably true of everybody, but perhaps of myself a little more so. As long as I can keep my mind occupied, I think I stand a better chance of avoiding a lot of the discomfort that comes with all this. In Los Angeles I can do that. Also, my brother is in Los Angeles and I like being where he is. My parents know I'm only an hour away, and that if anything serious happens my first move will be toward the airport. Naturally the whole idea of doing everything right medically is the most important thing. Everything else is secondary."

"How do you think it's going to work out to be in Los Angeles and to commute to San Francisco for your shots? Do you think you can handle it?" I asked.

"At first I was very optimistic. I was going to take my shot, be out for a day, and then be back at work, like the stories I've heard. But after the second shot, in December, when I found I didn't have the best reaction, I became pessimistic and thought perhaps I'd spend the 2 weeks that I'm on chemotherapy at home, and the 2 weeks that I'm off down in Los Angeles. However, now I'm back on the optimistic attitude again. Tomorrow I'll return to Los Angeles and try to conduct myself as normally as possible. Because this next week, when I'll be between the two shots, is going to be a gauge for me as to how well I can handle myself when I'm feeling uncomfortable."

"I think you have a good attitude. People somehow adjust. You had more reaction initially with radiation because of fear, and that fear may be having a similar effect now that you're beginning chemotherapy. But the drug you're on does cause gastrointestinal distress in a certain percentage of people. You might help to alleviate it by nibbling small amounts of food all day long, keeping your stomach full but not eating any big meals. Then, using the antinausea medicine and changing antacids, you might try different sequences of taking your pills. Try taking both at bedtime; or try one in the morning and one in the evening. You've survived the first course and that should give you a little assurance that you can make it through the rest. It may become routine in time."

"I haven't noticed it becoming routine yet. Routine is when I know when I'm not going to feel well, and for how long, although I feel quite well considering I just had the shot yesterday."

"That's excellent. I think that shows you can tolerate it. The next question is: can you tolerate the oral pills as well? The odds are you can, and you will get whatever you need as antinausea medicine."

"Actually my apprehension has decreased a little now that the first series is over. And this has lessened my father's apprehension also. He was at least as worried as I was, if not more so. The fact that chemotherapy doesn't occur every day, as radiation did, is also a help. My body may need 2 weeks off between the chemicals, but my parents also need 2 weeks off in between my discomfort."

"Have you noticed any other changes in your feelings or attitudes? Many of my patients have said they develop a new viewpoint while living with a malignancy. It's not that their basic personalities undergo radical change, but they say they perceive themselves and their relationships more clearly. They feel calmer, more certain about the things they want to do and what they want to eliminate from their lives."

"Since I've been home for Christmas, many of my friends say I've mellowed quite a bit. I used to talk a lot. There was a laugh-a-minute way about me. I'm still the same person. I laugh at the same jokes. But I seem to take things easier. I don't know whether that's because I don't have the energy or because I've really mellowed. I am tired more often than I used to be. I sleep more and I'm sick much of the time. I look forward to when I'll be finished with therapy because it will only be then that I'll really be able to sit back and relax.

"I've changed in one respect, however. Something that would have made me very nervous before—the rent being overdue or being late for something—I find I don't worry as much about these things because I've had something in my life that was really worth worrying about. I saw my friends during this last quarter at school panic when final exams came around, especially the premeds. I don't say this to their faces, and I don't know why I don't, but I wonder what disease they're going to get before they realize what's important. I find my own grade-point average is higher because of this attitude. I take it much easier, and I think that once this is all over, it will really have made an improvement in my life."

"How else are you different, aside from this ability to take things easier and this sense of what's really important?"

"I'm a lot more timid. My daring has been cut back because I'm worried about the physical repercussions. But as time goes on, my fear of the daring has become less. What I try to do is be daring in a pattern, a little more daring each time, to build up my tolerance."

"Do your parents worry about your being too daring?"

"Yes, but I understand why they feel how they feel. When they show concern, they're just covering all the bases. When they're overprotective, I can usually convince them that they are and they ease up. They'd like— everyone would like—everything to be written down, to follow a book. It would make things much easier if a person could anticipate each thing before it happens. But since that's not possible, I understand their feelings. If we talk to each other, we can usually find a point in between where we can understand each other.

"I even think my being in Los Angeles helps them. As long as I'm around, they feel a necessity to be overprotective. When I'm away, they forget about me for a while. Even then they call every other day to find out how I'm feeling, and they know my brother is there to keep tabs on me."

Darrell and I had talked before about the book I was writing for cancer patients and their families, and I asked him now if he thought such a book would have helped him.

"I don't think it would have helped me personally because I've had my parents and my brother. I've had other things to lean on. But I think for most people that may not be the case. The strong family tie is an oddity these days."

"Is there anything special that you would tell other people who have Hodgkin's, or a lung or a stomach problem—anything that's a threat to their existence, immediately or in the distant future?"

Darrell thought for a moment. "I'm offering the point of view of someone who's on the homestretch, who has a chance of cure—and I'm speaking as a 19-year-old—but my advice to anyone who is considering treatment is that there is nothing they can do to you that if it saves your life will be too high a price.

"As long as you have time, as long as you have the gift of a normal life ahead of you, there is nothing you can do wrong that you can't try to undo. Perhaps one of the worst things that could happen is that you couldn't undo something you'd done.

"Time is something man invented somewhere along the line, and it really is in some ways one of the greatest inventions; in other ways it's the scariest. It gives you a beginning and an end. If there's a chance of that end being premature, there is no gamble too great to get rid of your disease. You don't worry about whether the cure will be worth it."

"What is your feeling about death at this point in your illness?"

"Not to fear death now would be a mistake, after what I've gone through to hold on to life. But I don't think my fear lies in the childish fear of death, in fear of the unknown or of darkness or being alone. It's different. I've paid the price. It's like paying an exorbitant price for a piece of jewelry and then not getting the jewelry. That's my fear now. It's as though I don't deserve death now. I've bought from the devil. I've bought time."

"I understand. You want your deserts. You want to find your happiness."

"I'm not expecting immortality or anything. I expect comfort. I want a break. It isn't as if I haven't earned it."

"You've earned it," I confirmed.

"However, there's something still in me. It isn't disease. It's something that says, 'It isn't over yet.' Lately I've indulged in a lot of daydreams of you saying, 'I bet you never thought this would be over.' And it flows out of your mouth so easily. Each time I go to your office I expect to hear those words. Unfortunately, they haven't come out yet. I'm still waiting. I know the day will come."

"You've made your contract," I assured him, "and you're going to win."

DECEMBER 1974

After our conversation in January Darrell returned to Los Angeles and remained there until the end of the quarter, in early April, returning to San Francisco for a couple of days at a time to receive his shots. Although he functioned very well, despite some discomfort, he decided to skip the last quarter and to complete his chemotherapy at home in San Francisco. He told me, "School was a big thing in the beginning. I wanted to prove I could function, but that became less important as it became obvious that chemotherapy was something very debilitating."

Chemotherapy was completed by the end of May. Darrell remained at home over the summer, working part time, and returned to college in the fall, in good physical condition but aware that he was particularly susceptible to infections because of his Hodgkin's disease and his therapy.

The fall quarter went well, and when Darrell came home for the holidays we had several talks. Of the year from late June 1973 to the summer of 1974 Darrell said, "It was like having the flu for a year, a bad case of the flu.

"I could tolerate the radiation, but when it was time for the chemotherapy I actually dreaded it. I didn't have the strength to be nervous. I just didn't want to do it. I had been sure there was going to be a way out of it, but there wasn't. That intravenous stuff just blows you out. I didn't realize how debilitating it was going to be, even though you gave me all kinds of sedatives to minimize my psychological reactions. I'm still not up from it, although the nervous twitches and all the nervous energy is back."

"Yes," I said, "but you are slowly getting back your strength."

"I could be, but I haven't done the exercises. It's easy to say you want to go on a regular daily exercising routine, another thing to do it. Actually, I'd like to be playing basketball."

"Can you tell me about your nervousness and your anxiety?" I inquired.

"Yes. I wonder why things aren't different now. I have damned good reason for them to be drastically changed, and they're not. I wonder why I'm still able to drink an occasional drink or smoke an occasional cigarette when I know the farfetched possibilities of what could happen to me, just like anybody else. How come I eat food with preservatives in them? How come I'm not a health nut?

"Other things haven't changed either. I thought the whole time I was taking chemotherapy, 'Boy when this is over, those petty little things just aren't going to bother me.' That's true to a certain extent, but it's also true that when you get better again, you have the same anxieties and the same problems as before. You still have to cope with them. Disease in many ways is a way around coping with a lot of your normal problems, your inadequacies and insecurities. As long as you're sick, you can forget about them because, of course, the reason for them is that you're sick. When you're well, they'll be gone.

"I now think my so-called mellowness was a physical thing, fatigue. I think of it sometimes in terms of Scrooge. Did you ever think about what happened to Scrooge after his conversion? Did he stay the great sweet guy he became that night, or did he gradually fall back into his old pattern of being a schmuck? What happened to me was more in terms of mental anguish than what happened to Scrooge, yet I've experienced no outrageous changes. I'm still what I was before, with the same weaknesses."

"How do your parents feel, now that the ordeal is over? Do you worry about them?"

"They're not free of concern, and that does worry me. There's no way I can satisfy their need to have me around. Yet they're not stifling in any way. I'll be going back to school in 4 or 5 days, but I'm aware that my departure is more of a trauma than for any of my friends and their parents because of what we've been through. It's made a difference. Most people who say good-bye are sad, and say something like 'See you in 2 months,' but with me I sense there's something more."

"Is it hard for you, knowing your parents are so concerned?"

"Only in that I have always tried to control my own reactions. For instance, regardless of how rotten I've ever felt, I would still say, "Well, it was worse 3 weeks ago,' or 'It'll be over in a little while.' Simply, that was easier. I can avoid the emotional aspects within myself. It's harder to handle when I see emotion in other people, and hardest of all when I see it in my parents. I'm not shocked or surprised. I just don't know what to do and it makes me uncomfortable.

"I've always felt this is supposed to be hard on me; there's nothing I can do about that. But if there is ever anything I can do that will make it easier for my parents, then I have no qualms about it."

"Are you doing that now?"

"Yes. I keep a lot of my feelings of nervousness from them because I feel it's best for them that they think everything is great. It does me no good for them to think otherwise. It would just be another burden for me if I knew they were worried."

"That may be the only disadvantage to having such a close family," I said.

JANUARY 1981

"When I got my B.A. from UCLA in December 1977, all I could do was to phone home and say, 'They said it couldn't be done,' " Darrell smiled.

Today Darrell is cured of Hodgkin's disease, but he experienced one more ordeal before he was completely on the road to recovery. In the spring of 1974 he came down with herpes zoster (chicken pox). Although he subsequently recovered from the disease, he was once again forced to postpone his return to college. Herpes zoster is a common accompaniment to Hodgkin's disease. A patient must be kept under careful observation when it occurs because it can spread over the body and/or cause pneumonia. No standard therapy has yet been developed to deal with the disease.

Darrell was now home for the holidays, from UCLA once again, where he is only a few months away from getting his M.B.A. I asked him if he would discuss his cancer experience from the perspective of several years and also talk about some of his activities since that time.

"In March of 1978, I went to Japan for the better part of the next year. I spent half my time studying Japanese and the other half teaching English—a common combination. It's the way in which you pay your tuition at the Japanese school. It was a logical move for me to make because I had studied a lot of Japanese history and sociology in college."

"Did you have any medical checkups while you were there?" I asked.

"No. I was only gone 8 months. I saw you and the doctors at Stanford before I left and when I got back. It was just about the time of my return that my checkups were extended to annual occasions—which was a kind of graduation in itself. Now my checkups will occur annually ad infinitum. I remember only too vividly when they occurred every 3 months. Then I graduated to 6. Now, seeing the doctors once a year is almost like not having to see them at all.

"I have been on medication for an overactive thyroid gland but I recently had some good news. I'm off all medication. It's the first time in a long time I haven't had to pack a vial of tablets when I travel. It's not a freedom I missed having, but it's a freedom I'm glad to have now that I've got it!"

I then asked Darrell what his philosophy is now that he is cured.

"I don't think that philosophy is that big an issue when you're all right. Philosophizing about life is something that is more likely to happen in a crisis situation, so for me to define my philosophy right now and to pinpoint how I feel about my body and my vulnerability is difficult. I think I'm more aware of every ache and pain. There's a fine line between hypochondria and hypersensitivity, but one of the best ways I have ever thought of to describe hypochondria after you've had some sort of cancer is that you live a life in which there are no bumps—only lumps. And every little thing that gets raised on your body, you jump to the conclusion that it is in fact not a bruise or a swelling that comes from bumping your knee on the table but that it's some sort of growth."

"Have you recently made any choices that you might not have made without having had the cancer experience?"

"I have never been exactly sure when it was over. I still have lots of visual reminders. There are scars, but they aren't just the one on my belly from surgery. There are the eyes, which protrude as a result of damage to my thyroid from radiation treatments; and there's the balding hair on my temples, and the little patches missing here and there in my beard. I still notice these effects and have acclimated myself to them without ever really getting used to them.

"But as to whether I have made any decisions differently because of cancer, I'm not sure. I'd like to think that I think things out a little more carefully than I did when I was younger, but that could partially be a result of just getting older.

"The only thing I can really say that I have now that I don't think I would otherwise have had is: no one can confront me with a situation and say to me, 'There is no way you are going to make it!' I have confidence that any set of circumstances can be dealt with."

I then asked Darrell, "Do you think you now have a better perspective on the daily aggravations that we all experience?"

"All the promises you make to yourself in the last 2 months of chemo-therapy about what your perspective is going to be on the day it's over don't always come to pass. You think, 'Boy, if I ever get out of this bind, nothing will ever bother me again.' In fact, when you are well, everything is just as burden-some and there are just as many crises, and 'What am I going to do's?' for as many meaningless things as there were before. However, I like to think that in a real pinch I would feel that as long as I have time, I can straighten it out and that, comparatively, this crisis is not that bad.

"In theory, there is no question that I have a much better perspective than a lot of people; in reality, I have perspective when I'm thinking about it, but unconsciously I still freak and jump and buck—all the things that horses do when they don't know what is crawling around on the ground.

"These questions are like the ones they ask people like Jackie Cooper, who was a child actor: 'Do you think that as a child actor you led a strange life?' The answer is, 'Compared to what?' The only life he knew was that of a child actor. For me, I'm not sure what my life would have been like without Hodgkin's disease, so it's difficult to say it's changed my life. I'm sure that it has, but I don't think you have to have had Hodgkin's disease to have a good set of weights and measures of what's important and what isn't."

"You mention that your eyes protrude as a result of radiation. Specialists at Stanford are following this development very closely, but the change in configuration has made a difference in your life, hasn't it?"

"Yes. It's more difficult to have confidence about my appearance when I know that my eyes are protruding—or protruding less. I don't know what's going on. I just feel I would look better if I had my old eyes back. It's something I have had to think a lot about because there is some kind of surgical option available to me. I finally decided not to have it done. Unless something arises medically that endangers my sight, I prefer to go through life as I am than to go through surgery to change the protrusion. At first there was some question of whether I would need the surgery to keep my eyes from being damaged, but when that danger passed and everything stabilized, I discussed with the doctors the available options and what they entailed. Was it worth it for a 5% improvement in my eyes to spend 2 weeks recovering from stitches in my eyes, or to have radiation treatment to the back of my eyes, or to have the bones behind my eyes chipped a little bit to increase the size of the orbit? Was it worth it to improve my appearance by 'X' percent? I decided it wasn't."

"I know that you are job-hunting right now. Do you have any concerns about the effect of your physical appearance on prospective employers?"

"I don't think that's part of it. Even if my appearance had maintained from my 17-year-old level, I would still not be the pretty-boy type that a lot of these firms are looking for. My awareness of the problem comes and goes. I'm more sensitive to it when I'm in San Francisco because my father is more sensitive to it.

"I am beginning to investigate 'career opportunities,' as we say in the field. I've been talking to some people at advertising agencies, and with any luck I should land something in advertising. I don't really care what city I live in. Every city has its little corner that's worth living in, and right now I'm only interested in getting a job that will be good for me. I'd like to think I'm the cat's meow and that prospective employers can't wait to send me airplane tickets, but I'm finding out there are a lot of people out there who don't even answer the telephone. I've wallpapered my bedroom with notes that say, 'We're impressed with your qualifications and we're putting your resume on file.' So here I am talking about how I can deal with any situation that comes up, yet I wake up at 2:00 in the morning thinking, 'Maybe I should write a couple more letters.' I don't know what I'm going to do but perhaps, unlike my colleagues, if I don't have a job when June rolls around, I just won't have a job! I'll have to keep looking. I'm not quite as competitive as some of my classmates; and I don't know whether that's because Hodgkin's took the edge off my competitiveness, whether I'm characteristically a less competitive person, or whether I have a better sense of what is important and what isn't."

Thinking of the problems some people who have had cancer run into with prospective employers, I asked Darrell how he intended to handle this fact.

"I wish I had a chance to talk to a prospective employer about Hodgkin's disease during my interview, because I consider it to be one of my greatest achievements. Some people climb the Matterhorn and afterwards they want everyone to know about it and show them slides. In the same way, I'm sorry there's not a place on my resume to show I had Hodgkin's. After all, I did that a lot longer than I've held any job.*

"However, I think I understand the stigma that's attached to a sick person, both in his own eyes and in the eyes of the employer. For the prospective employee, it's rather like the person who is embarrassed about seeing a psychiatrist. He hates to show any weakness; it's humiliating. And even if he is free and open about it, other people will think of it as a weakness, although I think that these attitudes are less prevalent among educated people. So, with illness, a person who's looking for a job doesn't want anyone to know that they've faltered because there are people in the business community who have a certain view of success: they think you're born to it. 'Are you going to be a lucky guy? Are you a guy who lives a charmed life or are you going to be a loser? If you were just on the operating table for 4 hours, maybe you're a loser.' I look at it quite the opposite. I think that the winner is the guy who was on the table for 4 hours and gets off it.

"Therefore, if I'm ever in an interview situation, shooting the breeze, and I

---

*I suggested that Darrell answer the question on his job application about past health with the statement: "Hodgkin's disease: cured."

feel comfortable enough, I don't think I'll hesitate to bring it up when asked about the events in my life that have been really important. I'd wear it on my sleeve. But it usually doesn't come up, which reminds me of a problem I've gotten over in the last couple of years. When you have a disease like Hodgkin's, you tend to spill your guts to anyone who looks like they want to hear about it. This urge is immediately followed by a period in which you don't want to talk to anyone about it. Subsequently, you hit a middle ground."

"Now that you've been away from home for several years, how do you handle your relationship with your parents regarding, for instance, your decision not to do anything about your eyes?"

"I let them have their input but I do this after I've made my decision and explained my reasons to them. I don't keep them out of it—but in a lot of ways we have a problem that way. For instance, I like to deal with my annual checkups as being very unimportant. I just want to go in and leave as though I've gone to have my teeth cleaned, but my folks expect a long-winded, detailed report of what happened as though it were still 5 or 6 years ago. This prevents me a little bit from taking it all in stride."

"What factors do you feel made it possible for you to get better?"

"I chalk it up almost exclusively to the medicine. I view what happened to me as a malfunction, and I believe that the technicians pretty much corrected it. But if you want to know what enabled me to get better as comfortably as I did, it made it a lot easier to have my family around. I had people to feed me, help me walk around, and pick me up at the hospital. I was lucky not to be the guy who showed up for his chemotherapy on the 38 Geary bus and who then went back to his apartment alone in a cab. That doesn't mean such a person can't get well but it must mean that it's more difficult for him."

"Did you ever doubt that you would get well?"

"No, because you filled me in right away on what the statistics were for cure."

"The statistics have gone from 10% to 85+% in the last 20 years. It's one of the great medical achievements of our times."

"Was there any doubt in *your* mind that I'd get well, Ernie?"

"No. I treat for cure in everyone that I can—if there is a chance for cure. Otherwise, a doctor transfers his doubts to the patient. And if the patient has doubts, he is going to say to himself, 'Why should I go through all this treatment and get sick if I'm not going to get better?' "

"Yes. Well, what I picked up was that because of the level of Hodgkin's that I had, something would really have had to go wrong for me not to be cured. In that sense, I never dealt with a life-endangering disease."

"What ingredients do you think are important for living with cancer?"

"I think endurance is important. There is a method to being able to close your eyes and just *do* it. I don't know how you develop it, but all my life I've had little methods of getting through unpleasant things. Like when you wake up in the morning and you have to get out of bed. I have a swinging technique so that no matter what my whole mind and body say, I can get my feet on the ground. You're virtually out of bed at that point.

"The hot coals are there, and you just look at the other end. Somehow you just do it. You are looking at that spoon that's filled with God knows what, and you know you can swallow it. These are the kinds of endurance that take on uncommon importance when you have to go into one more radiation treatment. You focus your mind on being in the dressing room afterwards while you're taking off your clothes beforehand. You remind yourself of the last three or four times you were there and you think about getting dressed again. That's all you think about—not about going to the Bahamas when you get well.

"If you've been successful at everything you've done in life, and you have that kind of endurance, then maybe you will feel a little better about your chances of fighting cancer. But 'courage' is much too much of an intangible. I don't think a person ever has courage; I think it's attributed to him. So, I'm not sure what 'living with cancer' means."

"It means that you're living with disease for that period of time that you have it. It's living with the treatments, and living after the treatments, even if they fail. How do you define the 'will to live,' Darrell?"

"I think that the will to live is another crisis mechanism and that you don't know you have it until you need it. Part of the will to live is endurance and part is resourcefulness. But a lot of it has to do with having the imagination— when things are really bad—to divorce yourself from what's going on. You hear about people who are in a lot of pain who have this ability. When you want to live, you'll think of ways to work at it, no matter what the situation. It's the sprint for the runner who wants to win the race.

About 2 weeks after Darrell had returned to Los Angeles, I had the occasion to speak with Mr. and Mrs. Ansbacher about their feelings now that Darrell is well. Mrs. Ansbacher commented on some of her feelings as a mother:

"I wonder about the times when Darrell was young that I took him to have x-rays. I keep asking myself whether I did something wrong. Should I have had his tonsils out? Was I wrong to have him x-rayed when he had a stomach ache? Was I always a conscientious parent? I think crazy things that have no logic. As a parent I constantly think of things I might not have done had I known better. But we didn't know."

"I can assure you that the x-rays had nothing to do with Darrell's disease," I said.

"It's nice to know but, as I say, there is no logic to what a parent thinks. In former generations, parents were inclined to ask, 'Why are my children doing this to me?' But in our generation we say, 'What am I doing to my children?' "

"It's part of the Jewish guilt complex!"

"Part of it is that we have more time to concern ourselves with the psychological aspects of life. Life was hard for many people in the old days, and there wasn't as much time for introspection."

"It's the mezuzah!* In the old days they would check to see if it was in the wrong place because the house might fall down if it wasn't right. They had to

---

*A small parchment religious scroll placed in a case fixed to the doorpost by some Jewish families as a sign and reminder of their faith.

find a reason, and there is no reason. We haven't changed. We still look for a reason."

"You're right. But there's another reaction. Now that Darrell is cured, some of the outer, unimportant symptoms have started to become major ones, such as the way the back of his neck looks and his balding. Generally speaking, Darrell has made excellent progress, but he tends not to want to speak of the illness because it's remote to him now. He barely relates to it anymore. He has put it out of his mind unless he is reminded of it by others."

"Has your own—not Darrell's—life changed as a result of living with cancer?" I asked both Mr. and Mrs. Ansbacher.

Mrs. Ansbacher replied, "Of course, I'm more aware of Hodgkin's disease. I read all the articles in the newspapers and try to keep up with what's going on, although I don't think a lot about it because we had a good experience. However, I have been working as a volunteer in Patient Services at Mt. Zion Hospital. I find that when I visit patients I am much more conscious of what they and their families are going through than I was before. I try to talk to them about it but sometimes it's difficult."

"It's often very hard for people who have been through grief to go through it again by helping others," I replied.

Mr. Ansbacher then said, "One thing that has changed for me is that I have become more courageous when it comes to my relationship with doctors. I rarely go to a doctor, but when I do go, I'm apprehensive. Recently I went through a number of things—blood tests, tooth out, and my sinuses pierced and drained. But when the ENT man stuck that needle up my nose, I thought, 'If Darrell had his liver tested and all the things he's been through without complaining very much, who am I to complain?' At least I get a taste of what Darrell went through and feel I vicariously participate in the agonizing experience he has had.

"During Darrell's illness, I went through an enormous amount of agony and it was only because my wife could—at least externally—bear this much more than I could that I got through it. I could sit down and cry for an hour and it would make me feel good. She didn't do that and she comforted me.

"Whenever Darrell was sick after these chemotherapy regimens, I used to sit in my office and wait with bated breath until my wife would phone me and say she was home and that he was asleep. Then, we were relieved when you would come by at 6PM. Just your walking in the door would make us feel much better.

"Now that it's over, I try to put it out of my mind. In our relationship with Darrell, my concern is that we not treat him—even subliminally—as though he has some kind of invalid condition. This is why we were willing that he go to Japan a year after the conclusion of the treatments. Between us, we would have preferred him not to go because we felt he would be so far away from his doctors. He is now in the process of finding a job. We would prefer him to be in the neighborhood—not because of his former illness but because it's nice to have your children close by. He is going to New York and Chicago for interviews, but under no circumstances would I hold him back from that because we don't want him to get the impression that the reason we are doing so is because we are apprehensive about his physical condition."

Mrs. Ansbacher interrupted to say that she is not apprehensive and Mr. Ansbacher continued, "But I am. For as long as I live I will have apprehensions and I will continue to make a conscious effort not to demonstrate them in his presence. When he gets a cold, I ask, 'Have you taken aspirin?' Yet deep down I think, 'My God! Is he properly taken care of?' I am certain that if he broke his leg, I would think it had something to do with Hodgkin's, even though I would *know* that it didn't."

I reminded Mr. Ansbacher that people who have had cancer and who then have an ache or a pain that they would normally ignore, come to my office and ask, "Is this a recurrence of my cancer?" "This happens about 10 times a week. When you've had a serious disease, you are petrified and you always ask those questions."

"Well, the patient asks those questions," said Mr. Ansbacher.

"But you are like the patient. You act like that because you are so close to Darrell," I added.

Mr. Ansbacher also pointed out that Darrell himself seemed to have apprehensions a few days before his yearly tests. "I know he is tense. But then he goes to the doctor and it's over. For the rest of his life he will have this tension when he has to be tested."

"How else has your attitude toward Darrell changed?" I asked Mr. Ansbacher.

"Whenever I look at Darrell's appearance, I think, 'Suppose a young man like this—no matter what his qualities might be—were to interview for a job with me. I would look at his face and his very prominent eyes and I would be apprehensive.' Therefore, I am apprehensive for Darrell."

"You may feel that way, but Darrell has learned to live with his problem. He has made a miraculous adjustment," I replied.

Then Mrs. Ansbacher said, "The fact that he's had so much thyroid medication is another concern. We hope that situation is finished, too. We watch to see whether his behavior patterns are the same, whether taking the medication over a couple of years has made him a slightly different person."

"I don't think you need to worry. Darrell is active and alert."

"Yes, but we'll always be watching his eyes."

"I understand that. As parents you want everything to be right with your children. But we often worry more than the person whose leg is short. People learn to live with their problems because they have no choice. They make the kind of compromise we all have to make, whatever our deficiencies, and we think no one else will accept them. But they do."

I then asked Mr. and Mrs. Ansbacher what advice they would have for a family who is going through what they went through.

Mrs. Ansbacher answered first. "We have said it before, but I think it's worth repeating. You live what you're going through day by day. You don't anticipate problems. You take each day as it comes and try to be as positive as you can. If you try to analyze or anticipate what's ahead, it's much worse than actually going through the motions each day. So I would say to a cancer patient, 'Do as your physician tells you to do, and don't waste a lot of time thinking about what might happen. Also, don't listen to anyone else tell about aspects of his disease because it can only make you feel worse. Another person's condition is entirely different from your condition. Therefore, while waiting in the doctor's office, don't translate what other people say to your own case. Be concerned and helpful but don't think that what happened to someone else will happen to you just because you have the same disease.' "

Mr. Ansbacher added, "I think what you need is total and unconditional support between the parents and the child, between the parents themselves, and between the child and each of his parents. Absolute candor is terribly important. We never conveyed that what was happening was a burden to us because our lives had to change, too. We assumed whatever restraints were placed on us without any qualification. There was never a moment's regret that we had given up something because of Darrell. And he knew that."

• • •

Darrell received his M.B.A. in June 1981 and now works as an account executive in an advertising agency in the San Francisco area.

17

Magdalena Matunan

Magdalena and Teofilo Matunan were married in 1934 in the Philippines. In 1945 they emigrated to the United States with their three daughters and one son. They settled, with other Filipino immigrants, on a section of land on the southern perimeter of San Francisco, close to the bay. There they raised their children, worked hard, and saved enough money to buy their own home in the same section of town, close to their friends, in 1952. Their eldest daughter, Kate, was then 17 years old.

Kate is now 40, herself the mother of a 17-year-old girl and an 18-year-old boy. She smiles happily as she speaks of the years she and her sisters and brother spent in their parents' home. "The house was always full of people, and we always had pets. My parents shared the household chores because they were both working. Since my father liked to cook, my mother cleaned and did a lot of other things. She was never still for a minute. And she had a green thumb. I remember the windows were always full of African violets. My mother and father even fixed up an apartment for my husband, David, and me when we were first married. We lived with them for 2 years, until we could afford our own place and I became pregnant."

Victoria and Dely, Kate's younger sisters, are now also married, and each has three children. Victoria lives in Denver; Dely and Kate live within 20 miles of their old home. Their brother, Manuel, died when he was 12 years old.

When their children married and moved away, Magdalena and Teofilo did not seek smaller quarters. Their house remained a center of activity, a source of delight to their eight grandchildren and themselves. They also enjoyed visiting the homes of their daughters. Because they both worked—Teofilo at night and Magdalena in the daytime—these visits were limited to weekends, when they would drive about in their car, visit the grave of their son, and stop at their daughters' homes to talk and to play with their grandchildren. The three generations were in close touch.

The first hint of cancer occurred in June 1969, when Magdalena Matunan was 54 years old. Malignant cells were discovered in her right ovary, and she immediately had a hysterectomy. However, her cancer had been diagnosed early and her doctors decided against giving follow-up radiation therapy. Instead, she took hormones to replace those that her ovaries had once produced, and received a thorough checkup every 6 months. Life continued as before for Magdalena and Teofilo.

Then in early June 1972 Magdalena noticed a swelling in the lymph nodes in her neck. Although they gave her no discomfort, she quickly notified her doctor. A biopsy of one of the nodes revealed that Magdalena's ovarian cancer had spread to her lymph nodes on the left side of her neck, but there was no evidence of disease in her pelvis or elsewhere.

Magdalena was given local radiation on her neck for a period of 5 weeks. When this therapy was completed in the first week of August, the mass had been reduced. For the next $4\frac{1}{2}$ months her doctors closely watched her condition but were unable to discern any other evidence of recurrence. As a precaution they talked with me in November about the advisability of putting Magdalena on a program of chemotherapy. After studying her case, I felt we must be guarded in giving a long-term prognosis because her disease had recurred so far from its point of origin. But because she was otherwise in good health, had lost little weight, and showed no evidence of liver or lung involvement, I considered her a good candidate for chemotherapy.

Magdalena began a course of chemotherapy on December 24, 1972, 5 days after a palpable node appeared just above the area that had been treated by radiation the previous summer. She received her chemotherapy intravenously at first, and later in tablet form. In addition to the swelling that had returned to the neck area, she had edema in her right leg, so I also prescribed a low-salt diet and diuretics.

During January and February 1973, chemotherapy was successful in shrinking Magdalena's nodes, although by the end of March, with the completion of that particular chemotherapeutic program, it appeared that the neck mass was again increasing. There was also evidence of fluid in her abdomen and continuing edema in her right leg. In addition, her white blood cell count had dropped, making it necessary to wait until the count returned to a safer level before continuing with a second round of chemotherapy.

Magdalena's blood count was taken every Monday and Thursday, and toward the end of April radiotherapy was again prescribed. Her nodes were increasing in size, and her edema was worse, making her right thigh swollen and painful, and walking difficult. The second course of radiation therapy was completed on May 9, 1973, and a new round of chemotherapy begun shortly thereafter. Both legs were now afflicted with edema.

On June 20, with increasing evidence of disease in her neck and abdomen, and increased edema in her right leg, Magdalena was put on a new chemotherapeutic program. By June 29, I noted on her record, "Chances for improvement or control do not appear good."

Magdalena was one of the 50% of women with ovarian cancer whose disease fails to respond to chemotherapy, a tragedy for her and Teofilo and the rest of the family. I have, of course, seen many similar cases, and I have observed the ways in which families come together in support of a stricken member. However, the care that Magdalena now received from her family, particularly Teofilo, and the love and sensitivity shown to both

Magdalena and Teofilo by their daughters, sons-in-law, and grandchildren, will always be a vivid and touching memory for me.

Magdalena knew what was happening to her. She asked me many times how bad things were, and I always gave her a frank reply. Yet she rarely discussed her prognosis with her family. One of the rare occasions when she did refer to her impending death occurred just before Christmas 1972. At her parents' home Kate was helping her mother trim the Christmas tree when her mother suddenly said, "If anything happens to me, promise me that your dad can stay with you and David." Kate's first reaction was to tell her mother not to talk that way; then she quickly reassured her that Teofilo was always welcome in her home. Magdalena concluded the conversation, saying, "I don't want your dad to stay here by himself."

In July, Magdalena was finding it increasingly difficult to walk, and in early August, when she could no longer stand by herself, Teofilo retired from his job prematurely to take care of her. I told him Magdalena's prospects for long-term survival were poor, but how much he suppressed, or how much he admitted to himself, was difficult to ascertain. His task was to take care of Magdalena, pray for a miracle, and offer constant encouragement. They had their own silent ways of helping each other.

Magdalena could just make it to the car with Teofilo's help, and during the early part of August she would urge him to take her for rides. They always followed their familiar path, visiting their son's grave before going to Kate's or Dely's home, except that these days the girls and their families would come out to the car to chat with Magdalena.

By the middle of August Magdalena could no longer go out in the car. She couldn't even get out of bed. However, Teofilo was determined that she not be hospitalized; and when a family feels this way, I always try to treat the patient at home.

Teofilo took over the management of the house. He cooked food that would please Magdalena and kept the house spotless because she liked it that way. He slept on a cot beside her bed and awakened when she did. Yet during all this time he avoided discussing Magdalena's condition with his daughters and sons-in-law. They, of course, knew without being told that Magdalena was dying, but they could not guess what Teofilo was thinking. Was he protecting himself or Magdalena or his daughters with his silence?

Kate and her sisters agreed among themselves that by preparing himself in advance, Teofilo might find it easier to face Magdalena's death when it occurred, but they were wary of broaching the subject with him. Then Kate decided that I might be the best means of approach to their father. She phoned me one afternoon and first confirmed what she already knew by asking me whether her mother was dying. The truth was shocking, nevertheless. She then spoke to me of the family's concern for Teofilo and arranged that I make a house call at an hour when she and her sisters would be together at her parents' home.

A few days later, at the appointed hour, I went to the Matunan house. After a long talk with Magdalena, I stopped in the living room, where Teofilo was sitting with his daughters. As though for the first time, Kate quizzed me about her mother's condition. I tried to respond clearly and candidly. Teofilo listened, but Kate thinks he still did not accept his wife's impending death.

Kate and her sisters visited their mother daily, and helped their father, but he remained in charge of Magdalena's care. His daughters, in turn, tried to care for him. They brought him food because he cooked only for Magdalena. They arranged that one grandchild always be present as company for Teofilo. Kate's son, Sam, said, "I come here a lot and stay with my grandfather. It's natural for us to be sad and sympathetic. Just knowing we're here helps him."

When Magdalena needed a shot, the family even had its own supply of nurses. One was a cousin who worked in a San Francisco hospital, the other a sister-in-law of Kate's husband. When it was necessary to tap the fluid in Magdalena's abdomen, I always did it at home, because home was where she wanted to be.

Magdalena and Teofilo were Catholics who had been married in a civil ceremony. Again, with no more than the breath of a wish from Magdalena, a priest was summoned and Magdalena's brothers and sisters (all of whom had immigrated to the United States) were invited to the Matunan home. In early September, in the presence of all her relatives, Magdalena was married to Teofilo in a religious ceremony. Kate recalls, "It was like a party. My mother would beckon to her brothers and sisters, one at a time. She remembered everything they did as youngsters. She'd recall funny stories with each one."

Two weeks after the wedding, Kate remembers, her mother couldn't keep her eyes open. "When we saw she was resting, we'd leave her alone. When her eyes were open and she felt like talking, we'd talk. Sometimes I'd just sit there and hold her hands and pray.

"At other times she'd be her old stubborn self, and that was wonderful. It meant she was still alert. We'd be whispering in the kitchen about what to give her for lunch, and she'd suddenly say very loudly, 'I don't *want* chicken soup.'"

Magdalena's sons-in-law were as supportive and eager to help as their wives. Victoria's husband, Larry, who had recently been ill himself, drove West from Denver on his vacation to be with Magdalena. He said, "That's what families are for and I was never close to mine." Although Dely's husband, Jim, had just started his own business, he gave all his free time to Magdalena and Teofilo with the simple explanation, "When a person is ill, people should be there." Kate and David were quietly preparing a section of their home so that Teofilo might move in when Magdalena died. These silent acts of love were instinctive, the result of years of being together and enjoying each other.

The weaker Magdalena became, the more she needed Teofilo. He sat with her, massaged her, and helped her from her bed to the bedside commode. When she could no longer swallow easily, he prepared baby food for her.

One night he had to telephone Kate and David to come and help him. Magdalena had fallen between the bed and the commode. She weighed 10 extra pounds from the swelling and the edema, and Teofilo was too weak from his vigil to get her back into bed.

It was not long after that episode that Magdalena asked Kate why God was making her suffer so much. She wanted Him to take her immediately. Then she fell asleep and Kate tiptoed out of the room. Magdalena awakened an hour later and called for Kate's 15-year-old daughter, Mary. Teofilo kept a pistol in a drawer in the next room. Magdalena told Mary to get it. Mary, suspecting nothing, brought it to her grandmother, who said, "Now give it to me." As soon as it was in her hands, she tried to cock it and end her life. Kate said, "It's a good thing the pistol was hard to open and the trigger hard to pull. Of course my father was screaming and I was furious. My daughter was so hurt. Then my mother spoke, very quietly. 'Don't blame Mary. Blame me. It has nothing to do with her.' We were so mad at my mother, but at the same time we knew how she felt and how much she was suffering.

"But that was the only incident like that," Kate said. "So many times in those last months and weeks, my mother would call for Dad, and when he got to her room, she'd just smile at him and say, 'I just wanted to look at you and say I love you.' "

In early October Magdalena began to have moments of irrationality. I explained to the family that it was caused by toxicity from the disease, that it was like being delirious from pneumonia. I also assured them that people usually don't remember what they've said during a toxic phase.

Then one day Teofilo told Kate that her mother refused to take her pills. When Kate urged her to take her medicine, her mother was furious with both of them. After that, she refused to eat, and Kate knew it was time for her mother to go to the hospital. She telephoned her sisters. None of them wanted to suggest such a step to Teofilo. They waited a few days, to let him come to the decision on his own. Kate remembers, "It was a hard thing for him to do. He didn't want to let go of my mother."

I also tried to help Teofilo with his decision, as did Magdalena. I told him a family can do only so much and that there comes a time when special nursing care is needed. Magdalena agreed with the decision, and that helped him too.

During the week that Magdalena spent in the hospital before she died, Teofilo was there all day every day. He went straight to his wife each morning, returned home for lunch at Kate's pleading, and went back to the hospital immediately afterward. Kate or Dely or Victoria would join him there in the afternoons and evenings. Magdalena recognized them only intermittently, and her speech was no longer clear. However, to Kate's relief her mother apologized for speaking to her so angrily the week before. Kate had been worried that her mother would die feeling she had mistreated her.

Speaking of that time, Kate said to me recently, "At first I prayed for a miracle. But after seeing my mother suffer, I hoped it would happen fast. The suffering was too much for her and it was too much for the family.

"Then one day she went into a coma and you told Victoria she might not last the night. We sat by the telephone. It rang at a quarter to one. My father answered it. When he came back into the room he said you had called and my mother had passed away. It was a relief, and yet it was so painful because I knew my Dad would be lost without her. Even when she was in the hospital, at least she was somewhere."

Two days after Magdalena's death, Kate told Dely their father should go to Denver immediately. In 2 weeks he was home again, but while he was gone Kate and Dely had packed their mother's clothes into a box and stored them in a closet.

"Since that time he's stayed in the room we fixed for him," Kate told me. "But he didn't sell his house. My father is one who keeps things. He's sentimental and he likes to keep good memories.

"At my husband's suggestion Dad took a trip to the Philippines about 2 months after my mother died. His whole family is there and he hadn't been back in 28 years. While he was there I received a letter from my aunt saying he was quite depressed. They gave him lots of parties and tried to make him happy, but they understood. It was a good trip for him in spite of everything. He took a lot of movies that he now looks at every day."

It is now 15 months since Magdalena Matunan died. Although Teofilo stays with Kate and her family, he returns to his own home every day. He leaves at midday, visits the cemetery, and spends the remainder of the afternoon in the old house.

Kate says, "At first it broke my heart to see him go there and just sit and watch television. Then one day he said, 'It just makes me feel good to go home.' He feels as though Mom is at work and that she'll be back. I don't know how he feels when it's time for him to leave the house and come back to us. But if that's what makes him happy, nothing else matters.

"My father is a loner. He's at ease with other people, but he doesn't have close friends. He's a family man. He likes to spend his time with his grandchildren, and they're all very fond of him. It makes me happy when I see him smiling and joking around with them, especially my kids and their friends, because they're older and go places with him. He laughs a lot more lately. And he talks much more about my mother. He speaks of her with pride and laughs at some of the things she did.

"Last week he offered rooms in his house to my daughter, who is getting married this spring. It's like seeing myself all over again. I told him they would pay rent, but he got angry and said, 'If your mother were alive, she'd be furious. Are you crazy? Those kids are just getting started.' "

18

Robert Wong

MICHI

My husband, Robert, is the first person I ever knew who at 22 was living for the time when he would be 35 years old. In his fantasy, at the age of 35 he would be married, have children, live in his own house in Tiburon, and own a Maserati. He would practice law in San Francisco, where he would also be active in community social work. The car and the house were the extent of his material desires. Any further wealth he accrued would be given to a foundation which he would set up to fund public programs for the children and the elderly of Chinatown.

Then, when Robert found out in March 1976 that he had leukemia and was told he had 1 to 5 years to live, he went through a complete change. It wasn't traumatic for him to change; it was just a reality that he was able to deal with, that life doesn't all happen when you are 35—that all you have is the present.

Robert was always a clear thinker who knew what was important and what was not. He knew there were family and friends who were close to you, whom he called "SP's" (significant persons), and other people, "PP's" (peripheral persons). So Robert did not need to rearrange his priorities when he became ill. He just carried on with what he always knew was significant.

He was actually glad that he didn't have to go to law school. His primary goal was to serve the people of Chinatown, but he knew there were other ways in which he might do that—as a social worker or a businessman. Certainly he saw advantages in being a lawyer, and he may eventually have come to that decision on his own; but at that time he just felt that going to law school was not totally his decision. It was what his parents wanted for him. He later told his doctor,

I studied compulsively, up to 16 hours a day. All my energy was geared toward getting into law school, getting a high grade-point average and a high score on the law school aptitude test, and getting the best letters of recommendation. I was really scratching. So it was actually a release, a watershed of relaxation, to know I wouldn't have to go.

In the Chinese community, being a lawyer—a professional—is worth 100 points. My Dad would say, "You don't have to go, but it would be nice." And my uncle would remind me of the prestige and the things a lawyer can do. I'd hear about my cousins who went to Stanford and Harvard Law Schools, and "wouldn't it be nice to have another lawyer in the family?" It was a personal conflict for me because, being American as well as Chinese, I had a strong streak of individualism. I think what I was really looking for was freedom of choice.

Robert knew that life is too short—whether you live to be 22 or 92—to be frantic about, and spend energy on, things you aren't truly interested in doing. The stress that results from doing things you are unsure about or that you feel pressured into doing, isn't worth it.

Thus Robert was very together in his thoughts, even in the first days after he found out about his leukemia. He was upset and cried, of course, but he immediately went about taking care of his family and me by speaking with us individually. He told his mom and dad how he wanted very much for them to take care of one another; and he had private talks with each of his two sisters and with me about our futures.

Another illustration of Robert's balance at this time occurred when he and I went to Lake Tahoe for a weekend. We gambled, fished, and hiked to a snowed-in lake. Robert always liked action and total concentration; now it provided him with one of the few times when he wouldn't be thinking of his disease. More than that, however, because of this weekend we were able to establish early on that life wasn't going to change that much. We would continue to share our lives with each other and others.

Prior to Robert's illness, we had talked about getting married someday. I had always felt we had all the time in the world, and I had complete faith that our relationship would last; so I didn't feel any pressing need for the security of marriage. Now Robert asked me to marry him soon, saying he couldn't promise me a long time, but he could promise me quality of time. He kept that promise.

Robert's rational attitude faltered somewhat under the clinic setup at the medical center near our university, where several doctors were responsible for his case. Although they were treating him with chemotherapy, not one of them ever really explained to Robert what his long-term treatment regimen would be. Therefore, Robert would have preferred to have one doctor to whom he could really talk, especially when it became clear that the chemotherapy was not improving his condition.

No one at the medical center gave Robert support for living, or encouragement to do things. Instead, they did destructive things like tell him over and over again that he was going to die, although each person predicted a different life expectancy, ranging from 1 to 7 years. It seems that doctors feel they have a responsibility—even an urgent need—to express the worst, but it isn't clear to me whether they feel they have any responsibility for hope, as if hope and dying are not within their province.

Robert had always been a moody person, experiencing great joy but also deep depression. Now, with the traumatic experience of finding out he had a terminal illness, the failure of his initial chemotherapy and the side effect of hair loss, his mood swings were even more intense. In late May he became so morose that for 2 weeks he refused to see anyone except me. He wouldn't even see his mother, who knew what he was going through and therefore was understanding.

Robert did have a medical consultation in San Francisco with a medical oncologist at this time, because we were planning a return to San Francisco after graduation. This doctor felt that Robert's condition appeared stable enough for him to attend graduation and urged him to do so before reporting back to him for further diagnostic tests and treatments.

Finally, on graduation day Robert pulled himself together. I had considered cancelling our plans because of Robert's depression, but decided against it because both sets of parents were planning to attend. Robert not only decided to participate in the ceremonies, he really enjoyed himself. The event served as a happy opportunity to rejoin the significant people in his life. Moreover, after that depressed period, there wasn't a day when Robert didn't laugh or smile about something. He was always able to get out of himself and into another person, which gave him a reprieve from worrying.

When we returned to San Francisco in early June, the medical oncologist discovered that Robert actually had a different variety of leukemia from the one he was previously thought to have had and that his disease was progressing rapidly, with brain involvement. Robert then was admitted to the hospital to start a new program of chemotherapy.

At the same time the doctor called the family together to explain the severity of Robert's relapse, the exact progression of his disease, and his prognosis. The doctor also described his treatment plans for Robert and encouraged us to ask him questions.

There was nothing Robert's family wouldn't do to make him well. While he was in the hospital they brought him appetizing food from Chinatown and changed his sheets for him every day. Each family member was also available on 10 minutes' notice to give blood. This was especially important in Robert's case, because the family has a rare blood type. When Robert's blood count was low and he developed an infection, this often meant that a family member could spend 6 hours on a complex machine that separates out the different components of the blood. Such hasty action could avert the onset of further life-threatening complications.

Robert was on his new program of chemotherapy all through July. In early August the doctor told me, "It looks as though Robert is in a remission, but I can't promise you how long it's going to last. If you're going to get married, do it now." He made it clear to me that this was a respite, not a cure; and the idea really came through that no one can promise you tomorrow.

The doctor not only clarified my thinking, he also invited Robert, Robert's family (including a family confidant), and me to his house a few days later, because he felt there was a need for improved communications between Robert and his parents. His parents seemed to want to treat him as though he were well, and he wasn't well. At the meeting the doctor asked Robert what he felt he needed in order to get well, which gave Robert an opportunity to say things he wouldn't have otherwise have said. He replied that he didn't want to feel he had to live up to his parent's expectations. He said the stress of trying to get into law school and of doing things he didn't want to do probably contributed to his getting leukemia, and that he therefore was going to have to be selfish and do what he wanted to do if he was going to get better. This meant creating a life-style that alleviated stress—and part of the plan for this new life-style involved hobbies. He wanted a used sports car to work on and a small boat for fishing.

Generally, the doctor wanted Robert's family to understand that the future was uncertain, and he wanted to accelerate our marriage plans. Nevertheless, when Robert was finished speaking, his parents were very angry. Recalling that time, his mother says:

In my heart, I thought he was ungrateful. I thought of all the people who want to go to school whose parents can't afford it. But that wasn't what he meant. He just meant that all these people had been badgering him to go to law school and now he didn't want anyone telling him what to do. It wasn't his request for money that made me angry. It was the way he expressed himself.

Robert was hurt by my anger, but the next day we explained our feelings to each other. After that, everything opened up and we were very close. We worried so much about him and he worried about us.

Robert and I were married in a small private ceremony toward the end of August (planning later to have a Chinese wedding for him and a Japanese ceremony for me). It was a glorious event, in a garden. I didn't buy anything new, but Robert was so into getting married that he bought himself a trousseau—new suit, new hat, new shoes, new socks, and new underwear. He even wore something borrowed and something blue and was annoyed afterward to discover he had forgotten to put a penny in his shoe.

Once he said, "Your parents probably don't want you to marry a dying man." I could honestly tell him, "They don't think of it that way, and neither do I." My parents were very understanding. I will be forever grateful for their strength and compassion. It would have been awful if they had been against our marriage, because a person who is going through an experience like Robert's doesn't need any extra hassles.

We moved into our own house, given to us by Robert's parents. It was a time of great hope, because Robert was still in remission and out of the hospital. Because Robert is a gourmet cook, he prepared all our meals when we ate at home, but we also ate out a lot, especially at one restaurant where Robert liked to flirt with a special waitress. We went to shows and visited friends and family; and Robert bought a used Classic sports car, which he hoped to recondition and sell at a profit; he also bought new components for his stereo and some books on business. His plan was to spend 2 years getting well before dedicating all of his time to his father's business and to social work. To this end he was reading books on management and the worker, modern Japanese organization, and decision making.

One day toward the end of September I came home from a trip to the grocery store to find Robert sitting in a chair, totally shattered. His doctor had telephoned to say a blood sample taken that morning had revealed he was beginning to have a recurrence of his leukemia. The doctor asked us to come right over to his house, where he explained his next treatment plan for Robert. Knowing there was an immediate plan of action was comforting. It helped Robert to regroup his forces to reenter the hospital and to cope with all the fears and discomforts such a move entailed.

The method of coping that was most natural to Robert was one of talking things out, and he felt best when he was able to talk to people who he felt had some understanding of their own life. He needed to hear all the arguments for a particular point of view and then to make his own decision. It was also essential to him that there be a mutuality of caring in any relationship.

One of the SP's with whom Robert now chose to share his experience was his Catholic priest, Father Anthony, who later was to baptize Robert the afternoon before he died. They were really good buddies, as Father Anthony explains:

It was easy to relate to Robert. He was warm and kind; and he was open about himself, which enabled other people to be the same way. He was interested in everything. We wouldn't necessarily talk about God or religion when we were together. We would try to reason why this was happening to him, why he was chosen to suffer.

I remember times when Robert was so emotionally and physically drained from chemotherapy that he didn't have the energy to talk to his sisters or his mother or me. He was so within himself and fighting so hard in his own way that it was all he could do just to keep going. It often happened that on such a day I would be in the next room and hear the phone ring. Robert would answer it, and suddenly I would hear his voice booming with energy and life because he was talking with Father Anthony. Their dialogues were very important to him.

Robert had similar dialogues with Rabbi Joe Karasic, who also had leukemia. They laughed and traded stories, and had philosophical discussions, and simply cared about each other when one or the other was depressed. All the unspoken trials of having cancer—the lack of dignity, the loss of autonomy, the fear of dying—tend to alienate you from others and from yourself; and I think it is just these alienating aspects that are responsible for the emotional bond that exists between cancer patients. In their brotherhood, there is an unspoken assumption of mutual support and comfort.

Another important new friend in Robert's life was a clinical psychologist at the University of California Medical Center, whose major concern is with people who are facing death. He and Robert got to know each other in September when Robert returned to the hospital following his loss of remission. With this man Robert could not only express his thoughts about dying and his concern about his family, but about how to do the best he could for himself in trying to get well without hurting their feelings. For instance, Robert needed privacy and some control over whom he saw. He was tired of being given advice. The psychologist also gave Robert the feeling he wasn't alone, and that he would be all right, whether his ordeal resulted in living or in dying.

People like Robert who have a severe illness need to have options in terms of support people. They need friends outside the family who can provide them with opportunities to express themselves and share their lives, because life *alone* is meaningless—and they know that. I could see the energy Robert derived from talking to people.

Another way in which Robert coped was to cry. He said,

I get depressed and I'm cynical, but that's me. I also cry a lot, but afterwards I feel better. When I'm finished getting upset, it's time to get in gear and stick out my arm and say, "Now it's time to get well."

Robert also got angry. One day while he was in the hospital his medical oncologist walked in and jokingly said, "How many push-ups did you do this morning?" Actually, he wanted Robert to walk around the room so his muscles wouldn't atrophy. Robert took him literally, however, and felt the doctor wasn't appreciative of his efforts to get well. I happened to be there and took the doctor's side when Robert asked my opinion. Then I had to leave the hospital to attend my classes.

The doctor later apologized to Robert, telling him he realized he hadn't been sensitive to Robert's feelings and to the effect on him of all that he was going through at that time. In the meantime, however, Robert was extremely depressed by the episode. He felt he was trying hard and not getting any credit for it. It was all he could do to let people stick him with needles, give him lumbar punctures and bone-marrow tests.

Later the same day three different nurses attempted to irrigate his IV tube, which was a painful process. Robert's despair grew. He needed to talk. It was the psychologist's day off, and Father Anthony couldn't be reached by phone. A fourth nurse entered his room and attempted a fourth irrigation, whereupon Robert screamed, pulled out his IV needle, and announced, "I'm getting out of this damned place. I can't stand it anymore."

A pass was arranged, and Robert came home for a few hours. He could have quit doctors and chemotherapy right then. We could have gone to Europe and Robert would have died eventually without fighting for the chance of another remission with chemotherapy; but he made the decision to return to the hospital. As he later explained,

Emotionally, I wanted to stay at home, but rationally I knew that for me to get well I had to return to the hospital.

Sometimes your springs break down and you have to force them back up again. You have to take a rest from fighting, and then regroup your forces and start again. I call it resiliency. But my doctor didn't understand that at first. He would come in rah rah, full blast, always getting me to try harder. I'm not a person who has ever been full blast about anything, unlike my father, who, like the doctor, is rah rah 24 hours a day.

In order to come into the hospital and accept what is going on, you have to compromise. You can say to yourself, "I don't care if I live or die, but there is a lot to live for." That's a compromise in terms of being positive and wanting to live.

Robert had majored in the social sciences and had no scientific background, so he often had no idea what the doctors were talking about. My major had been child development, which had included natural sciences, so I was able to explain words such as "metabolism" or describe cell structures to Robert. I could repeat what the doctor had said when Robert was too frightened to hear the words; and I could allay his fears about being kept alive artifically. With Robert's oncologist's encouragement I slept with Robert and helped him with his baths at the hospital. I also learned to administer his shots and to regulate his IV at home. Acting in this way as Robert's interpreter and nurse-advocate gave me a real sense of purpose. Instead of feeling like an impotent observer, watching him die, I was an active participant, helping him live. I was helping him fight for that outside chance that he would get well.

All of us, including Robert, were enhanced by the interaction that occurred when he let us do things for him. We never viewed these acts as obligations, and he knew that. They were gestures of love that he allowed us to perform.

Robert was out of the hospital in November and December for his favorite holidays—Thanksgiving and Christmas. It is a tradition in the Gee family to donate to charitable organizations, especially at this time of year. Their donations were never just a question of dollars but of preparing food and giving presents, such as robes for the elderly and the chronically ill at a city hospital. Last Thanksgiving was no exception in their tradition. Robert phoned St. Anthony's Kitchen (a charitable organization that provides free Thanksgiving dinners to the needy), found out what they wanted and, together with one of his sisters, delivered the food. When they arrived with pies and turkeys, they met other people who were donating food and flowers, which made the experience a particularly gratifying one.

Thus Robert just kept on enjoying everything, such as single-handedly preparing Thanksgiving dinner for the entire family, going to his first professional basketball game with his dad, and spontaneously inviting friends to our house for a party on Christmas Eve. On Christmas Day Robert was so happy he was like those images people have of little kids on Christmas. He put on the new corduroy suit I had bought him, a new hat and shoes, and we went to his parents' for dinner. The next day we went to the movies, and the day after that we drove to Bodega Bay to spend a couple of nights. The week continued like that with gaiety and visiting relatives until New Year's Eve, when Robert developed a fever and entered the hospital. He died there 6 days later; yet in the interim he even made phone calls concerning how he could help someone from a Chinese community organization.

Living was Robert's whole experience; even in dying, he was living. He wasn't frantic, and he didn't live in constant fear, which makes me think that perhaps I can do it and other people can do it. I think that how you live prior to getting an illness may be an important factor in how you choose to live and grow afterwards. Robert's personal tradition was to be out of himself and into others, so that during his illness he got the most enjoyment from talking to other people. He said over and over that if he hadn't gotten leukemia, he wouldn't have met a lot of wonderful people—the doctors, the nurses and his other new friends. I feel the same way. Out of any experience, good or bad, you have the option of choosing your attitude.

For instance, Robert was always very much aware of our pain and felt that if there was any justification for our suffering, it was that we would become better people for having had the experience. He looked for the good in a potentially fatal experience and was able to get some meaning and comfort from that. What I learned from Robert and never want to forget is that you have a choice in how you live and how you die, and that it is important to do what you want to do. Those who care about you may not always like what you do, but they will love you for taking care of yourself.

19

When staff and fellow patients become the family

For the past 9½ years I have been associated with a unique hospital that has recently been closed because of administrative changes within the hospital and because the premises did not meet the earthquake requirements of a new state building code. This was the Southern Pacific Railroad Hospital, founded in Sacramento in 1870 and relocated in San Francisco in 1899. The hospital, the first in the world to be built by a railroad for its employees, became a major diagnostic and treatment center for railroad employees. Both young and old employees, retired workers, and many members of their families used the services of the Southern Pacific's prepaid health plan. In 1966 the hospital was renamed the Harkness Community Hospital and Medical Center, and its scope was enlarged to serve private patients from the surrounding community.

The hospital building I worked in was built in 1909, after the 1906 earthquake destroyed the earlier one. Despite its antiquity, the medical facilities, the diagnostic and treatment procedures, and the quality of patient care at Harkness Hospital were excellent. However, its most unusual feature was not its medical excellence but the camaraderie that existed among the patients and between the patients and the hospital staff—nurses and doctors alike. The nurses were devoted to the hospital and some of them had been there for 30 years. The doctors were closely allied and felt little rivalry with each other because they were employed as a group by the hospital association. Among patients who used the medical center frequently, many long-lasting friendships were made.

Harkness patients who had cancer usually returned to the hospital every 1 to 3 months for a reassessment, staging, and/or therapy. It was the policy of the Oncology Service that any time patients felt their illness had progressed or that immediate attention was necessary, they could admit themselves to the hospital. All they had to do was go to Admitting and explain that they were oncology patients on my service. Thus cancer patients treated at Harkness could feel secure in knowing they would never be denied admission and would receive care whenever they needed it.

The patients were from all over California and often from neighboring states. Those from out of town who came for a diagnostic evaluation or reevaluation were admitted to a boarding ward for 3 or 4 days. The nurses and other personnel on the boarding ward were friendly, and the meals were excellent. Family members who came to San Francisco with a patient were helped to find accommodations in the immediate neighborhood.

Patients were usually housed on open wards consisting of 12 to 15 beds. Private rooms were also available, for a modest additional sum, to those who requested them. On occasion, private rooms were used for patients with communicable infections, and sometimes they were used for patients who were doing poorly, so that families and friends could visit them frequently and stay as long as they wished. Most patients, however, seemed to prefer being on the wards. There they and their families exchanged stories about the old days on the railroad and shared their present concerns as well. Patients would call back and forth to each other: "What kind of tumor do you have? What kind of drugs are you taking?" or "Don't get an IV or a bone-marrow from Dr. So-and-so. He's lousy." They were never reticent about grading the performance of their doctors and nurses.

In this friendly, candid atmosphere, the hospital staff, patients, and families became a family for each other. This was especially helpful for patients who had few relatives and friends or who were far from home. Being in the hospital offered a change from a possibly lonely existence. It was a place to go, to be helped, to enjoy the friendly interest of others, and to be regenerated with courage by other patients and the medical staff.

One patient who gave warmth and courage to his fellow patients was Willard Whitmore, a 60-year-old man with Hodgkin's disease. Willard's cancer was discovered in the spring of 1973, but he had learned to live with cancer in 1949, when his wife became ill with cancer of the intestinal tract. Although she survived a serious operation, she and her husband were told that she did not have long to live. They wondered how soon death would come. This was when Willard decided they must learn to live one day at a time. He recalled, "I told Alice there wasn't any sense worrying about the future because you couldn't tell what it held for anyone. She was very nervous at first. But we made ourselves pay attention to individual days. We walked by the river, got up early to see the sun rise, and sat on the patio to watch the colors change at sunset. Each day there was something special to enjoy."

Twenty-four years later Alice was alive and doing well; Willard was ill. But he announced, "When I told Alice she had to live one day at a time, I learned to do the same thing myself. When you do that, it doesn't make sense to worry about accumulating a lot of money. You don't worry about time or death, either. Everything is destined to live a certain time, like the seasons of the year. When it passes, something new is born. Since that's the way it is, why worry? Besides, worry and fear inhibit your ability to fight disease. As a matter of fact, worry and fear kill more people than disease."

After having his spleen removed, Willard remained in the hospital for a few weeks and then began to commute to San Francisco from his home near Sacramento for radiation therapy. He would stay at the hospital from Monday night until Friday morning, then spend his weekends water-skiing and fishing. Although he had temporary radiation side effects of hair loss and loss of appetite, I never heard him complain. He was gentle and philosophical with everyone, and a sympathetic listener. He wandered through the wards cheering up patients and staff alike. I remember especially a day when he was teasing a friend, Joe, who had just had a lung removed. Joe was terrified and bemoaning his fate when Willard inquired innocently, "Joe, did someone die?"

Joe reminded him that he had lost a lung, whereupon Willard asked, "You mean you don't have a lung left?"

"No," Joe explained further. "They took one lung. I still have the other."

Willard winked and looked perplexed. "Well, what are you complaining for? The time to worry is when you lose the other one."

Willard gave each patient the benefit of his wisdom, on subjects from acupuncture to water-skiing, from being able to discern which doctor gave painless injections to the advantages of living in the country.

Occasionally there was a patient whom not even Willard could reach. Roger Cook was such a person. For him the hospital was just a place to go. In addition to being a retired railroad employee, he was a veteran of World War II and therefore had a second option of going to a veterans hospital. We know little else of Roger's past beyond a few facts on his medical record and a short acquaintance with him in the hospital. Born in 1912, he told us he had lived alone since being discharged from the army in 1945. In 1943 he had gotten a divorce after a brief marriage. He then became a ticket seller for the Southern Pacific Railroad and remained in that job for 20 years, retiring in 1968 in Los Angeles.

Roger seemed to have minimal contact with two surviving sisters, but apparently he had been close to a brother who died in early July 1971. A week after his brother's death, Roger was admitted to Harkness for the first time, suffering from depression and severe headaches. Two months later, in September, he was readmitted for the same reason. Although Roger denied feeling depressed and having thoughts of suicide, he did admit that he often stayed in bed most of the day, going to bed at midnight and arising around 11:00 in the morning, sometimes not bothering to get up until late afternoon. A report by the psychiatric consultant stated that Roger was depressed and that his depression was being manifested through physical symptoms.

Two years later, in June 1973, Roger returned to Harkness for a reevaluation in the Medical Service. He said he had lost 30 pounds in 6 months. On physical examination a mass was found in his right flank, and an exploratory laparotomy revealed a large mass in his right kidney, with superficial invasion of the liver. Roger was subsequently seen by the doctors in the Oncology Service, where we explained his diagnosis to him and began treatment with hormone injections. He either did not understand or refused to acknowledge his problem and the desirability of continuing hormonal therapy, and did not follow our recommendations for continuing treatment when he returned to Los Angeles. We did not see him again until 3 months later, when he asked to be readmitted to Harkness. By then he had lost an additional 10 pounds and complained that his right leg was swollen and tender.

When I arrived on the ward the morning following Roger's readmittance, he was lying on his side, awake. His body was bent and worn, his thin face covered with a stubble of gray. He was frightened and in pain. We talked for a little while. I asked him whether he knew what was wrong with him, but he didn't want to say. I told him he had a tumor, but his only response was, "You fix up my leg and I'll be all right." Such a comment is not unusual. A patient will often be more concerned about what is hurting at the moment than about his major medical problem, which in Roger's case was metastatic cancer. I told Roger we would treat his leg and that we could help relieve his pain, but I also tried to convey to him the gravity of his disease. He began to cry. He then asked to be transferred to a veterans hospital in southern California, near one of his sisters, though he admitted that he had not seen or corresponded with her in years.

We began to make the necessary arrangements for Roger's transfer. In the meantime he rarely spoke to anyone, although he never took his eyes off the doctors as we made our rounds and talked with other patients. He never asked questions except to inquire in a belligerent manner, "When will my leg get better?" He also watched very closely a patient across the room whose family visited frequently. This family and other people, including the house staff and the nurses, would try to talk to Roger. He seemed terrified of being alone and of dying, yet he was unable to respond to their many gestures of friendship. He continued to cry intermittently. He was in pain but he refused medication, saying there was no point in taking it.

We explained and offered to Roger the available cancer therapies and assured him that we would do everything possible to make him comfortable if he would give us his cooperation. He was furious that we could offer him so little, and convinced that he would receive more effective treatment at the veterans hospital. Yet before we could complete the arrangements for his transfer, he announced one morning, "What's the use," packed his belongings, and, barely able to walk, departed for Los Angeles. Before he left, we told him there would always be a bed for him at Harkness if he wasn't satisfied with the veterans hospital. We never heard from him again. A follow-up phone call to his sister revealed that Roger had died in the veterans hospital a month after he left us.

It was Roger's choice to live by himself. However, when he became ill, he needed help, and after the death of his brother there appeared to be no one with whom he could share his problems. When he was finally offered support and friendship at Harkness, he was unable to accept them. That he could not talk about his sadness and his fears was a sorrow to those of us who tried to reach him. He seemed not to have the capacity to participate in the unique system of group therapy and mutual help that had evolved at Harkness.

20

The cancer patient who lives alone

When their condition permits it, many patients prefer to receive treatment as outpatients, so that they can remain at home. This is not difficult when home consists of adequate living facilities and friends or family members who can help out when needed. Unfortunately, not every patient has such ideal circumstances at home, and it is not easy for a doctor to know which of the patients may need more help than they are being given. This was my experience with Arthur English.

Once a robust man, Arthur, at 62, had metastatic colon cancer with bladder involvement. He had a colostomy on his abdomen and a urinary catheter attached to a bag on his thigh. He had been referred to me a year after his surgery, and in the year and a half since then I had found him cheerful and outgoing, despite his cancer problems. Talking with him was always a pleasant experience.

Although Arthur lived alone in a hotel near the financial district in San Francisco, I never thought of him as a lonely man. He had many concerned friends who would phone me frequently to find out what could be done to help him. Arthur was from Oklahoma and still had close relatives there, but he frankly admitted that they irritated him after a short time, so he limited contact with them to occasional brief visits.

While Arthur was under my care, he always preferred to be treated as an outpatient for his therapy and his blood transfusions. He said he had been hospitalized too often in the past. However, on one of his visits to my office for therapy, I found that Arthur was very run-down—anemic, exhausted, and unable to eat satisfactorily. As these symptoms increased, he was less able to tolerate chemotherapy, and I suggested that he be hospitalized so we could rebuild his strength. Arthur said he would think it over, and we made an appointment for him to come to my office again the following week.

When Arthur failed to keep the appointment, I phoned him. He said he needed some rest and would come the next week. Once again he failed to appear. This time Isadora phoned him and reported to me that Arthur sounded sad and depressed. She also said he hesitated and did not give a clear answer when she asked whether he would like me to make a house call. He muttered something about being fine. That evening I decided to visit Arthur to make sure he was all right.

I had known that Arthur lived in a somewhat shabby residential hotel, but I was unprepared for some of the physical hardships he had to endure in addition to his cancer. He lived in one room that contained a bed, two dressers, two wooden chairs, and a washbasin. A blender, a coffee maker, some packets of instant breakfast, and other items were crowded onto a table next to a hot plate. On the hot plate was a frying pan with a small amount of dried-up food. A clean quilt was thrown across the bed where Arthur lay, and his favorite books and cherished possessions were on top of the dresser and stacked around the room.

These accommodations would have been bearable if they had not lacked a private bathroom. At best it must have been difficult and distressing for Arthur to perform colostomy irrigations in the shared bathroom at the end of the hall.

Arthur explained that he had not been back for chemotherapy because he had been weakened by a severe attack of diarrhea after his therapy 2 weeks earlier. He hadn't mentioned his condition to me on the telephone. Even now he wasn't complaining; he was merely telling me in a matter-of-fact voice what the trouble was. He then apologized because his room was in a state of disarray and had not been cleaned while he was sick. I had been acquainted with Arthur long enough to know he was an orderly, fastidious person, immaculate in dress and in the care of his colostomy. He was a man of great dignity, proud of his self-sufficiency, and was now embarrassed to have me see how he was living.

After I examined him we talked again about the possibility of his being hospitalized, and he agreed to let me send for him in a few days. The reason for the delay was that he wanted to put his room in order. I then realized that Arthur had no telephone either, and that whenever we called him he had to walk to the hall phone and talk standing up. A few days later, according to our agreement, I arranged hospitalization and sent an ambulance for him.

There are many people who live alone and who, like Arthur, are either too proud to accept help or simply don't want it, even though their illness has incapacitated them and brought upheaval and disorganization to their lives. Doctors may not realize how often this situation occurs, or what other essentials of home care may be lacking. I did not realize until I visited him what Arthur went through when he had diarrhea and had to care for his colostomy several times in one day. I also did not realize that he could have used help with cleaning and cooking from time to time. I am certain Arthur's friends would have been glad to help him, but Arthur, like many other people, did not want to ask. I can understand such reticence and admire the obvious courage it implies, but that attitude is not realistic. If patients who prefer not to ask family or friends for favors will at least be candid with their doctor about their needs, the doctor may direct them to one of the social service agencies whose function is to provide assistance in such matters. Their help can make a substantial difference in the basic everyday comfort and convenience that are needed to make living with cancer a little more tolerable.

PART SEVEN

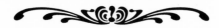

The will to live

21
Anthony Verdi

"I had a total conviction that I would be all right. I never once considered myself a leukemia victim. I never bought your philosophy, Rosie. You said I had to respect the disease, but I said, 'No way. I don't respect it at all because the moment I do, I'll be afraid of it, and fear is the greatest enemy in this thing.'"

"But you acknowledge that you had leukemia," I reminded Anthony.

"Yes. I had the disease. I created it and I got rid of it."

"How does chemotherapy fit into your philosophy?" I continued.

"Chemotherapy was a crutch, and I was willing to go along with all the crutches. I was willing to use any means available until I was able to do it myself."

"You know I don't agree with your theories, Anthony, but I won't fight them either. It will be many years before research will supply us with answers to some of the issues you raise. Whichever of us is right, one of my rules is 'Don't knock success.' Some people would agree with you, however, and others would be interested in what you have to say. Would you describe your experience with leukemia—your medical treatment, and your own views on the cause and control of disease?"

"I'd be glad to."

The symptoms came upon me gradually, just after I turned 26. In March 1970, about 6 months before my diagnosis, I began to feel tired more easily than usual. By summer my fatigue was even more pronounced. I was bleeding from the gums, but I reasoned that that was because of a baby tooth that had never been replaced.

The discovery of my condition was even postponed by a couple of coincidences. In August I had to go to an army summer camp and I was supposed to have a blood test the day before I left, but I didn't know that I was supposed to fast before a blood test, so they didn't give it to me. I spent 2 weeks in the camp and felt pretty good although I was still somewhat tired. The only other unusual physical symptoms were blood blisters on my feet that failed to heal.

The blood test that I missed was rescheduled for September 12, after my return, but I had to cancel the appointment because I was an usher at a wedding. I didn't have the test until the next Saturday. That day I noticed the first hematoma on my right arm. By the next night I had four or five hematomas on other parts of my body. Monday morning I consulted my internist, whoreferred me to you.

During the previous week I had taken a leave of absence from my job to attend law school full time. However, I noticed that I was taking three or four times longer than usual to make decisions or to function in any way. To check out all these symptoms I looked through a layman's handbook on medicine the night before I saw my internist, so I already guessed that I might have a blood disease of some sort. I just didn't know which one.

I entered the hospital for tests on Tuesday, September 21. Blood and bone-marrow tests were performed. When the diagnosis was confirmed, you and your Fellow took me into the nurses' room. You both looked grave. You told me I had acute leukemia.

I experienced a momentary panic, during which I thought, "Why me?" That didn't last more than a second or two because at the same moment I decided I was going to lick it. The reason for the quickness of my decision and the stabilization of my emotions is that I had been practicing a way of thinking, a way of life, for many years. This philosophy has an approach toward cancer, as well as other diseases, that is based on the belief that every disease, although real, is psychosomatically induced. There are no exceptions. The emotional and mental state of the individual triggers the germs and viruses in the body that create disease. I therefore knew I was responsible for creating the climate that allowed leukemia to develop and that I was just as responsible for changing that climate in order to conquer it. I also subscribe to the notion that anything can be done if you believe in it strongly enough, and this includes the eradication of disease. You can even kid yourself about what you believe as long as you realize you're kidding yourself—just so there's no internal conflict. There are no defeats, only wins. Even the defeats have an element of win in them. You have to concentrate all your attention on that one little element of win and drop the rest.

I knew why I was vulnerable to leukemia. My marriage had recently broken up and I was very depressed. I was depressed because the relationship was destroyed, not because I was particularly in love with my ex-wife at that point. I was also having problems at work. The people there were bugging me. I had been given extra jobs to do, and I was being criticized for not being able to do them as they wanted me to. Therefore there was a series of resentments and rejections that had a lot to do with my emotional state.

Another thing that calmed me down when you gave me my diagnosis was that I said to myself, "I don't care whether I live or die." This also helped eliminate volcanic emotional eruptions because I then went on to think, "Okay, but there are some worthwhile things to live for." Then I began ticking them off. "This would be nice and that would be nice." Going through this process cleared me of panic, and I was able to think calmly, "Let's hear them out." The technical term for my acute leukemia was promyelocytic. I was told I had two alternatives. I could do nothing, or I could take chemotherapy. I decided on the latter, which was what you recommended. I was also to receive blood transfusions.

You told me a little about chemotherapy, how the drugs were strong but that they were no longer experimental. We decided to begin the next day with a 5-day course of multidrug chemotherapy. I had never had my veins punctured in any way, except for an occasional blood test, and that became a traumatic new experience, because it was done more than once or twice a day. However, you and the Fellow had told me about the advantages of giving chemotherapy by IV. You also tried to reduce the number of blood tests per day, and you drew the blood and serviced the IVs yourselves in order to save my veins.

I was never afraid while receiving chemotherapy, but as the drugs entered my body, there was a cold feeling. It wasn't necessarily clammy or distasteful, just a cold feeling that lasted anywhere from a few minutes to half an hour. Although I felt subjectively that my temperature had been lowered, I know that wasn't the case.

At that time my blood counts were extremely low; I had about 300 to 500 white blood cells, as opposed to a normal count of over 5000. I had no platelets, and I had many immature, or blastic, leukemia cells. You also told me I was to receive an anticoagulant, because with my particular form of leukemia there was clotting in my blood vessels. I was also bleeding internally, and I was tired.

The 5-day course of chemotherapy was followed by a 10-day rest, and then the cycle would be repeated. The objective during that initial phase of treatment was to destroy the malignant cells in the bone marrow. Of course, the longer I was on chemotherapy, the weaker I got. During the 10 days that I was off the drugs, I often had a fever.

You were a tremendous boost to me at that time. You were cheerful in front of me and conveyed great hope, although privately I think you felt I was a lost cause because you had seen so many similar cases. I didn't pick up any negative thinking, however; I was too busy trying to convince you and my parents that everything would be all right. You showed your faith and optimism when you phoned the law school and asked for a leave of absence for me and arranged that I could go back the following year.

As I look back, I believe my basic determination to get well never left me. Not once. During the first 3 or 4 weeks, when I wasn't completely wiped out, I was very cheerful, bantering with you and the nurses, and trying to cheer up my parents and friends. Then the fevers began to get worse. In fact, during October and November I had fevers of 104° and 105° daily for a 3-week period and was in a semicomatose state. You controlled my fever with an ice blanket, ice packs, and antibiotics and other medicines. I became delirious and also had a mild stroke. I had extremely heavy headaches, which you thought might be due to a small brain hemorrhage. Also, I lost my hair bit by bit. I was put in reverse isolation several times so I wouldn't pick up infections.

One of the funniest things was that when I had my stroke I was convinced I was all right and hadn't had a stroke. A neurologist came in and examined me, and even though I was wiped out, with no bone marrow, I performed feats like jumping on one foot and running up and down the hall, through sheer willpower, to prove to him that I was all right. Brain scans, EEGs, and other tests were made, but the exact cause of the stroke was never determined. You said it could have been from bleeding because of the low platelet count or from the toxic effect of the drugs.

During that 3-week period of high fever and delirium a friend came to visit me who shares the same ideas I do. He looked at me and said, "Gee, Anthony, that's a marvelous game you're playing." That's all he said. The next day my fever came down to 99, and from then on I was fairly stable.

That autumn of 1970 I was in the hospital for 3 months, from September 21 to the end of December. During that time I received 105 units of blood. They consisted of platelets for bleeding and red blood cells for anemia. When my leukemia was announced where my dad works, and at law school, which I'd only attended for a week, there was a spontaneous offering of blood donations. The blood transfusions produced a rushing feeling. It must be like the rushing feeling people speak of who are on amphetamines or STP. It was a very uncomfortable sensation, as though things were rushing through me. I later had hepatitis, probably from the blood, because my serum liver-function tests were abnormal.

Within that 3-month time span I did sink into moods similar to depression, but they were mainly apathy. My thoughts were always positive, though. I knew—I didn't just hope—that everything would be okay. I remember telling you that in January 1971. You said, "Why didn't you tell me in September?" and I replied, "You wouldn't have believed me."

While I was in the hospital my parents were there morning, noon, and night. Dad and mother would both take time off from work. They were completely devoted parents. After I had been there 2 months I could no longer eat the food, either for taste or for psychological reasons. My mouth was full of sores and I could only eat pureed food. So Ma would fix pureed food for me. I am from Argentina and we have a Spanish-Latin American tradition of very close family ties, so although such acts of devotion aren't necessarily expected, they just seem like the natural things that parents do for children. No sacrifice is too great for any member of the family. So to me it was not an unusual thing for my mother to do that, although everyone was commenting on it, saying, "You're being spoiled. You're depending too much on your parents. It's an unnatural relationship."

One thing that helped me a lot during those months was the number of people with whom I became involved. It was fascinating, because people that I'd never met before, total strangers, would come in and want to talk to me. Of course I always went out of my way to make them feel comfortable and welcomed in my room. I was also extremely touched and flattered by their warmth and friendship because I knew they really cared for me. One of my favorites was a nurse from England, a brilliant guy named Fleur Stanley, who did a great deal for my morale. He was a no-nonsense individual and very witty. He was a positive person with lots of determination. He had a psychological plan for me. He visited me at a certain time each day, and we would have a 15-minute talk on some subject of interest. We'd discuss these ideas back and forth, and of course he'd never believe anything I'd say, and I'd tease him.

Once or twice I had a problem with the other nurses, however, because they would get too emotionally involved with me. I think this tends to happen especially when a patient is young and seriously ill. There was one particular student nurse who spent too much time in my room. I was asked whether she was bothering me and if I wanted her transferred, but I said, "No. She can stay." She was transferred to another floor anyway. I had told her myself many times, "Look, you've been here long enough. You'd better go do your other duties." I think this kind of problem arose because I didn't give a damn about what anybody thought of my ideas, and I seem to be a person that people like to tell their problems to. In turn, I would give them the benefit of my philosophy and tell them what they could do if they wanted to. This young nurse listened to me, was impressed by what I said, and apparently became infatuated.

At the end of December 1970 I was shocked to find out that I was in remission, because that meant that I had to leave the hospital. The hospital had become my home and I didn't want to leave. I was happy that the remission had come about as I had wanted it to, but going home was less exciting than being in the hospital, where people are more apt to visit you. I wanted that attention, and I think that feeling fostered the problem I some times had with the nurses. Anyway, I had formed a lot of fast friendships in the hospital, and I didn't want to lose the daily contact. The support of these friends meant love, that people really cared about me. And that was another factor in what I believe induced my illness. I had wanted everybody to love me. I no longer feel this way. Before, if anyone showed any kind of ill will or reaction against me, I instantly thought he or she hated me or didn't like me, and this would totally depress me. I didn't spend my time peering around every corner to see if people liked me, but there were certain times when I felt that way.

Those reactions have been diminishing for years, as I have learned to handle such feelings on my own. It was part of a pattern of thinking in which I felt that at some point the environment was at fault for things that happened to me. In other words, *they* did it to me. I now believe the opposite is true, that anything that happens to me I have caused in some way, even if it is a razor-thin responsibility on my part. My share of the responsibility may only be the fact that I was there to receive the stimulus from the outside. I am responsible for being there, for receiving it, and finally for how I react to it. With anything that has a cause outside myself—even if it's someone menacing me, or acting as if he hates my guts—it is still within my power to react one way or the other and in that way to exert control over my own life. That is to say, I can believe the game that guy out there is playing and respond with either "How terrible. He hates me" or "What the hell is bothering him so much that he has to feel that way about me?"

At home during the month of January 1971 I spent most of my time on my back because I was very weak. I had gone from 192 pounds down to 150 since September. The disease and the drugs had weakened me so that running across the street was enough to make my knees collapse. In fact I fell down one time. But even though I was weak, I was in partial remission and I felt clean and purged inside.

Between January 1971 and June 1971 I went to the hospital for 1 week each month for chemotherapy and would be off for 3 weeks. In May I came down with a fever and an infection. I don't know what caused it, but I was admitted to the hospital for 4 days in reverse isolation. My white blood cells were down to 500 again, and I was given a blood transfusion and antibiotic therapy for the infection. It lasted approximately 7 days, but this time when I left the hospital I no longer felt I was leaving a nice place. In 5 months I had adjusted to being out of the hospital and had no desire to return.

My total remission came sometime during that year, 1971. I reenrolled in law school in September and was put on maintenance therapy, a reduced chemotherapeutic program. I would spend 3 days in the hospital every 4 weeks, to receive the intravenous part of the therapy, and would complete the cycle by taking tablets at home.

I continued in this way until January 30, 1972, when I had a coronary and had to spend 18 days in the hospital. My cardiologist, Dr. Gordon Katznelson, felt that the tension of going back to law school would aggravate my heart problem, so he phoned the school and arranged for another leave of absence. I can understand his reasoning, but if he hadn't done that, I would probably have faked it and gone back and finished with no problems. He didn't understand the way I felt about things. I never explained my philosophy to him.

From that time until I returned to law school the next September I kept myself busy seeing friends and doing all kinds of things. I took the real estate license exam and I went to Argentina for 35 days.

I continued with a maintenance dose of chemotherapy, but on a schedule that allowed me more independence than before. Then, Rosie, you would insert a small IV tube in my vein that would remain for several days, and I could go home and inject the chemotherapy into the tubing myself. I also continued with the chemotherapy tablets. You would see me once a day for 5 days each month, to check my blood and supply the drugs for the next injection. This program of chemotherapy lasted until August 1973, when I decided I didn't want any more. You discussed the possibility of immunotherapy or brain radiation, but I had a negative reaction to both suggestions. I don't know how much you were aware of my feelings. I hope I was diplomatic, but I felt I didn't need any more therapy. I felt fine.

Therefore, in August I went off chemotherapy of all kinds. I also stopped taking the oral antibiotic that I had been on for 3 years to guard against skin infection. It is now May 1975, and I've been off chemotherapy for 20 months. I'm feeling marvelous. I remember when I quit, I said to myself, "At last you had the courage to go off that stuff."

"Anthony, that was an accurate account of the last 3½ years, but you forgot to mention that you got married 6 months ago to one of my favorite nurses, that you have graduated from law school and taken the bar examination. But back to your decision to stop therapy. I did not agree with that decision, but I also did not have an exact answer on how much longer we should continue some form of therapy. You were in a fortunate state to stop treatment when you did, and it worked. Since August 1973 we've watched you closely. At first we performed bone-marrow tests every 3 weeks, then at 6-week intervals; and now we only do a test every 2 months. We're relying on your body to take over and defend itself, but if there is ever a recurrence of your leukemia we'll treat it as we did before. How would you feel if you had a recurrence, Anthony?"

"No problem," was his prompt reply. "If I got a recurrence, I'd know I created it. If I'm willing to play that game again, then what the hell am I doing, that's all. But I certainly would not panic."

"You say you didn't respect your disease, but when we explained to you how we wanted to treat it, you were cooperative, and that was important," I said. "You and I have been talking about the desire to live that is in all of us. Our philosophies about how to accomplish a cure are different, but we both know the will to live makes a difference, and that patients who have this desire to survive fight harder and do better medically than those who lack the drive. It's an intangible, unmeasurable force that makes a difference."

"I believe it makes all the difference," Anthony replied. "If you have the faith that you're going to make it, if you have the will to win, you'll make it. And if you introduce any doubts, you've had it."

I nodded. "But many people *say* they're going to beat their disease."

"The difference is, they don't believe it. In the back of their minds they're saying, 'You fool. You're really kidding yourself.' "

"Are you being completely fair about that?" I asked. "The will to live is important, and if a person is convinced he will get well, that's even better. But we know of no specific effect on cancer cells that is caused by a positive state of mind."

"I know you don't agree with some of my ideas," Anthony said patiently, "but I know that even when I kid myself into feeling something, once I acquire the feeling, it's a true feeling. It's the feeling you're going to be okay. You convince yourself. You know you have something, and you say, 'Well, I'm going to have something else instead, something that's healthy. What would it be like to feel healthy right now, even though I'm sick?' In that way you begin to create a future for yourself. When you do that, you're not thinking about how you have this dread disease that will kill you. You shift your focus, your concentration, away from the disease, even though you are still aware of it.

"That's just my understanding of health in me," Anthony added. "It might not apply to someone else's way of thinking. I was totally convinced. It's that simple. I knew, just as I know that the sun is going to rise tomorrow, even if I don't see it—I knew that I would be healthy again."

JANUARY 1981

Almost 6 years have passed since Anthony was last interviewed for this book. During that time he has earned two M.B.A.s in addition to the law degree he received in 1975. He worked for 2½ years with a general practice law firm, another 2½ years as an advisor on international tax matters for a bank, and just recently Anthony joined the tax department of a major construction engineering firm to advise on individual, corporate, and international tax matters.

Anthony has not changed. When I asked him how he felt about his cancer experience, he replied, "I am no longer living with cancer. It's no longer a relevant part of my life, and I can't understand why in hell we're doing this interview! And by the way, the drugs didn't cure me; they had nothing to do with it. Shall we go on?"

But he continued, "On a daily basis, cancer is a memory that is fading quickly. I am not afraid of it—never have been, except for that second or two when I was told what my diagnosis was. The actual experience from 1970 to 1973 was one of the more fantastic experiences I have ever had. It taught me a lot about life and myself—and about other people. I think that having cancer accelerated the maturation process. I felt more a member of the adult community. It opened my eyes to lots of things I wasn't aware of before, such as other people and the way those people were more tolerant than I am of what I consider to be idiosyncrasies in others. Or perhaps they made me aware of things I hadn't paid attention to before because I had been concentrating too much on myself and my own reactions to the world. I was able to understand others a little bit better and to deal with them more effectively—and perhaps more lovingly."

"I gather that you still feel you were responsible for causing your disease," I ventured.

"Yes. I was responsible. Wow! That shows my ability to cause either health or ill health in my body. Rather than feel guilty about this, I congratulate myself for *doing* something. Among the general populace, what I did—getting cancer—is labeled bad, and I ultimately don't believe in labels. A thing is what it is, and then we interpret it and color it with feelings, emotions, and ideas. I felt that if I was creative enough to cause it, I could be creative enough to "uncause" it. I could say, 'I've had cancer up to this point. Now I'll move in this direction where I don't have cancer.' But if you feel guilty or you blame the environment, then you can't act. You can't decide to drop it and take up something new. It's interesting to me that I continued to apply this philosophy of what I was trying to do with myself even when I was unconscious for periods of time. The feeling never left me that I was going to take care of the problem eventually—using medication as a crutch, of course."

"Your philosophy would be hard to translate to another person because it's an internal process."

"Absolutely. You have to have a background in it. I was fortunate, and sometimes I wonder if I didn't plan the whole thing in the first place for the experience. I believe that life is a game, and in a game there are various roles—various things can happen—and there are rules. And that's life. Life is a role."

"Could you lecture on this subject?"

"No. There would be a communication problem. The audience could not duplicate the image that I have in my mind about this thing. I could do it with someone over a period of years as someone else did it with me. He introduced me to these concepts; we sounded them out and exhausted them to the point where I understood what he meant by being responsible, by being the doer of what happens to your life.

By the way, your chapter about me was entitled 'The Will to Live.' That has never been an accurate concept in my mind. What I am talking about is above willpower; it's *knowing*. And when you know something, it *is*. You don't have to convince yourself, whereas willpower implies an effort. My idea is that you just know it and do it even if you have to delude yourself, as I explained in my chapter. If belief involves a little self-delusion, so what? Who are you hurting if you are deluding yourself? If you have to kid yourself into something until you believe it and the results are positive, so what? That may be my subjective evaluation of my experience, and someone else may say, 'Well, the medication helped you.' That's fine, too. I will let anyone who thinks that think it. I won't fight them on it. Tritely, it's called individual salvation, and it has to be done by each and every one of us at some point."

Then Anthony laughed and added, "I guess you have the same unanswered questions you had the last time we talked."

"I can appreciate your ideas," I replied, "but they remain yours. Nevertheless, they helped you have endurance and to maintain your courage. They made it possible for you to complete your therapy and return to active life."

22

Alexander Jones

On my fiftieth birthday, I really felt elated. I thought, "Jesus Christ, you've reached a half a hundred years. You're sort of remarkable." I felt I should receive a citation, and I put signs all around the house saying "Happy 50th Birthday."

I thought my friends would share my elation but they didn't seem to want to talk about it. Some of them had achieved 50 or were damned close to it, and they weren't enamoured by my enthusiasm. They resented the chronological exposure and felt compromised.

I think I was pleased to have reached 50 because I got there without encountering anything I couldn't surmount. Along the line I was besieged by a series of tragedies. I lost my entire family and had numerous disappointments and reversals, so I felt rather good that I had risen to the occasion, that I had been able to endure and prevail. I was scarred, but I wasn't bowed and I wasn't emotionally crippled.

My friends take the same attitude of denial toward my lung cancer as they did to my reaching 50. If they can't bestow longevity on me, they can't bestow it on themselves. Therefore, not one of them wants to face it. They say such things as, "It's going to be a mistaken diagnosis"; "More than likely you're going to be cured"; or "You can still live to be the oldest person in the world." This approach makes them feel more comfortable and secure, death being one of the mysteries people tend to shy away from if they possibly can. I've learned to go along with all of these diverse opinions and not to pursue them to the place where it makes my friends uncomfortable.

Another reason people find it difficult to accept that I have lung cancer is because they prefer not to think of me as having emotional or physical needs. I have only one friend who understands that I have wants and needs of people. The rest think I'm self-sufficient and have never needed anyone. Therefore, they have rarely taken my problems seriously. Yet, at the same time—and especially now—I have always found my friends to be unselfishly supportive.

I think that one reason people felt I didn't have needs is because I have always led a somewhat solitary life, even when I was married. Lately I have been able to maintain this isolation at home by keeping my place in constant turmoil through endless remodeling. After all, you shouldn't be in the midst of things if guests are coming; they should be comfortable and they deserve your undivided attention. This ploy was more subconscious than conscious, and I've only come to recognize it for what it is in the past couple of years. I think that's because I have become more secure and don't need it anymore. Lately, I have developed a real desire to have people in, but unfortunately, I don't have much physical stamina to complete my projects as rapidly as I would like. My knees are pretty well shot from arthritis, and I need two joint replacements.

The decline in my strength and ability has also led me to neglect my volunteer activities. I have always worked in one organization or another teaching typing, social responses, and creative writing, including poetry. Although I don't have a formal academic background, I feel I am sufficiently conversant with literature to meet the needs of my students. And I always know that if any problem arises with an exceptional student, I can call on one of my academically trained friends to give me advice.

In addition to teaching poetry, I have also written poetry for many years. I find it interesting to observe how, in different ways, I expressed the same philosophy at 18 as I do now. I was amazed then as I am now at how the human being, screwed by circumstances beyond all belief, can manage to stand up despite the unmitigating bullshit that presses down upon him. I'm talking about mankind, and about people like myself—the survivors and the contributors—the people who I think have become successful human beings. When I was 18 I wrote:

> Trace the affinity
> Of the will to be
> with the ability
> To be no longer
>
> Ah . . . such a narrow way divides.
> And yet, in the precarious clime
> Of this most eccentric inch
> A world of men have lived
> Triumphant!

I believe in man, but God is unrelated to me. Man created him. God is too much like man and very little like God; he doesn't seem to be too well insulated from anger, disappointment, gullibility and nastiness. Or insensitivity; that seems to be a great part of his career. He's godlike only in his longevity; moreover, he doesn't seem to be as nice or as understanding as many people I know. And he certainly is contradictory as all hell.

I never thought much about a right way to live. I don't think there is one. And I don't think you always have to look good to be a successful human being. A person can look good on the surface and have as much humanity as a snake; another person may be a bastard to get along with, but his basic response is one for mankind.

I do believe in choice, however. When I was younger, I went through a period where I thought all things should be permissible, and all things should be forgiven. Then I reevaluated. I don't believe that anymore. Although I don't condemn or feel harshly, I feel there are some people you have to scratch. You can't rehabilitate them. They had a choice whether to be fundamentally decent, and they decided not to be. I don't care if their mother was a prostitute and their father was a thief. At some point they could have decided that's not a cool way to live and taken responsibility for their own lives. They have a right to be, but I have a right not to be bothered with them.

There's a second category of people—the dependents—and these are people we have to carry. They may not have it spiritually or mentally or physically; they'll never be independent. Whether they are morally good or bad is irrelevant. They're not competent, and we need to take care of them. Some are charmingly helpless; others are helpless in a way that elicits no pity. But we have to carry them all and to contribute to their well-being.

A third category is composed of the stumblebums—the rest of us. They do the whole gamut: They're nice, they're good; they're bad, they're different. They fail, they falter, they succeed. And they need help.

Everyone needs help at some time, regardless of their age or stage of maturity. It's normal—the human condition. It's like saying someone needs love, a meal, or a favor. Some people may need more help than others; they may need professional help where a certain service is provided and then they can be put on their own and be independent again. Any one of us might be in this position at one time or another.

Although these categories of human beings can overlap, I don't believe people can change very much. The decision to be a decent person is made rather early, and I can dredge up few excuses for those who choose otherwise. Youth is no excuse for unkind or immoral behavior, nor all the derogatory and delimiting aspects of living in the ghetto. For myself, I never worried about being poor or black. On the contrary, poor people don't have any illusions about the facts of life, and poor kids are pretty goddamned good psychologists. They develop a degree of sophistication that doesn't come to other people until much later.

Even drugs cannot be blamed. There is no way kids can be tricked into drugs or anything else today. Information about the results is too well disseminated throughout the culture. Not even the worst liar says you can beat drugs. Thus the decision on the direction to be followed is made early, and basic change is unlikely. Age and maturity may enable us to manage better or to be better at what we do, but that's not change.

It's much harder for me to discuss my cancer. I'm not intensely interested in the mechanics. All I want to know is the outcome. How long is the cancer going to give me to live and what is it going to do to my physical and mental abilities? I just want to know my limits, so I can work around them.

I feel no need to learn the medical terminology. The names of the chemicals are the doctors' problem. I'm just for anything that makes me feel better, especially if I can swallow it. Besides, most cancer patients are amateur pharmacologists. If they dabble in the medical aspects of their disease, they're going to come up with a lot of disconcerting answers that are going to make them unhappy. So, why bother with it when you aren't even going to become mildly well informed? The doctors don't even know that much.

What I do know is that you can learn to live above and through pain. You may not have the happiest hee-haw life, but you can learn how to husband those few moments when you aren't in as much pain as you were before. You also learn how to transcend it and how to move across the room, even if it's painful. Pretty soon you can do a great number of things, the pain notwithstanding. Like my knees. I need joint replacements, but I don't know whether I want to be crippled for a month or two from the operation; and I don't even know if the replacements would work. My knees hurt a great deal, but I don't notice them as much as I did at first. I just keep moving and creep down the stairs if I have to.

This is not because I'm particularly valiant or strong. That's not my thing. I'm not one of those great heroic personalities, I just think pain is awfully overrated. It's a thing we all fear. But when we eventually face it, we do what we have to do, and we aren't quite as disabled as we thought we would be. Great numbers of people move around in tremendous pain.

The only thing that concerns me is money. I've held a rather responsible position, but who cares about that? I was beginning to feel like an anachronism at work anyway because I was never going to get my point across. Yet I couldn't afford to quit because I didn't have any particular skills or formal education. Now I understand I can go on disability and receive 40% of my salary. I'll probably do that, but you need money for more than food and rent. You need money to give presents or to loan a friend $5. If you can't do that, you don't feel very good.

I just don't want to end up on the dole. If I'm invited to dinner, I want to be glad to go because of the joy of sharing dinner, not because I wouldn't otherwise have been able to eat. I don't want it to come to that.

On the other hand, I can use the free time. I'd read, paint, and write more. I'm not a good writer or painter, but I think more people should paint and write and sculpt. Even if we all had a lot more skill, we still wouldn't be good. Few people are. A famous painter, Juan Gris, once said to Gertrude Stein, "The little painter has all the things the great painter has. He just isn't great." He's just as meticulous, just as intense a craftsman, tries just as hard, puts as much passion and pain into it. He just isn't a great painter. But, all the other externals? He does everything Picasso did — suffers, enjoys, works, is dissatisfied.

This sounds a little stupid and pompous, but if I had more free time, I'd think more. One of the joys of being in the hospital was having time to think. I don't mean I'd have time to be profound. I'm not trying to change the world, and I'm not trying to change myself. It's just a matter of having the leisure, the luxury, to think anything at all.

I'm not afraid of dying, but I've been afraid of being a living dead person. What concerns me is the quality of life. If you have 6 good months, it's better than 16 frightened years. In 6 months you can pack a hell of a lot of living, if you do it right. Thus, other than the fact that I've lived a half a hundred years, time has never impressed me. It's what you do with it. It's the same way with money. It's what kind of mileage you're able to get out of your money or your life. Having large amounts of either one is neither here nor there.

This isn't foolish bravado on my part or that I'm too stupid to catch the importance of longevity. It's just that I think I'm intelligent enough not to give it an improper value, and to consider it for what it's worth, which is certainly something. It's nice to live long, if you can *live* long.

Even some brilliant people, leaders in their time, have ended up with no intellectual interests. That has always mystified me, but *that's* the kind of thing I'm afraid of, or losing my mind, or becoming a vegetable.

Those are the only circumstances under which I could condone suicide, when all the chips are down, and nothing can be done, and no one is going to be harmed by it. When your life-support machine does not allow you to involve yourself in the business of living, then I think you should pull the plug. If you can never again make a contribution, and you are an object of pity, a nothing; you shouldn't have to endure such debasement. I think these cases are rare, however. I think there are few states of disability in which it is impossible to become involved, because as long as you have your mind, or even some vestiges of will and speech, you can still be a great listener. You can still be a person whom people call, even if you're in a respirator. People can come and unburden themselves to you. There are still contributions you can make.

It seems to me that the majority of suicides are carried out by people in deep despair who have exhausted all their spiritual and emotional resources. That must be a dreadful moment. I don't feel sorry for them because there is nothing I can do to prevent it. They have created their situation, and even if they don't commit suicide eventually, they commit living suicide. They become the living dead.

A few people will make a stab at suicide at one time or another. I certainly contemplated it and even attempted it once, but I also aborted it. One of the things that took me away from it was the thought of how dreadful this would be for my friends. It would be a terrible letdown after they had put so much into their friendship and love for me. It seemed like a rotten repayment for the comfort and solace they had given me from time to time.

I feel I'm still in the ball game if a friend comes to me with a big problem and upsets me, or if he comes to me with a great happiness and makes me feel glad. Either way, it means I have a sincere friend who wants to share a real part of his experience, good or bad, whether it's tears or laughter.

I'm looking for the same answers I looked for at 18. I haven't changed, but I do know that even with the odds tremendously against you, in spite of all the oppression, most of us manage, somehow, to make it.

> The vulgar splendor of a noise
> Contents the appetite of ears
> Insensitive to subtleties.
> The really loud occurrence falls
> without the benefit of sound
> How silently are these:
> The awakening to love,
> The audacity to dream,
> The will to live.

PART EIGHT

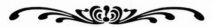

Supportive services

23

Nurses

The nurse is one of the first people a patient meets after being admitted to a hospital. She may be wearing a white uniform or cap or, as in many hospitals today, she may be dressed in a brightly colored uniform or smock. Today, "she" may even be a "he," as there is an ever-increasing number of men entering the nursing profession.

The routine of the orientation period for the person just entering the hospital will vary only slightly from hospital to hospital. After greeting a new patient, the nurse usually checks weight, blood pressure, temperature, and pulse. (In some hospitals, an LVN—Licensed Vocational Nurse—or nurse's aid will check these vital signs.) A new patient is asked about dietetic likes and dislikes, about allergic reactions, and any other special information that may help a nurse to make the patient's stay more comfortable.

Nurses also perform another important function. They are the principal people to whom patients regularly communicate their needs, frustrations, fears, and delights. The principal nurses assigned to each patient within a 24-hour period (usually three nurses on 8-hour shifts) communicate to each other as they change shifts all the things each has learned and observed about the patients in their charge. In this way, patients can be sure their personal needs, desires, medical history, and status have been communicated from one nurse to the next.

Nurses are responsible for approximately 80 to 90% of the patient care in a hospital. With few exceptions (e.g., in a few public hospitals), a nurse will not prescribe medications, initiate tests, or make changes in a diet ordered by the physician without his or her express permission. In most other areas of patient care, the doctor relies on the knowledge and judgment of the nurse to make patient-care decisions.

I interviewed six nurses* who work exclusively with cancer patients. I was

---

*Kim Drucker, R.N., Oncology Nurse in private office practice, San Francisco, California.
Mary Lawton, R.N., Oncology Nurse, formerly at Mount Zion Hospital and Medical Center, San Francisco, California.
Lizabeth Light, B.S.N., Patient Care Coordinator, Marshal Hale Memorial Hospital, San Francisco, California.
Becky Moore, R.N., Oncology Nurse, Mt. Zion Hospital, San Francisco, California.
Eileen Shepley, R.N., Oncology Nurse, Claire Zellerbach Saroni Tumor Institute, Mount Zion Hospital and Medical Center, San Francisco, California.
Fleur Frederick Stanley, S.R.N., O.N.C., West Middlesex Hospital, London, England, Nursing Administrative Supervisor, Mount Zion Hospital and Medical Center, San Francisco, California.

particularly interested in finding out how they feel about cancer nursing after several years of experience, and how they deal with their own emotional responses, as well as those of the patients and their families.

ER: Why did you go into cancer nursing?

Eileen Shepley: I think it's one of the more satisfying kinds of nursing. The patients are fantastic to work with, despite their anxieties and fears. In comparison with the average internal medical patient, cancer patients have fewer pretenses. They readily accept the side effects of therapy because of their will to live, and they are more responsive to the support and encouragement of doctors and nurses. Another reason I like cancer nursing is the feeling I have of being needed.

Mary Lawton: I came to cancer nursing in a roundabout way. My prior nursing experience had been one of defeat, and I thought it was something I never wanted to encounter again. I was depressed. I had found it difficult and painful to work with patients who were ill, undergoing therapy, or dying. Then, because of a series of circumstances, I found I needed a job, and Memorial Hospital in New York City was the only place with an opening. I thought, "Necessity has brought me to something I'm not going to be able to handle." Instead, I found I was very comfortable at Memorial Hospital and liked it enormously. I'm not sure why. Perhaps I had reached a level of personal development that made it possible for me to relax and face all the problems that had once seemed so overwhelming. Also, I began to realize that cancer nursing was the most rewarding kind. Before I went to Memorial Hospital I was bored with nursing. In contrast, although emotionally taxing, cancer nursing is challenging and gratifying.

You can do so much for cancer patients that doctors don't have time to do by offering them something personal. To follow through after receiving a doctor's orders isn't enough. There are many situations in which a doctor may say, "You take care of it. You know more than I do." For example, when a patient has a colostomy, a nurse can teach him how to take care of it. A colostomy can be a traumatic experience for a patient. The help he receives from the nurse is real and useful.

ER: Mrs. Shepley, what qualities and skills do you think are most essential in a good cancer nurse?

ES: I used to think that a concerned nurse needed only a good theoretical and practical background in communication and interpersonal relationships. Now this view seems superficial. Nurses are taught communication skills and the importance of good interpersonal relationships, but herein lies the problem. Feelings of empathy and caring inherent in communication and interpersonal relationships cannot be taught. They come from the heart and from a lifetime of personal, satisfying experiences. Touching, just being there, and the use of other therapeutic communication techniques are meaningless gestures when a nurse does not feel genuine concern for a patient and his family. She must want to become involved with the patient's problems and be willing to give of herself even though this means she will be hurt if the patient suffers a relapse and dies. However, she will also share the joy when a patient does well.

Being able to maintain an optimistic outlook is vital, even when prognosis is less than favorable. I'm constantly surprised at how well some patients do when statistically they shouldn't be doing well at all. It's impossible to predict which patient will "beat the odds," but the nurse's conveyance of hope contributes to the well-being of all patients.

A good cancer nurse also has to have a broad background of knowledge and skill. She needs experience in specific procedures such as colostomy and tracheostomy care. She must be skilled in doing procedures because cancer patients are very good at detecting indecision and lack of skill. They often equate getting well with how efficiently a procedure is carried out, whether it involves an IV, chemotherapy, or another kind of therapy. If a nurse is not adept, a patient may think his chances of recovery are reduced.

ER: How do your patients respond to you?

ES: At first most patients are fearful and anxious, but after we've worked together for a while they become more relaxed. A large part of a nurse's job is to help alleviate anxiety. Hers is a supportive, sharing role. She must be able to interpret and integrate a patient's problems into the plan of medical therapy and acknowledge the feasibility of what can be done for him.

ER: Mr. Stanley, you're a nursing supervisor on a floor where the majority are cancer patients. Would you describe a typical day and some of the problems that may arise?

Fleur Stanley: When I come on to the floor each day, I look through the patients' files and I see what changes have occurred and what notes have been made. I also talk with the nurses who are going off duty and find out if there are any new problems from the day before. When I have analyzed the data, I have a good sense of what I want to do and set up the plan for that day.

Often a nurse will tell me that a patient has asked me to drop by his room if I am "not too busy." Then I know that the patient has something on his mind that he wishes to discuss with me. This kind of visit is of critical importance. The patient needs an opportunity to voice his pent-up feelings. He needs a person who will encourage him to blow off steam without taking what he says too personally and becoming defensive. A nurse should know that a patient who is irritable or irate is rarely angry at her. More likely, he is angry with someone else—a relative, perhaps, or at his illness—but is unable to admit his frustration. He has to do something with his anger, so he directs it at whomever is around. If the nurse can accept this bitterness and anger and talk with the patient about it, she may enable him to explore what's really on his mind.

Other tense situations may occur. The person with cancer is often apprehensive. Any treatment he is receiving is a major issue because he feels his life depends on it. When he puts on the light that summons the nurse, it must be answered immediately. For example, if a patient is on intravenous therapy and the IV should become empty and need replacement, the patient will turn on the light and call the nurse. "The IV is out! You know that's important to me. I need it. You shouldn't have allowed it to happen." He's really saying, "Look what I'm going through!"

The daily menu provides another object for the ventilation of frustration and apprehension. A patient may become extra sensitive regarding any item of food that doesn't come up to his expectations. That everything be properly done is essential because he must get well. Each slight inconvenience becomes a major event over which he can express his constant fear of being neglected.

ER: But the patient isn't the only one who presents problems.

FS: Certainly not. In some cases the nurse can be the cause of a problem. One afternoon I went into a patient's room and sensed immediately that something was wrong between the patient and his special duty nurse. Afterward, I took another nurse aside and told her to ask the patient, when she was next alone in his room, what was wrong. It turned out that the patient's morning nurse completed her duty at 3:00 but that the afternoon nurse was always 45 minutes late. The morning nurse resented having to stay until her replacement arrived. Animosity had built up between them and it was making the patient uncomfortable. Naturally, he was reluctant to speak about it in front of the nurse who was causing the trouble. Asking him while she was out of the room enabled us to find out quickly what was wrong and to replace her.

ER: When a patient is admitted to the hospital, the staff's first concern is whether he has been informed of his diagnosis, or, if he has been informed, whether he has accepted it. Occasionally, too, as you have all experienced, a patient may not have been given an adequate explanation of his illness. In such a situation, a patient is puzzled or fearful and may ask the nurse if she knows the answer to his medical problem or the meaning of his diagnosis. Even when a patient has been told his diagnosis, he may ask the nurse for confirmation and explanation. She, of course, cannot give that explanation without first obtaining the permission of the patient's physician. What has been your experience with uninformed, or inadequately informed, patients?

FS: Very often a patient who is not adequately informed about his condition has a doctor who doesn't want to become emotionally involved with him or his family. You can tell which doctors are like this by watching them with a patient. They will practically run into the room, have a quick chat, and depart as soon as possible to avoid a direct confrontation with the patient. I have often observed this pattern of behavior and sometimes try to help the patient by telephoning the doctor and asking him, "Did you explain the problem to the family? Does the patient want to know his diagnosis?"

ML: Most patients, of course, are told their diagnoses, but doctors vary as to how well they explain it or how frank they are with a patient. I think most nurses are disappointed with doctors who are not sufficiently candid. A lot of doctors feel that once they have told a patient he has cancer, there is no need for further discussion. For most people this is a shattering experience. They need to have the details repeated several times before they can begin to comprehend and accept their situation. I think the reason some doctors don't want to talk about the diagnosis in detail is simply that it makes them feel helpless and therefore uncomfortable. They just don't want to communicate bad news to a patient.

A doctor's reluctance to talk openly can initiate a cycle of isolation and noncommunication. A triangle develops, with the patient thinking his thoughts, the nurse her thoughts, and the doctor his thoughts. This can cause resentment in the patient, who is, after all, the person who matters most. He probably knows what he has and how bad it is, but there is no one with whom he can talk. Thus, in addition to suffering through denial and depression, he will also feel alienated from the health professionals who should be building his trust and confidence.

A lack of communication can also interfere with treatment. A patient who has not sufficiently understood his medical problems and prospects may be reluctant or afraid to undergo therapy.

ES: In contrast to inadequately informed patients, sometimes patients can be informed about their prognosis when they're not ready to hear it. I'm reminded of my aunt who was diagnosed as having lung cancer. I cared about her and wanted to reassure her that someone cared. Soon after the diagnosis, I conveyed to her the need to get her affairs in order. She resented this advice because she didn't believe she was going to die. Because my approach and timing caused such negative feelings, we were never able to discuss her feelings about terminal illness.

Here's another example of well-meaning but poor judgment. One of our patients—a young woman in her 20s—had melanoma metastatic to the lymph nodes. She had been free of the disease for 5 years when, a short time ago, a mass was palpated in her pelvis, and confirmed by diagnostic tests. She was told that this was probably recurrent melanoma and was scheduled for surgery. A nurse who was trying to be helpful asked her what her plans were for the remainder of her life, hoping to encourage her to make the time "meaningful." Until that moment, the young woman had coped very well with the new threat to her health, but the nurse's words were too much for her. She checked herself out of the hospital. Fortunately, further testing showed the mass to be a benign ovarian cyst and surgery was not needed.

I wonder what patients really think when we advise them to enjoy the time remaining to them and to do what they have always wanted to do. I suppose the reaction to such advice is an individual one, but we as nurses should be more careful what we say.

Kim Drucker: People differ in their reactions, and a nurse should respect these differences. Some people deny what they have and it seems to work for them for a while. I don't want to break down that defense. I can't say to someone, "You've got to face life and make something out of the time you have left." Each person has his own defense mechanisms and each family has a way of coping with these defenses. The nurse and doctor can only treat a patient medically, and try to minimize side effects and physical complications while maintaining sensitivity to his psychological needs.

FS: It's not always a matter of whether a patient knows his diagnosis or of how well it's been presented to him, but of whether he wants to know it and has accepted it. Usually, if you listen very carefully, the answer is apparent. Sometimes a patient will refer to his "symptoms," his "complaint," or his "illness." Eventually he may enlarge on that and say, "I think it's a tumor." He may even refer to his malignancy as "cancer." When he reaches this stage, you realize he not only knows but accepts his diagnosis.

However, there are some patients who will tell you outright, "I don't want to know. Don't tell me." If that's what a patient wants, it's perfectly all right, although even this patient inwardly knows the truth. If you watch him carefully, you'll see his knowledge manifested in depression, anger, frustration, or a need for attention. Comments such as "The food's not good enough," "It's too hot," "It's too cold," "It doesn't taste right," or "I can't sleep. My bed's uncomfortable" reveal his state of mind. Once you actually sit down and talk to such a patient and help him understand his diagnosis, his behavior may change.

ER: Mrs. Shepley, how do you reduce anxiety in a patient and/or help him accept his diagnosis?

ES: It isn't so much what I do as how I interact with a patient that reduces his anxiety. I can communicate my warmth and interest simply by being with him. I follow no rules. Sometimes I find a point of common interest. It may be family life, children, sports, travel, or whatever. As we become better acquainted with each other, it becomes easier for him to talk. It's also important that I be relaxed. If I can convey a degree of calm and serenity, a patient who is uptight may relax and begin to express his feelings. I may touch a shoulder or pat an arm. It depends on the patient but almost all of them like a feeling of closeness. As I said before, a patient associates the cancer nurse, as well as his doctor, with his hope for recovery.

ER: A patient who has difficulty confiding in his doctor may have more courage to speak to his nurse. A sensitive nurse will be alert to such a dilemma and consult the attending physician as to how they can best handle the situation.

At other times a patient may never have had the opportunity during his doctor's routine visits to ask him all the questions that bother him. Again, the nurse can be an effective intermediary between patient and doctor. Mr. Stanley, how do you go about finding out what's really troubling a patient?

FS: I find it best not to ask direct questions. When a patient appears upset, there's a tendency to ask him "What's the matter?" or "What's bothering you?" The form of the question suggests that there's something wrong with the patient or that he's behaving badly. Patients suffer enough indignities without receiving additional insults. I find that an indirect statement that doesn't require an answer is most effective in encouraging a patient to share his feelings. "You seem to be upset about something" or "I can tell there's something on your mind" indicates to a patient that I'm aware of how he feels and offer him a choice as to whether he will share his thoughts at that time.

ER: Such a patient may be afraid, among other things. In what ways do you detect fear, and how do you help a patient who is afraid?

FS: One of the most common feelings a patient conceals is fear. Although some people will be quite frank and tell you, "I'm scared stiff," most people don't like to admit they're afraid; and many are afraid without knowing it. Concealed fear may be expressed as depression, withdrawal, or a need for diversion. The most common reaction to fear is withdrawal, where a patient just sleeps for long periods of time. Diversion includes any ordinary behavior carried to an extreme. Some patients read voraciously, day and night; others play their television or radio at high volume for hours; and some joke continuously and refuse to talk about anything serious. These same people are subject to the complaints, outbursts of temper, and other signs of emotional strain that I mentioned. When we have such a patient on the floor, I take time to go into his room, sit down, and talk with him. At some point in the conversation I ask him if he is frightened, and why. He may deny his feelings, but more often he will admit he is afraid. I may then tell him I think I would feel as he does.

I do the same thing with the family. I may see the wife of a patient crying. She will apologize, saying she can't help it, and I will tell her, "This is a normal reaction. You don't like to see your husband this way. You're hurt." It usually works. The wife is relieved of the pressure of having to control her feelings, and she is less reluctant to talk about them.

ER: Miss Lawton, how do you relate to the families of patients?

ML: This depends in part on how the members of a family interpret the nurse's role. Some people see the nurse as an authority figure, while others see her simply as a worker. When the doctor isn't available, one family may be content with talking to the nurse. Another family may say "No" very emphatically when I ask whether I can be of help. Still other families never even ask to speak to the doctor but seek all their information from the nurse.

ER: Mr. Stanley, what do you see as the advantages and disadvantages of a family's presence and participation in the hospital care of a patient?

FS: Relatives are frequently in a highly anxious state and may have a pronounced effect on the patient. It's not unusual for them to spend enormous amounts of time with him, to the extent of sleeping in his room. Often they feel responsibility or guilt for the patient's illness and try to assuage it with overattentiveness. This diligence may express itself through impatience with the hospital services, or through a sense of urgency similar to the apprehensiveness expressed by the patient himself.

The mother of a young boy with Hodgkin's disease practically lived in her son's room and was constantly critical of the nursing care he was receiving. Once she asked me to get her son a mouthwash, and when I did not reappear with it instantly, she ran into the hall, grabbed my coat, and shook me, screaming that I was ignoring her child's needs. I took the woman's arms, held her firmly, and said, "Calm down. I'm going to get the mouthwash in a few minutes. Now, please sit here in the nursing station and drink a cup of coffee." I wanted to reassert a sense of priorities so she would realize that a mouthwash was not an acute medical necessity.

An inexperienced nurse may tend to view relatives as impediments and try to work around them. She will acknowledge their presence and try to accommodate them without compromising her duties. However, she will soon learn that a family's participation in the care of a patient can be advantageous to herself, the patient, and his family. The family's ability to do things for the patient frees her for other duties, gives the patient a sense of family warmth and support, and gives the family itself a feeling of participation and usefulness. Once a nurse appreciates the complex feelings behind the relatives' behavior, she will have much more empathy, patience, and understanding.

ER: Are there any particular problems or areas of conflict concerning the nurse-patient-family relationship that occur more frequently than others?

FS: Yes. Some of the most difficult problems for the nurses revolve around the children of older patients. One often witnesses the culmination of long-term conflicts when a parent is seriously ill. A child who feels he has neglected his parents may try to compensate for this during the illness of one of them. He may externalize his guilty feelings by accusing the nursing staff of neglect. Obviously the nurses shouldn't take these accusations personally. They should understand that he is merely berating himself.

The family conflicts that surface in the hospital have usually been present for years, and a nurse would be naïve to think she could help solve them with a little attention and discussion. Child-parent conflicts can be deep and painful. Sometimes the parent perpetuates the suffering by refusing to accept his child's offer of help, saying "It's too late." The parent implies that he will carry his child's "crime" unexcused into the grave, and the child feels he can never atone for it. The nurse and the doctor must appreciate how powerful this experience can be and, when feasible, try to play the role of mediator. I have seen adult children engage in a fistfight in the hospital room when one accused another of not giving their parent the attention he needed.

ER: How else can a family create difficulties for the nursing staff?

FS: The family of terminally ill people can also be difficult if they have not accepted that their loved one is dying. This is hard on the patient, whose natural withdrawal into himself is contradicted by his relatives' refusal to let him die. This is more common when the patient is fairly young. The wife of a man in his 40s, dying of advanced cancer, was so anxious about her husband that she woke him up every 20 minutes to find out his level of consciousness. She brought the children into the room and they prayed for an impossible recovery for hours each day. They prayed and cried for so long that when the end approached we had to bring in a special nurse to support them in case they became uncontrollable when he died. They did manage to cope with his death when it occurred, but their holding on made his dying more difficult for everyone, especially for him.

ER: Do you have any suggestions for achieving closer family cooperation with the hospital staff?

FS: A good way to sort out a lot of problems is for the doctor to call a family conference, and include the patient and the nursing staff. Then everyone is in the picture. Each knows what the other knows, and no one is being protected. It eliminates a lot of frustration. It eliminates pretense. A daughter needn't say, "Oh, mother, you're looking much better today," when both mother and daughter know she is actually looking a lot worse. Such a conference also provides the family with an opportunity to communicate directly with the doctor and the nursing staff. A nurse who is caring for a cancer patient becomes involved with the entire family, because the family and the patient go through the same agony.

ER: Mrs. Shepley, you've spoken of your involvement with your patients and of your own hurt when one of them suffers or dies. How does this affect your own family?

ES: My family is involved in my work. I talk about the problems of patients at home, because the patients are a part of my life. My family sympathizes with me when I need sympathy and supports me when I need support. When I go through a period of anxiety about a patient who has developed new metastases or a low blood count, my family suffers with me. I don't want to just be a clinical nurse while I'm in the hospital and then go home and forget about it. On the other hand, I don't let it dominate my life. I have plenty of activities and other involvements. I think that's very important.

ER: I wonder what all three of you feel about the limits of treatment. Should vigorous treatment ever be stopped, and when should it cease?

FS: I have strong feelings about that. The cessation of treatment is the doctor's decision, of course, but his decision affects the nursing staff. I have often seen a patient who is not responding to treatment. He may be breaking down with bedsores, mouth ulcers, and weight loss. Everything seems to be going against him, yet some doctors will still feel they must carry on treatment as vigorously as possible. Quite often I'll say, "For what? Why all this?" and the doctor may reply, "Well, there's always hope." I realize that no one wants to give up hope, but I feel that it would be better if doctors would get together with members of a family and say, "The time has come when we literally can do no more." However, some doctors seem to think the family's minds will be eased if the patient has a nasogastric tube and intravenous fluids. Also, I find that many doctors cannot accept death because they interpret it as a failure on their part. Many nurses also have difficulty in coping with a patient who is dying.

ES: A short time ago I helped care for a 45-year-old man who had recurrent colon cancer. He was on chemotherapy. We saw him once a week, and each time he was depressed, dependent, and totally dejected. Then one day his personality seemed to change. He sat up straight, seemed confident, and in a firm, clear voice announced that he didn't want any more chemotherapy, that it wasn't helping him, and that he was ready to die. He stated that he no longer liked his body and that he didn't like the kind of person he had become. He seemed relieved that he had reached this decision and had shared his feelings with me. His condition at that time was not really terminal, but to everyone's surprise, he was admitted to the hospital the following week with extreme weakness and died 2 days later.

I had asked him if he was frightened of a painful death because I wanted to reassure him that we could use medication to reduce his pain as much as possible. He said he was not afraid of pain, but that he didn't like the idea of IVs and other tubes. We also discussed his right to refuse treatment.

FS: I recently had a similar experience. I admitted a 72-year-old patient with a leg ulcer. There was a form on the front of his chart which said that in the event of his having a heart attack, he did not want any heroics. He didn't want any cardiac resuscitation. He just wanted to be allowed to die in peace. That was the first form I've seen in this hospital, and I showed it to the staff. I said, "At last we're coming down to reality. Medical personnel are actually facing the fact that when the time comes, a patient should have the choice of how he is to die."

Peculiarly enough, the refusal of treatment is much more common in females than in males. They will say, "Oh, for goodness' sake, leave me alone. Let me die. Take that IV out." I'm sorry that in such a case my response must be, "You'll have to discuss this with your doctor." I have known two patients who said to their doctors point-blank, "I don't want any of this. Leave me alone."

ER: What did the doctors do in these cases?

FS: They had to accept their patients' wishes. A patient has the right to refuse treatment. Not long ago a patient with complete renal failure hadn't passed urine for a whole week. He had a cardiac problem as well as a malignancy. The doctor sat down to discuss the situation with me and said, "As far as I'm concerned there's nothing more we can do for this man." I said, "I wholeheartedly agree with you. We'll do what we can to make him comfortable." I came back the following day and the patient was again receiving intravenous fluids. When the doctor arrived, I asked him what had happened and he replied,

"Believe it or not, his son said I had to continue the IVs." The patient lived 4 more days.
ML: People want to live, but everyone has his own set of conditions, and these conditions have to be respected. Some people would rather be dead than deformed or dependent. On the other hand, a lot of people sit around and say, "Boy, I wouldn't want anyone to have to do that for me." But if they become sick, they feel differently. Then they say, "I remember when I was well I thought I'd rather die than be in this condition. But now that I'm like this, I still want help. I still want to live." A patient has to be able to examine his own feelings, and we have to try to determine what he really wants.
ER: Kim, will you comment on your role as an office nurse? What can a nurse in an office situation offer a patient that is not available in the hospital?
KD: As an office nurse, I'm in a situation of being the coordinator to help solve the problems patients encounter at home. I'm the one who telephones them frequently and makes sure they know they have someone they can turn to whenever they're in trouble or when they're down and just need to talk. My role in the office setting is a psychological one as well as medical.

An office nurse can help meet the need for familiarity and continuity. When a person is in the hospital, he has various nurses on three daily shifts. The office nurse is the steady person he knows will be there. Therefore, when one of our patients is in the hospital, I can act as a listener and also as a liaison between him, the hospital staff, and the physician.
ER: Liz, you've been involved in home care as a nurse coordinator. How do you think you can help patients and their families develop a good home-care program?
Lizabeth Light: If a patient feels well enough to take some responsibility for his own care, we help him learn what to do. For a patient who doesn't have the physical reserve to care for himself, it's important to let friends and family assist. However, patients are often reluctant to let family members get involved; and sometimes the family is timid and insecure about their ability to care for the patient. The more we as nurses can do in the hospital to start teaching home-care procedures to family and patient, the more successful the transfer to home care will be. By training family and patient in the hospital, we can evaluate their skills, reinforce our teaching methods, or even arrange for some supplemental assistance at home, if that seems appropriate. Most patients would prefer to go home, so if you can identify their needs early in the hospitalization and involve family and friends in the learning process, home care can be accomplished smoothly.
ER: In the office we see chronically ill patients who are more depressed than they would be if they were in the hospital. By living at home and coming to the office for treatment, they are facing the reality of what their disease means to their normal life. What is the best approach a nurse can take to help alleviate this natural depression?
KD: To the extent that a patient has nonmedical problems that have arisen as a result of the disease—such as a lack of communication with family members or the inability to do something in particular—we can try to find a way to help in that situation by talking to the patient and family members, together or separately, and then work for a mutually acceptable solution.
ER: You handle a lot of questions and answers from patients and their families on the telephone during the day. What advice do you give them to help them cope?
KD: It's different for each person, but basically I receive a question such as, "How am I going to deal with this situation at home?" "How am I ever going to live a normal life?" I try to help that person see that although they have a problem, they have faced it. They are dealing with it. They are doing everything they can by getting the appropriate treatments.

I advise a patient to be as active as he can—to go to work, if that is possible; and, if he can't work, to spend as much time with his family as possible, if that's what he wants; or to indulge in his hobbies. A person who has cancer knows he has this overwhelming thing and that he has a choice in how to deal with it. The doctors and nurses are there for support—to listen to them and their families. The support systems are set up and any problems patients and families have can be dealt with. It's not impossible. Nothing is impossible.

LL: I agree. It's really only in the past few years that there has been a bit more emphasis on cancer as a chronic illness. Hopefully, this aspect of the disease will receive more emphasis in the future. Many people have cancer and they live with it for a long time.

Becky Moore: It's true. People increasingly look at cancer as a chronic disease. However, a lot of people are still dying from it, and I take care of many dying people. I think that to make it clear to someone that they are never going to be deserted while they are dying is very important. I remember a patient who had a slogan on her wall that said, "Face your fear and it will disappear." It became inevitable that she was going to die and she wanted to talk about what was going to happen to her when she did die. She needed to talk about her fear of death. When you open up the whole subject of death to someone who's clearly dying, he may be incredibly relieved to finally have someone to talk to. So often he doesn't want to scare his family; it can be traumatic to talk to a loved one or family member about specific fears of death. But a patient can ask concrete questions of a nurse. I find that people who go into cancer nursing are especially sensitive to identifying with such patient needs.

ER: What effect have new medical techniques had on your role as a nurse?

BM: There are changes being made that have really benefited the cancer nurse in a hospital setting. For example, most large hospitals now have oncology units specifically designated to take care of cancer patients. When I started nursing, oncology patients were mixed up with other patients on the medical-surgical floors, and little attention was paid to their specific needs. Also, the nurses who took care of them often didn't really want to take care of people with cancer. Many had cancer phobia.

Consistency and continuity in nursing care is important to both patient and nurse. One thing that can enhance continuity is to provide more outpatient services to enable people to be at home rather than in the hospital. For example, in our unit, we do outpatient blood transfusions and outpatient chemotherapy. It's a real morale boost to us as nurses to see people we've taken care of when they were acutely ill walk into the hospital after work, get a blood transfusion, and then walk out to go home. That gives *us* a lot of hope. We are able to see that people aren't always acutely ill and sick in bed. Cancer nursing is a lot less depressing when we see people functioning in the world and coming to us only for periodic treatments.

ER: What are the recent changes in cancer nursing?

BM: The changes that occurred in cancer nursing are mainly clinical ones. Nurses receive more specific education in the technical skills, such as the administration of chemotherapy, with the result that cancer nursing has become even more of a specialty area than it was before.

However, I don't think the direct care of patients has changed much. People who go into cancer nursing have always done so not because of the technical skills they will develop but because of the emotional aspects of taking care of people with cancer, and the special kind of continuity that they can have with such patients. By continuity I mean that you see them throughout all the phases of their illness, from diagnosis through treatment, and sometimes when they are dying. I think that the people who are going into cancer nursing now have to make a firm commitment to maintain such continuity— to share in the whole process that their patients are going through.

LL: One of the major changes I've noticed in the 7 years I've been in nursing is that patients and families are much more informed today. I now see my role as being expanded to that of teacher, because patients are taking more responsibility for finding out about their disease and treatments so they can make more informed decisions about their therapies.

I also feel that I've become more of a patient advocate. Patients sometimes get into situations where they're afraid to ask their doctors for information or they're afraid to bother the physicians or the nursing staff with certain problems. I like to think of myself as helping them set up dialogues with their physicians and helping the physicians know what their patients need.

BM: Patients should decide what their needs are and be assertive about having them met. A nurse can help them articulate these needs. After all, they are in the hospital, lying in bed. They feel sick. They may have had some devastating news given to them, and they are trying to make a decision about what they want to do about it. They often need a nurse to help them figure out what their plan of action is going to be. That's the first step. When they have decided such things as what treatment to have or whether to go home, we can help them implement their plan. We often see patients pushed by their physician or their family into doing something against their will, so I think it's important for a nurse to help patients to be assertive and stick to their guns. Too often patients adopt the attitude, "I'm in your hands, doctor. Do whatever you please." What the doctor wants often isn't what the patient really wants; at the same time, the patient wants to be a "good patient" and to please his doctor.

ER: The nurse is now playing the role not only in educating patients but in educating other nurses and participating in physician programs. What do you consider to be the future role of the cancer nurse?

LL: I've been impressed with all the cancer nurses I've met—not just here in the Bay Area, but across the nation. Cancer nurses seem to be a highly motivated group of people who are interested in learning more about their profession and keeping up with what is happening in cancer research and treatment.

As for new directions, we now have an international oncology nursing society, a dynamic group involved in all aspects of cancer care, including nursing research. When I did my training, we didn't even have a special course on cancer nursing; most schools have now added such a course to the curriculum. That's why I see good things for cancer nurses. We're getting more organized. For instance, in the Bay Area, we've established a network for the exchange of information. If someone in the East Bay has developed a protocol for extravasation (a chemotherapy leak into the skin), we're close enough so that we can share that information with each other. It's exciting to participate in these changes, to see our specialty grow, and to support one another.

24

Social services

Social workers who directly assist cancer patients are usually affiliated with hospitals, government agencies, or independent organizations such as the American Cancer Society. They evaluate, plan, coordinate resources, and support patients in a variety of ways, depending on the administrative structure and purposes of their organization. Their overall goals are the same—to help the cancer patient, emotionally, financially, and/or with material goods.

To show the breadth of their activities, I interviewed an official of the American Cancer Society and two medical social workers associated with major medical centers: Mount Zion Hospital and Medical Center and Stanford University Medical Center.

John Caton, M.S.W., M.P.H., Director of Health and Rehabilitation Services of the San Francisco Unit of the American Cancer Society speaks of the San Francisco Unit's services, which are similar to ACS services in other parts of the country.

Irene Harrison, L.C.S.W., Clinical Social Worker with the Claire Zellerbach Saroni Tumor Institute and Oncology Unit of Mt. Zion Hospital and Medical Center in San Francisco, believes patients should be made aware of the services of the social worker early in their diagnosis.

Patricia Fobair, M.S.W., M.P.H., Department of Radiation Oncology, Stanford University Medical Center, talks about changes in patient attitudes and issues critical to the person who has cancer: employment and life and medical insurance. Formerly associated with Mt. Zion Hospital and Medical Center, Ms. Fobair also discusses her experience in forming a discussion group for cancer patients.

JOHN CATON, AMERICAN CANCER SOCIETY

JC: The emotional and financial impact of a cancer diagnosis is overwhelming for many of us. Due to financial hardship, emotional distress, or lack of information, we often cannot easily find our way through the myriad of physicians, specialists, hospitals, clinics, home-care agencies, and social service organizations. Getting the right kind of help at the right time is made more difficult by co-deductibles, exclusions, financial means tests, and home-care limitations that are characteristic of most public and private insurance.

We at the American Cancer Society in San Francisco believe that everyone in our community should have equal access to health care and a right to make their own decisions. With this in mind, we encourage people to look toward us as a central resource for information about a variety of cancer-related issues. We urge them to call us regardless of their questions. Typically, the average caller has many questions concerning diagnosis, treatment alternatives, financial matters, concrete services, and emotional concerns. To assist persons in dealing with these multiple issues, our staff must have a high degree of listening and counseling skills and a knowledge of community resources.

When someone calls, we try to assess their particular situation. A simple request for general information often leads to a discussion of the person's individual concerns. A woman who initially asks for a pamphlet on breast cancer treatment will not get all the information she needs if there is also a personal reason for making a request. She may be experiencing a symptom that worries her, or she might be currently under treatment and need information about alternatives. Perhaps she is calling on behalf of a relative or friend and wants our advice on how to talk to that person. Whatever her concerns might be, we use our knowledge and experience to help her make her own decisions and take action. We know quite a bit about health care and community resources, and we also have practical experience with the intricate workings of the various hospitals and clinics in our community. We never give medical advice, but we always give whatever medical information is available to us.

We often are involved in a longer relationship with people beyond the short-term counseling, information, and referral. If the person isn't able to handle their situation by themselves, or if the extent of their illness requires complicated decisions about medical and nursing care, then we will offer counseling assistance. There are a great many people in San Francisco for whom we provide either counseling or concrete services.

Our counseling is individualized. We visit persons at home if they are unable to come to our office. Sometimes the counseling involves coordinating medical care or assisting with financial matters on a continuing basis. Often, however, the counseling deals with the emotional and psychological effect the illness is having on patients and their families.

The American Cancer Society also sponsors and encourages the development of group counseling programs. It currently sponsors various "I Can Cope" programs throughout the country. "I Can Cope" was developed by the Minnesota Division of ACS and combines patient education with group support in an 8-week course that emphasizes information and positive methods of coping. The course is open to both patients and their families and is usually cosponsored by a hospital or community organization.

The American Cancer Society also has a number of concrete services it provides to persons with cancer. The exact nature of these services and their method of delivery varies in each community since each local chapter has its own way of doing things.

The concrete services are really meant to allow persons to convalesce at home and avoid costly and inappropriate hospitalization. Patients served by the American Cancer Society discover that a number of services are coordinated by staff to ease the physical, emotional, and financial burden of their illness. Our assistive-device program provides for the loan or rental of wheelchairs, walkers, commodes, hospital beds, overbed tables, bedpans, or other such equipment for use at home. The kind of loan item varies in each community, so it is wise to check with the local ACS office on the availability of specific items.

We also provide gift items that people can keep. In San Francisco we can occasionally provide blenders, nutrition handbooks, nutritional supplements, incontinent supplies, sterile dressings, and ostomy supplies. In addition, we may provide prosthetic devices such as electrolarynxes for laryngectomized persons, breast prostheses for women with mastectomies, or wigs for those who need them.

The American Cancer Society recognizes that traveling to radiation or chemotherapy treatment can be difficult for many people. We provide transportation to these treatments, usually through volunteers. The San Francisco office has a paid transportation program that utilizes local cabs and mini-vans from Canon Kip Operation Transportation, a community-based organization.

We are a voluntary nonprofit organization and, as such, we pride ourselves on volunteer action. Volunteers assist us in all of our service and rehabilitation programs. Our nonsterile dressings, laryngectomy bibs, and temporary breast prostheses are produced and donated by the volunteers of the Order of Eastern Star. They also assemble rehabilitation kits for our volunteer visiting programs.

Volunteers who have recovered from cancer make visits to persons facing illness through the American Cancer Society's Reach to Recovery, ostomy, and laryngectomy rehabilitation programs. The guiding philosophy behind these programs is that a person who has experienced and overcome cancer can provide invaluable emotional support and practical advice to someone else. We're really fortunate to have a number of dedicated volunteers whom we either train ourselves, or who come to us from self-help organizations like the United Ostomy Association and the International Association of Laryngectomees.

People who have mastectomies, ileostomies, colostomies, urostomies, or laryngectomies usually have important rehabilitation issues to deal with, and they often must wear a prosthetic device. Volunteers from the American Cancer Society, United Ostomy Association, or International Association of Laryngectomees offer practical assistance without giving medical advice. They show through their personal example that complete recovery is possible through early detection and proper medical treatment.

In all our services we try to make sure that everyone in our community has equal access. This means that we often reach out to those who ordinarily would not ask for help. San Francisco is a city with great diversity, composed of neighborhoods defined by culture, race, age, income, and life-style. Yet within these very neighborhoods are pockets of poverty and isolation. We have a responsibility to all residents of the city in making sure that our services reach them in a way that respects their individual and cultural integrity.

Ernest Rosenbaum: Is everyone eligible for counseling, information, and volunteer rehabilitation visits?

JC: Yes. These are free services.

ER: What about the cost of assistive devices?

JC: We usually look into other financial sources available to patients first and help them take advantage of their private or public insurance coverage. If they have no source to pay for these items, then we supply them.

ER: Are there limits to your transportation program?

JC: Yes. We can transport persons in San Francisco only for radiation or chemotherapy. However, this is significant since radiation therapy patients usually go to treatment daily.

ER: There is also a unique program available in San Francisco. Could you describe it?

JC: Through the use of two trusts administered by the San Francisco Foundation, we provide attendant care for homebound San Francisco residents and assistance with room and board for out-of-county patients who undergo treatment in San Francisco. Known as the Miller-Bunting Program for Cancer Patients (provided through the Doris

Martin Miller and Virginia McCormick Bunting trusts and administered by the San Francisco Foundation), this project coordinates a variety of casework services for patients receiving attendant care. The American Cancer Society pays for a director and an assistant to administer the program. Both of these people are professional medical social workers.

Attendant care involves personal care and/or household services as part of a medical and social plan allowing patients to remain at home. Attendant care services range from homemaker service to personal care performed by a skilled or semiskilled person. Patients can receive a maximum of 40 hours each week. Once patients are admitted to service, we are committed to assisting them through the entire course of their illness, even though they may initially need only minimal care.

Attendant care is provided by a core of more than 50 self-employed home-care attendants with varying skills. The desirability of home-care is assessed by professional American Cancer Society staff, who determine the total nursing and social needs of patients. In making this assessment, they consult with the patients, their families, physicians, hospital social workers and discharge planning staff, visiting nurses, and others responsible for providing care. The Miller-Bunting staff also provides counseling to home-care patients and families through regular home visits aimed at assisting them with the psychological impact of their illness.

The room-and-board aspect of the Miller-Bunting Program for Cancer Patients is designed to help pay the living costs for people who come to San Francisco for outpatient treatment. We generally make arrangements for them to stay at a guest house near the hospital.

ER: Your services sound very comprehensive.

JC: Yes. Typically, one patient may receive multiple assistance from the San Francisco office: home care, counseling, hospital bed, wheelchair, incontinent supplies, or nutritional supplements.

ER: Are you sometimes forced to turn down requests?

JC: We try to evaluate a person's entire family and financial situation. Generally, we offer assistance to those who can't get help elsewhere. The demand for attendant care, assistive devices, and transportation has increased dramatically over the last few years. These supportive services that enable people to remain at home are not provided to any great extent by public and private insurance, which are institutionally biased. This means that the American Cancer Society needs to examine its priorities. The voluntary health movement has an increasing responsibility in direct service, particularly as it relates to home-care needs.

ER: So you think finances are a big factor for many people with cancer?

JC: Yes. I personally believe that adequate medical care and supportive services should be a right, not a privilege. No one facing a chronic life-threatening illness should be denied the right to treatment because of financial hardship. A recent statewide patient-needs study conducted by the California Division of the American Cancer Society revealed that cancer patients with annual incomes under $15,000 delayed seeking treatment, had less access to medical care, and experienced higher stress.

ER: What programs of the American Cancer Society do you think are most valuable?

JC: The public-education and service programs that emphasize individual prevention techniques, early detection, and assistance in obtaining medical treatment are the most valuable programs. In the future, I hope the American Cancer Society will increase its efforts to eliminate known carcinogens from the general environment and from the workplace through public education and legislative advocacy.

IRENE HARRISON, MT. ZION HOSPITAL AND MEDICAL CENTER

ER: What do you perceive to be the effect on the public of all the information that is now available concerning cancer?

IH: With the increase in information about cancer available through the media, there is also a tendency to come to simplistic conclusions. Cancer is an umbrella term that includes many different types of malignancies. What they have in common is the fear they evoke.

Although the public is more informed today about cancer and available services, and although patients are encouraged to be active participants in their health care, the impact of a cancer diagnosis on an individual continues to be minimized by medical personnel as well as by members of the public. Studies show that cancer has a tremendous impact on the individual and the family.

ER: What can the social worker do to relieve this situation?

IH: Through interviews with cancer patients, we have learned that many of them would have liked to have been helped at the time of diagnosis but that they didn't know about the availability of the social worker's services. In some cases, patients weren't able to verbalize their needs and in other cases there were no social workers available.

However, these interviews have helped us to identify typical critical stress periods such as the time of the original diagnosis, entry into the hospital, the period of therapy and, for some people, the terminal phase of illness. With diagnosis comes shock; after that, people tend to mobilize their energies to participate in treatment. This is followed by an effort to forget cancer and go on with the business of living. If there is a recurrence, a cancer patient experiences a new but different crisis state. The final stage of illness occurs when treatment is no longer effective. The patient is then confronted with another psychological task.

We know that along the cancer disease continuum, strong feelings are evoked and that these feelings need expression. Family life is frequently disrupted. Priorities have to be reset. Problems of self-esteem, sexual functioning, social, financial, and vocational concerns are common, but frequently not openly discussed, creating additional tensions.

What we do know is that it is difficult for people to ask for help with emotional and psychological concerns. It is considered a weakness. Frequently, physicians are in collusion with this attitude, making it even more difficult for patients and their families to seek help and advice. It would therefore be helpful if the clinical social worker were to provide routine evaluation and assessment of every cancer patient. The social worker could then intervene as early as the period of diagnosis if she or he perceived the need. Trauma could more easily be dealt with at an early stage and future problems anticipated. Even though the intervention might only be periodic, the patient and his family would have a familiar person to contact when problems or questions arise.

The person who is ill needs to be viewed in his social context, which means that attention should be paid to his family and friends. There are some special services directed toward the family and friends to give them an opportunity to discuss and share their concerns.

To achieve comprehensive care, the health care system needs to make the services of the social worker available to all patients, especially during critical times. With advances in medical knowledge and the increased complexity of the health care system, it is essential that we also increase the medical system's sensitivity to the psychosocial needs of patients.

PATRICIA FOBAIR, STANFORD UNIVERSITY MEDICAL CENTER

ER: Before you joined the staff of the Stanford University Medical Center, you were associated with the Claire Zellerbach Saroni Tumor Institute at Mt. Zion Hospital and Medical Center. While there, you initiated a discussion group for cancer patients that is still functioning. How did you happen to do this?

PF: The first meeting of the staff-patient discussion group at the Claire Zellerbach Saroni Institute took place in February 1972. The idea for forming the group came to me when I noticed that a number of patients were lingering around the Institute after completing their course of radiation therapy. Though their disease was in remission, they seemed lost; they didn't know what to do with themselves. I thought they might need to talk about what that meant in terms of present strain and worry.

At an Institute staff meeting I introduced the idea of bringing these patients together with staff members for informal discussions. A resident and two staff members were willing to participate on a trial basis, so the first meeting consisted of these three people, six or seven patients, and myself.

ER: How did that first group of patients respond to the experience?

PF: They came to the meeting because they liked the idea, but they were also apprehensive. They didn't know exactly what was going to happen, and they weren't certain that they wanted therapy sessions. However, they soon relaxed and began to talk.

They first discussed their angry feelings toward their physicians. They vented a lot of anger about what had happened to them during their diagnostic and treatment periods. Later they discussed problems in their personal lives. These were usually related to employment, family relationships, and the broader issue of their own mental health.

ER: What did you feel were the sources of their anger, especially toward their physicians?

PF: There were several factors. Some patients were angry at themselves for having acquired the disease. They felt their bodies had let them down. They couldn't understand this or answer the question, "Why me?" Others were angry because there had been a delay in obtaining a diagnosis. Whether this was their own fault or that of a doctor, the resulting frustration had to be integrated with their other feelings.

Several of the patients had problems that originated in the doctor-patient relationship. A doctor is in a position of great importance, a Godlike figure. Few patients feel themselves to be his peers. Instead, they have toward doctors some of the parent-child feelings that accompany reverence for authority. The patients in the group needed a chance to reassert themselves and equalize the score. Being a patient meant submitting to medical care and going along with someone else's program, and they were reluctant to do that without offering some resistance. Their entire medical experience was a regressive one that they were partly able to overcome by releasing emotional tension in the group discussions.

ER: The group was successful, then, in helping them to think through their problems. How did they actually accomplish this? What steps were involved?

PF: They went through a number of stages. They began, as I said, by telling their medical stories and talking about their unhappy feelings. After a few weeks they were less depressed. Then they began to talk about their personal problems. They got a lot of support from the other members of the group and they soon began to take more responsibility for directing their lives in areas over which they had some control. For example, a widowed lady with ovarian cancer used the group for 1 year. She had had a distressing surgical experience at another hospital and was able to reveal her feelings about that, the hospital staff, and her disease. Eventually she began to talk about her relationships with her son and daughter, and the difficulties the three of them had shared after the death of her husband. She also discussed her relationship with her sister, whom she had always envied. After sharing her feelings about these experiences for several weeks, she suddenly began to talk about her hobbies and interests and about new activities in which she might participate. Within a year of joining the group, she had planned and successfully taken a trip to Europe, changed her place of living, and started a new life.

ER: Did some patients fail to benefit from the group, and, if so, to what do you attribute their failure to use the group to their advantage?

PF: Over a period of months and years there were patients who entered the group in the hope of finding something for themselves but who discovered they could not work out their problems or get support from the other patients. To try to find out why this occurred, I developed a questionnaire that I circulated to all the patient participants. I observed that if a patient comes into the group when he is very sick or in a deeply depressed state of mind and does not find someone else in the group with whom to identify, he finds it difficult to make a connection with the group as a whole. A group tends to operate on the basis of identification among its members and the projection of one's own problems onto others. Also, some people choose to withdraw at critical moments in their lives rather than to talk about their problems. But I discovered that people who are willing to talk, and who use talking as a way of relating to others and solving problems, get the most out of this kind of therapy.

The willingness to speak about having cancer is also important, but not all patients feel it is helpful to communicate openly about their disease process. They feel that it will seem worse if they talk too much about it, and they prefer to try to put it out of their minds between treatments.

Some patients have such strong emotional support within their families and such good prognoses that they have no need for the group.

ER: Do you think that some patients who didn't feel they benefited from the group were people who were failing medically and who expected the group to solve some of their medical problems?

PF: Yes. It was common for a patient to have a fantasy that the group could solve his medical problems. He would say, "I wish the doctor . . . " or "I wish the group could solve my cancer problems."

Our group was composed of 50% patients with cures or good remissions and 50% patients with progressive disease. The latter patients joined the group when they knew they were not doing well medically but when they were still active physically and eager to participate in group discussions. Later, when they became weaker, and showed physical deterioration, they were able to use the group for support. Quite a few of them died while still members of the group.

ER: How did the other members of the group feel and how did they behave when such a person was failing?

PF: They felt very sad. It's important, in a group process, for members to share with the failing member their own feelings about his impending death and to ask him how he wants them to act.

A person with rectal carcinoma that has metastasized has used the group as a source of energy and a means of maintaining his activity level. He's a person who believes in communicating. Now that he's going downhill, he is asked by the others at the beginning of many of our sessions how he wants us to respond to him. Does he want us to ignore the fact that he's failing or does he want us to talk about it and give him feedback? He says he wants us to be honest and direct with him, and he also is able to let us express our feelings for him. However, when I told him I was sad about the way he looked, he said, "I'll forgive you this time, but I really don't want you to feel sad for me." He still wants people to feel as though he is going to make it and to help bolster him. I suspect that should this particular patient die, a number of us will go to his funeral because of the intensity of our feelings for him. We've also been involved with his family because his wife and children have used the group.

ER: Did the families of patients participate in the group?

PF: Yes, quite a few spouses came. It was up to a patient to invite his or her spouse and the spouse was free to accept or decline the invitation. The group was very open-ended that way.

ER: What was the average number of participants in the group?

PF: We averaged 8 to 14 patients, plus 2 or 3 staff members, per session. We had as many as 17 to 20 patients at one time, but that proved unwieldy. We met once a week for 2 hours.

ER: How many relatives usually came?

PF: It fluctuated. The maximum number of relatives who attended a particular session was three.

ER: Have you heard of groups similar to the one you had in any other part of the United States?

PF: The first group I heard about before ours was at the University of California Medical School in the maxillo-facial unit, where Doris Ordway had a group for cancer patients who had undergone head or neck surgery. Since then I've been told about groups at Memorial Hospital in New York that consist of postoperative mastectomy patients and their relatives. Stanford University Hospital has a group especially for new cancer patients and a group for patients with advanced breast cancer. Other groups are being formed in San Francisco. Kaiser Hospital has started a group that is attended by a social worker, an oncology nurse, and a psychologist.

I think our group was unique because it included patients with different diagnoses, ages, stage of disease, and family situations. Also, we focused on rehabilitation. A patient in our group was encouraged to do all he could to adjust to his disease and not let it ruin his life.

ER: In other words, you were helping patients to develop a way of life rather than an approach to death.

PF: Yes, but we did discuss death, of course. Nevertheless, the group was most valuable in helping people to live with their disease. The patients defined this as their focus and I certainly concur. Their attitude was, "First you mourn and grieve your condition and then you figure out what you can do to improve your life."

The group was a place for patients to talk over the problems of cancer that affect daily living. We encouraged them to be frank with their doctors and not to let the hospital, as an institution, get the best of them. They were encouraged to defend themselves, to fight if an employer laid them off their job; and, if they did not succeed in such a situation, to find new employment.

ER: Some time has passed since you began the group at Mt. Zion. You are now with Stanford University Medical Center. What changes have occurred in the intervening years?

PF: So many new ideas and concepts have entered the cancer patient's arena that one can say there is a new stage now forming, with the patient more in central focus working with physician in greater equity. The picture of the cancer patient as an uninformed, pitiable victim relying heavily on the physician as rescuer has now shifted to a scene where the person with cancer learns as much as possible about his diagnosis prior to or during treatment, where he participates in decisions regarding alternative forms of treatment and asks for social services and group support. In other words, an important change has occurred in the physician-patient relationship and in the patient's desire for additional social service.

Another important change has been a shift in perspective from looking at cancer as a fatal disease to viewing it as a chronic illness with ongoing needs. These needs include patient education and support from physicians and other care givers. This new attitude has emerged because cancer patients are surviving beyond their initial estimate of prognosis as a result of better medical detection and treatment. Thus there is more interest among patients and professionals in the quality of life of cancer patients.

There is now evidence of recognition by national agencies such as the National Cancer Institute and the American Cancer Society that psychological issues are important areas for behavioral research. During the late 1970s the National Cancer Institute funded psychological research, thereby laying the groundwork for a data base on which future research could be developed. This year (1981), the American Cancer Society convened the first National Workshop on Psychological Social and Behavioral Medicine aspects of cancer and is making plans to fund research in this area.

A number of health-related movements have had an impact on concepts in the cancer field.

The surge of interest in death and dying led by E. Kubler-Ross, M.D., stimulated public interest and discussion on the subject of cancer. The stigma of cancer has been challenged further by the holistic health movement, which has added educational and psychological concepts to the treatment of cancer and encouraged cancer patients' involvement in helping themselves gain control over the disease along with medical treatment.

Encouraged by the self-help movement and the American Cancer Society's "I Can Cope" program, cancer patient discussion groups have expanded in hospitals and communities throughout the country. The patient's desire for education and self-help tools has led to a whole new literature for cancer patients to assist them in the illness experience.

Cancer rehabilitation is just beginning to take shape as an integrated form of rehabilitation. Physical rehabilitation has many more options to offer patients than was true a few years ago. Breast reconstruction, limb salvage, and the improvements made in prosthetic devices mean that a greater number of patients will be able to experience themselves as less damaged by therapy than they would have several years ago. There is greater involvement of physical and occupational therapists as well as clinical social workers and nurses in the patient's hospital recovery process.

The many questions about the quality of patient survival will be examined further in research to be funded by the American Cancer Society during the 1980s. Personal needs and quality-of-life issues, such as the need to continue working or to have the option to change jobs, are now becoming an area for greater focus for patients and health care professionals.

ER: What are the employment problems of cancer patients?

PF: There are two problems related to employability for cancer patients: keeping the current job he or she has held over the years; or finding a new job following the completion of therapy. Many studies have examined the question whether there is discrimination against employees returning to work following completion of cancer therapy. In one study, by Frances Feldman, 20 to 25% of adult patients reported severe employment difficulties. Other studies by Feldman and Foster looked at the problems of younger patients and found that 70% had difficulties in retaining or obtaining a job. However, this is a complex area requiring further examination. Sometimes job difficulties result from factors in the employment system, and sometimes they result from changes within the person with cancer.

One way of looking at work-related problems is to ask a large group of cancer patients if they had problems returning to work. In studies conducted by Frances Feldman for the American Cancer Society in 1976, 1978, and 1981, 50% of 138 white-collar adults experienced general work-related problems, such as difficulty in obtaining a promotion, whereas 2% suffered gross difficulties such as maintaining their position. Among 114 blue-collar workers, 84% experienced general problems; 50% had greater difficulties such as holding their position or experiencing at least one job rejection. Among 83 younger patients, fewer were employed, yet 25% had serious problems with employers.

Another way of looking at possible employment problems of cancer patients is by the percentage of patients who return to work by diagnostic category. In two different studies, Barofsky and Ashenburg, 70 and 85% of patients with breast and uterine cancer were able to return to work, whereas 42 and 68% of colon-rectal cancer patients returned to work.

While the rehabilitation act of 1973 classifies a cancer patient as a handicapped person and permits such persons to file formal complaint, only a small percentage of actual complaints are filed by cancer patients. Yet job discrimination is an everyday event. It occurs in personnel selection, in promotion evaluation, among workers, and by supervisors as they go about their day-to-day activities. As such, the process is subtle and difficult to document.

Unfortunately, as Barofsky reports, there is currently insufficient data to indicate that cancer patients are victims of institutional job discrimination. What the cancer patient faces is discrimination that comes from limitation of action or opportunity, some of which is treatment- and disease-related, some institutional, and some self-induced. Some 25 to 30% of cancer patients eliminate themselves in some instances from the job market, perhaps anticipating that (1) their disease may recur; (2) they will have difficulties with the employer; (3) they are fearful of physical effects of working, such as loss of energy; or (4) they wish to retire. Some people may also accept the stigma of the disease. Many of these people need not have stopped working.

ER: Can a patient with cancer buy life insurance and health insurance?

PF: According to N. J. Ashenburg, patients with nonmetastatic disease can purchase life insurance by paying an extra premium temporary flat fee. The flat fee may now be $20 per thousand. Within recent years some companies began to use data from *End Results,* studies from the National Cancer Institute, where significant reductions in mortality have been observed for cancer of the uterus, rectum, stomach, bladder in women, and lip in men, thereby justifying reductions in insurance premiums.

Some malignancies have been accepted as a lower risk group, including cancer in situ of the cervix, papillary cancer of the thyroid, Stage I Hodgkin's disease, and most nonmelanotic skin cancer. At present, all persons with metastatic disease are ineligible for life insurance.

The best way for cancer patients to remain covered (or obtain coverage) with health insurance is to seek or remain employed in a large firm with group health insurance coverage. Several studies support this finding, among them a study by N. J. Ashenburg, who writes:

Hospital, surgical and medical, comprehensive and major medical insurance is available to persons with a cancer history through group insurance programs. Currently, about 80 percent of the health insurance written is group insurance. The basic question then is whether the person with a cancer history can secure a job where such insurance protection is available. On an individual basis, health insurance is less readily available to persons with a cancer history. Most companies require a 10-year waiting period from the date of treatment. A significant extra premium as much as 50 percent over the standard rate is assessed.

A study that examined the effects of cancer, heart disease, epilepsy, and diabetes in group health coverage was carried out for the U.S. Department of Labor by Opinion Research Corporation (1980). They make some additional points.

Four carriers in five (85% of 149 insurance carriers) interviewed say most of their contracts have clauses pertaining to preexisting health conditions; however, only 10% say an employee would be excluded from health, life, or disability coverage due to a history of heart disease, cancer, epilepsy, or diabetes. No direct evidence was found that carriers have policies or practices that would prevent employers from hiring candidates with a history of serious illness. Forty-nine percent of the carriers surveyed in 1978 required some evidence of insurability before enrollment of a new employee in an insurance group plan.

A local claims representative for a large insurance company in Northern California told me: "An employee must prove to be employable and able to do the work. This does not mean he needs to reveal his cancer health history. Once accepted for employment, a person's cancer health history would probably not form the basis for termination. If he is capable of doing the work, medical bills related to the cancer would be absorbed without special notice, especially in a large firm (over 500 employees) where the risk pool is larger."

This viewpoint appears to find support in the Opinion Research Study, where medium-size companies (26 to 100 employees) were most likely (75%) to require evidence of insurability and large companies with over 500 employees were least likely (17%) to require evidence.

The Opinion Research Study report summarized its findings with this statement: "There appear to be hiring barriers in some instances; some of these barriers revolve about insurance company policies involving greater cost to the company." But they point out that what is not currently known is how employers interpret the policies of their insurance carrier.

In sum, some employment difficulties result from cancer patients seeing themselves as "less than before" and leaving the world of employment prematurely. In other instances, insurance company requirements also pose problems for employees. Thus problems with employment and insurance and with cancer patients appear to be multi-causal, derived from problems within the economic-employment-insurance system as well as within the individual with cancer.

25
Volunteers

Volunteers, like social workers, nurses, and clergy, must be sensitive to the needs of the people they serve. Their goal is to complement the skills of these professionals and to offer patients one more means of emotional or tangible support. Their efforts can often fill a need for nonmedical support to aid in a patient's recovery. Volunteers who work with cancer patients may have a specific, clearly defined goal, as the women who work for the American Cancer Society's Reach to Recovery Program do, or they may function within flexible guidelines, like those who have joined the Patient Service program at Mount Zion Hospital. This chapter contains excerpts from interviews with a former volunteer executive of the Reach to Recovery Program, the Assistant Director of Service and Rehabilitation of the American Cancer Society, the Chairman of the Patient Service Program at Mt. Zion Hospital, and a volunteer in the Patient Service Department at Mt. Zion Hospital.

THE REACH TO RECOVERY PROGRAM OF
THE AMERICAN CANCER SOCIETY* †

ER: In 1969 the Reach to Recovery Program became affiliated nationally with the American Cancer Society. You helped organize that program in California and served as Volunteer Coordinator for the state from 1969 to 1974. How did you become interested in Reach to Recovery?

Rhoda Goldman: Twenty-four years ago I had a mastectomy. While I was in the hospital I received visits from two friends who had had the same operation. I could see that they had resumed normal lives, and that gave me courage. I am now convinced that the only people who can offer that kind of encouragement and inspire that kind of confidence are women who have had similar experiences.

Sometime after my surgery I became aware of the Reach to Recovery Program through a friend of one of the founders,‡ and events moved from there.

ER: What is the primary message carried by volunteers of Reach to Recovery to women who have just undergone mastectomies?

RG: Our message is that there is no reason you cannot continue your former life-style

---

*Rhoda Goldman, Volunteer Coordinator, Reach to Recovery Program, American Cancer Society, San Francisco Unit: 1968-present; California Division: 1969-1974.

†The American Cancer Society also sponsors a rehabilitation visiting program for ostomy patients and cooperates with similar programs of the United Ostomy Association and the Lost Chord Club of the International Association of Laryngectomies.

‡Reach to Recovery was originated by Terese Lasser in 1952.

exactly as it was before surgery. You should not think of yourself as different or as a person apart from the community.

ER: Can anyone who has had a mastectomy become a volunteer?

RG: No. We screen our volunteers very carefully and train them under professional supervision. I think this is one of the strongest points of the program. This means that a woman who visits a new mastectomy patient doesn't just go into her room and say, "I've had a mastectomy and look at how well I'm doing. Everything is going to be fine with you." On the contrary, in the training sessions volunteers are taught what they should and should not say. For instance, they never discuss medical matters. They urge a patient to save those questions for her physician. However, they can relieve a lot of anxiety by answering the many small questions that have begun to loom very large. They are taught to think in terms of an individual's needs and to offer advice that is appropriate and supportive for a particular person. We try to match volunteers and new mastectomy patients in terms of personal experience, particularly with regard to age and marital status.

ER: How many times does a volunteer visit a patient?

RG: A volunteer makes one visit, which she follows up with a telephone call. This is usually sufficient for most patients. We are wary of creating a dependent relationship on the part of a patient toward a volunteer, or vice versa. Occasionally a further visit or telephone call can be made where advisable, upon request.

ER: Does that mean that most doctors support your program?

RG: Most, but not all. Some physicians have resisted using our services, even though the California Medical Association has approved the Reach to Recovery Program. These physicians who resist do it out of ignorance of our goals or through fear that a visit by a nonprofessional will cause emotional disturbance to their patient. They may also just be concerned about interference in the doctor-patient relationship.

One thing we are trying to do that may help win physician support is to arrange that Reach to Recovery have a base in each hospital. A liaison person in the hospital would contact a Reach to Recovery volunteer whenever a mastectomy is performed. This would not only ensure that each mastectomy patient would have the benefit of a visit from a volunteer but that the visit would be made at the ideal time, which we have found to be between the third and sixth postoperative days. A visit during that period seems to offer the most encouragement and to stimulate the strongest desire for a good future adjustment.

ER: How well do you think most women adjust to a mastectomy?

RG: I'd say that over 90% make a very good adjustment. We encourage a woman to face it, cope with it, and do whatever she can to help herself to recover. We tell her that her family and friends will take their cue from the way she reacts. She is encouraged to discuss her thoughts and emotions with those close to her.

Sometimes there is a need for further counseling, however, either for the woman herself or for a member of her family. For instance, a husband can often benefit from talking to someone about his own and his wife's feelings toward the mastectomy. The adjustment of the husband or children and other family members or friends is very important to a woman's recovery. Therefore, the availability of counseling for all these people is an essential of good care. For this reason, a volunteer will often ask a woman, "Would you like us to talk to your husband too?" or "How is your husband taking it?"

ER: What is the most prevalent fear among women faced with the possibility of a mastectomy?

RG: A lot of people are afraid they will be mutilated. The fear of mutilation is strong because our society is so breast conscious. Women worry about their future sex lives. We have created an image of the physically perfect woman, and a woman facing a mastectomy thinks, "I won't match up any more." That is why we emphasize in our Reach to Recovery literature that femininity and womanliness aren't dependent on a few ounces of flesh.

Considering the trauma that most women undergo in having a mastectomy, I think that some kind of preoperative consultation should take place with the doctor. For that matter, there should be a dialogue between a doctor and his patient before any kind of surgery, even before a biopsy, so that people can be helped to face reality.

ER: I agree. Such discussions would remove some of the fear of the unknown. We also need to attack the fear that women have of self-examination and the possibility of discovering a lump. Does the Reach to Recovery Program do anything to encourage self-examination of the breasts?

RG: Those of us within the program have been advocating the adoption of such a policy for years. I feel it would give the program an added dimension if Reach to Recovery volunteer visitors were among those who participate in teaching breast self-examination. The willingness of Mrs. Ford and Mrs. Rockefeller to share their experiences with American women not only saved many lives by encouraging women to examine themselves and consult their physicians, but they helped bring the whole subject out into the open. Too many women in the past have felt ashamed and wanted to conceal the fact that they had had mastectomies. In my own case it was basically a matter of life or death. There was never any question about the operation. I received the very best treatment and was given a lot of emotional support by my doctor, family, and friends. I never felt ashamed, and I never felt it was a deterrent. On the contrary, I think I'm basically a better person for it. This is the way I am, and the important fact is that I'm living today and leading an active, involved, and satisfying life.

ER: What is your hope for mastectomy patients in the future?

RG: I hope that in the future everyone who has a mastectomy will receive a visit from a Reach to Recovery volunteer, since our primary concern is for the quality of life after surgery.

SERVICE AND REHABILITATION:
AMERICAN CANCER SOCIETY*

ER: What's happened to Reach to Recovery in the last several years?

Helen Crothers: In California Reach to Recovery has emerged as a multifaceted service program in the last 5 years. Recognizing the growing complexities of breast cancer treatment facing women today, Reach to Recovery saw the need to update its entire program. Newer areas of program support are as follows:

- A service of Reach to Recovery women is now available (upon a physician's request) to make a first visit to a patient during the time *between* biopsy and definitive treatment, when a two-staged procedure is planned. This extra psychological support has produced excellent results in the attitudes of patients.
- The issue of reconstructive surgery was examined in 1979 through a pilot demonstration program. This led to the formation of a statewide breast reconstruction support program. It was so successful that it received a National American Cancer Society Service Award.

*Helen Crothers, M.S.W., Assistant Director, Service & Rehabilitation, American Cancer Society, California Division.

- Support groups have been established in areas throughout California under the guidance and direction of skilled professionals to help patients and families cope with the diagnosis and treatment of (breast) cancer.

ER: What is the future role of Reach to Recovery?

HC: As long as there is an established community need for support and assistance to women experiencing breast cancer, Reach to Recovery will be involved. We feel Reach to Recovery's new service programs will be instrumental in providing support to women as they explore treatment and rehabilitation options. Studies have shown that early intervention can improve subsequent ability to cope. Therefore, referrals to this program should immediately follow the diagnosis of breast cancer.

In view of our personal experience and professional training, we offer a unique supplement to the total patient-care team. More physicians should refer patients to our program—for without this type of support, patients almost predictably will turn to other forms of support that may not be in their best interest.

ER: Considering two of the treatment options for breast cancer, have you any information on the women who elect radiation therapy over surgery?

HC: Reach to Recovery is currently involved in studying the needs of women who choose radiation therapy. We receive many requests for information and assistance forwarded to us through local American Cancer Society offices. These women are looking for the same type of help they have requested in the past—a dialogue with other women who have experienced similar treatment. To offer appropriate information and support, Reach to Recovery is working with medical professionals to determine what women in these circumstances want and need.

ER: How can Reach to Recovery help women deal with the controversies over treatment?

HC: We assist women in thinking through and articulating their concerns because they are often too overwhelmed to do this following the diagnosis. As trained volunteers, we provide an experienced "ear" and try to help the patient use existing resources more effectively. We acknowledge the complexities and can refer women to additional sources of information (most ACS unit offices have lending libraries and resource materials). We do not give patients medical advice but rather help them formulate and feel confident in posing questions to their physicians.

ER: What books do you suggest that women read?

HC: If You Find a Lump in Your Breast, by Martha McLean, 1980, Bull Publishing, $2.95. Reference copies are available through local offices of the ACS. An excellent bibliography included.

Breast Cancer Digest: a guide to medical care, emotional support, educational programs and resources, N.I.H., 1979. D.H.E.W. Publication #80-1691. No charge. Available from National Cancer Institute.

Why Me?, by Rose Kushner, New American Library, Signet Press, 1977. $2.50.

Choices: Realistic Alternatives in Cancer Treatment, by Marion Moira and Eve Potts, Avon Books, 1980. $8.95.

THE PATIENT SERVICE DEPARTMENT: MT. ZION HOSPITAL AND MEDICAL CENTER*

Shirley Selby: At Mt. Zion Hospital and Medical Center there is a unique volunteer program called Patient Service. It is composed of carefully selected, well-trained

---

*Shirley A. Selby, Chairman, Patient Service Department, Mt. Zion Hospital and Medical Center.

volunteers who feel comfortable with direct patient contact. These volunteers are available as an additional support system to the patient and the patient's family and have special training to be with critically ill, chronically ill, and dying patients.

The Patient Service program was originally started in 1969 to provide a number of small services and extra comforts to patients. In the fall of 1974 I expanded the Patient Service program by initiating a series of noontime meetings that were attended not only by volunteers but by other interested hospital staff—nurses, social workers, and interns. These meetings caused a change in direction for the program from a basically patient-visiting program to a well-trained volunteer service that emphasized working with the critically ill, chronically ill, and dying patients. This concept might be viewed as an in-hospital hospice program, except the volunteers are there as a support system for all patients in the hospital.

The primary goals of this training program are to help patients, through our additional support system, to be more comfortable and accepting of their situation, and to encourage patients to communicate openly with their families and friends and with the medical and nursing staff.

ER: Mrs. Selby, how does a person become a member of Patient Service, and can you tell us something about the training program?

SS: Prospective volunteers are first screened by the Director of Volunteer Services. If they appear qualified for, and interested in, the Patient Service Department, they are referred to me for a further interview. The particular qualities we seek are awareness and sensitivity to others, the ability to listen, flexibility, and a willingness to be objective and nonjudgmental. Patient Service trainees receive the usual orientation training from the Volunteer Department and also receive an extensive training experience that includes viewing a 21-minute videotape that is an outgrowth of this program. Participants in the videotape include experienced volunteers, physicians, and nurses who have been a part of the Patient Service program at Mt. Zion Hospital.

ER: What do Patient Service volunteers actually do, Mrs. Williams?*

Laura Williams: Most volunteers spend only 1 or 2 days a week at the hospital. On arrival we go to the nurse on the floor to which we've been assigned and ask the nurse what special tasks need to be done that day. During the time we spend at the hospital we may accompany patients to x-ray, relay messages from patients to nurses, feed patients (only at the request of the nurse), run errands for the patients or the nurses, take care of patients' flowers, or change their drinking water. We also just visit with patients. Volunteers play card games, do crossword puzzles, read out loud, discuss anything from the patients' feelings about his disease and his treatment to politics and baseball. Or we may silently hold a hand, or sit quietly and listen.

Listening to a patient is the most important thing we do. It helps us more than anything else to gain understanding. We learn to interpret subtle changes in mood or train of thought. Often, by the time a volunteer has performed some simple task she will be able to determine whether a patient wants to talk or has an unspoken need. An anxious look may reveal whether the patient is saying, "I don't feel like a visit today," or "I want to tell you something." Sometimes it is the wrong moment to approach a patient. Sometimes the volunteer is simply the wrong person to make such an approach. The members of Patient Service recognize that, because of personality differences, they will not be acceptable to every patient, and they are aware that another volunteer may succeed in comforting a patient where they have failed.

---

*Laura Williams, a volunteer in the Patient Service Department, Mount Zion Hospital and Medical Center.

ER: Mrs. Selby, do you discuss medical information with a patient?

SS: No, we don't. Patient Service volunteers are not aware of the medical history and problems of the patients they see; they feel more comfortable that way. We are there as a friend to let patients tell us what they want us to know. We *never* ask questions.

Patient confidences are respected at all times. Volunteers are told many things of a personal nature that could later be an embarrassment to the patient. We keep those confidences.

ER: What do you consider the most important factor in achieving success with a program like Patient Service?

SS: The marvelous acceptance by the nursing and medical staff of volunteers on the nursing stations! There is a mutual respect and cooperation with one another, particularly the nurses with whom we work so closely.

ER: You have been invaluable to both the nurses and the patients. From my own experience, I know that the most important need of a patient, after medical care, is the availability of a sympathetic listener.

26

The clergy

Men and women of the clergy occupy a unique position. Whether Protestant ministers, Catholic priests, or Jewish rabbis, they have authority and respect in the community. One of their many functions is to comfort the sick, at home or in the hospital. The patients they visit in a hospital are not necessarily limited to members of one congregation, or even one religion. Some patients may no longer have any religious affiliation. Yet the clergy can still be welcome figures, sympathetic listeners, sources of emotional and spiritual sustenance.

Many people under the stress of illness or dying call upon God to help them. Severe stress and fear may also cause them to revert to previously held religious views. For these people, as well as for regular members of church, temple, or synagogue, the clergy represent faith, salvation, and the authority of God. They are expected to have special insight into the mysteries of life and death.

I interviewed representatives of three faiths—Chaplain Laursen, Father Shanahan, and Rabbi Asher*—to ask them how they approached individual patients and how those patients reacted to them. What follows is not a comprehensive discussion of religion; it is an attempt to understand the role of the clergy with regard to the patient who has cancer. In spite of the many differences among the three faiths, in both concept and practice, I found that in dealing with the cancer patient the three clergymen differed only in style. Their objectives were similar—to help people to live, and also to die. In this respect their roles do not differ from those of doctors, nurses, social workers, and volunteers.

John Shanahan: There are, of course, certain expectations, somewhat vaguely conceived, of what a clergyman should do. He is expected to minister to the patient, to provide the opportunity for sacraments and prayer, to bring comfort and solace in some way, to deal with spiritual problems, to lift the patient's morale, and to spread comfort and cheer. In the popular dichotomy, the doctor cares for the body, the chaplain cares for the soul. The clergyman has the opportunity to make a unique and valuable contribution to the spiritual, mental, and emotional well-being of the sick, the seriously ill, and the dying.

---

*The Reverend Elmer Laursen, D.Min., Chaplain and Supervisor, Clinical Pastoral Education, University of California, San Francisco; the Reverend John D. Shanahan, formerly Roman Catholic Chaplain, UCSF, presently Pastor, Star of the Sea Church, Sausalito; and Rabbi Joseph Asher, Temple Emanuel, San Francisco.

As a priest in a hospital setting, I am, among other things, acting as a representative of our religious community. The patients don't know me personally. They come from various parts of the Bay Area. They are separated from their families. My being there says, "We care about you. We want you to get well. How can we help?" Maybe these people haven't seen a priest in a long time. But my presence might remind them of a time when they attended church and thereby give them strength for the present. On the other hand, some people with tenuous ties to our religious community don't care about seeing a priest, so my visit to them will not be supportive. Each patient reacts differently. Therefore I don't have a planned approach.

Slowly and painfully I have learned one general approach. I think this approach helps me, as a priest caring for the seriously ill, to listen, and I hope it has helped the patients I visit. Unaware of the dynamics behind the emotional stresses or moral disorders in a man about to die, with not the faintest idea of what to say, I listen. I have learned to hold my tongue, learned what not to say. I try to show sincere interest, to reflect understanding of the person's feelings. I try to accept the man as a fellow human being. As a listener, I have learned that I can create an atmosphere of solicitous permissiveness in which the troubled patient feels free to share the burden he is unable to carry alone. I try to be compassionate, to touch the emotional pulse of the patient by identifying in some personal way with his anguish, his bewilderment, his interior conflict. I try to understand. I need hardly say a word. Someone is interested; someone understands; someone is in no hurry to run, to belittle, to disparage or explain away the worry or trot out pious clichés. I am, primarily, a listener whose contribution is a wholehearted acceptance of the patient. I try to create a climate in which the sick man feels he may speak without fear.

Joseph Asher: I feel that my function is to try to be an empathic person who relates to people not as a rabbi but as a friend. The only rabbinic component of this kind of relationship is that perhaps the person has more respect and regard for me because he recognizes that I have seen other people in his same situation and may even have some direct communication with the divine. But I don't have that. I really don't think I have ever contributed to a person to the extent that I have evoked resources of strength he did not have before I came. The best I have been able to do is maybe to awaken resources which this person was planning to set aside or was unaware he possessed.

I may say to a patient, "Now look, every day that you live is one more opportunity for an improvement in your condition, because with medical science the way it is today, what is impossible today may be possible tomorrow." I also explain to him that much of survival, and this may be impression rather than fact, depends on a person's will and a person's desire to survive.

Recently a member of my congregation had a stroke and simply did not want to live. He would not participate in such therapy as was available to him and after a period of months he just died. The physician who took care of him told me that this man could have lived longer and could have lived an active life. This man simply did not want to live. So what I can do, as a rabbi, is constantly reassure a patient that a great deal of his recovery depends on his will to live. If I can help strengthen that will to live, I have made a contribution.

Nevertheless, I'm terribly aware of my impotence in these things. It's very difficult for an outside force to have any effect in a situation like this. People's lives cannot be influenced to such an extent that a person can say, "The rabbi was here and he told me I'm going to live. Therefore I'm going to live. I'm going to try harder than I did before he came in." The person may do this for 5 minutes, in my presence, but if his nature is inclined toward giving up, that's what he's going to do.

However, I think we often underestimate both patients' ability to cope and their need for comfort arising from an apprehension of the truth. We always think they need to be babied when they are in such situations. It is really more the function of the rabbi to relate to the family, to help them accept the inevitable with grace and with a certain amount of consolation. They in turn convey this composure to the sick person. The entire Jewish tradition teaches us to confront reality. If a person is about to die, then we have to recognize the fact that this is about to happen. We do not, under any circumstances, encourage a kind of covering up of what is about to occur, nor do we hold out a description of a life beyond. That is why it's sometimes much more difficult for a rabbi to comfort a family, particularly when a death occurs that is out of the ordinary. In such instances the family's first response is often, "How could God let this happen to us? What justice is there from such a God?" I tell them that God is not doing something to hurt them. The untimely death of the person they love is simply one of the malfunctions of nature to which we are exposed from time to time. Death before one's time is a malfunction of nature just as much as an earthquake or a hurricane.

Elmer Laursen: Patients have fear of cancer as a disease, and they need to share their fear and anxiety with someone who will listen. Many physicians and nurses listen to patients, but a clergyman may do it in a different way. He comes to listen to their questions, which often include "Why did this happen? What did I do?"

Our objective is to support patients in the most appropriate way. We try to keep hope alive, but not to foster false hope. We share the bad times that depress patients. We try to help them accept illness as a part of their life instead of just to fight it. We try to emphasize the positives in their lives, but when there are few or none of these it is harder to help them.

I attempt to console and share and be alongside of people during their suffering. I listen to their questions in a supportive way, helping them tap and enlarge upon their religious resources. I listen, and sometimes in silence I give aid and comfort. Frequently my main function is just to be there. I try to hear patients' verbal and nonverbal cries and concerns and, if possible, to help them achieve a new perspective. It seems to me that by sharing I contribute the important element, which is to help them feel less alone and less deserted.

When there are family members, relatives, and friends who are a part of the supportive system for a patient, I can at times also help them with their feelings and enable them to be supportive rather than hindering to the patient.

I have become increasingly aware that in our work with people and their problems, we need not pretend to have any great answers for them. They sometimes find answers for themselves, or at the least they find someone with whom they can share their questions.

While as a chaplain my desire is to work closely with the physician, he is not always ready to involve me in patient care. Often I am able to minister effectively in spite of his reluctance to include me. However, we both do a better job when we can work together.

The acceptance of the problem of illness and the incorporation of that acceptance into one's life and trying to deal with it is a process, an upward process. People who learn to accept and reconcile themselves to dying often seem to live more effectively. Given the opportunity to vent their anger at God in the presence of an understanding clergyman, they may be relieved of their guilt feelings. It is normal to be angry, curse, or swear at God and ask, "Why?" Eventually they learn that they can be as angry as they wish at God because He is big enough to handle it. Then they can begin a more dynamic process of living for their remaining time. Somehow, it is helpful to most of us to be able to accept that death is a part of life.

The process of learning how best to support a patient is long and arduous. It involves going into a patient's room, letting him say whatever he wishes, and then helping him to look at what is going on, to reflect on it. I feel it is unnecessary to confront a person too heavily or bluntly. I have better ways of being with a patient than saying, "You know, you have to take a look at this for your wife and family. You can't just give up." Rather, I try to help him take hold of the problem and deal openly with it.

Finally, the time arrives when all I can do is to help a patient to die graciously. In doing that I believe I am helping people to live right up to the last moment.

The appropriate use of Holy Scriptures and prayer by sensitive and well-trained clergymen can also be of inestimable value in the total ministry of the ill.

ER: The three of you have a similar concept of the role of the clergy in supporting a cancer patient. You help by supporting, encouraging, listening, empathizing, and giving both faith and hope to a patient, his family and friends. You absorb the anger of a patient. You can be trusted with confidences and yet remain unshocked and uncondemning.

Ritual is often followed in ministering to patients. Father Shanahan, do you still administer the last rites to a patient who is coming to the end of his life? If so, what effect does this have on him?

JS: There has been a change in the administration of the sacraments that makes them more meaningful. The Sacrament of Extreme Unction is now called the Sacrament of the Sick. It is administered frequently and quite normally when a person is ill but not about to die. Last rites is a term reserved for the use of the funeral liturgy.

ER: Rabbi Asher, how does the Jewish ritual help people to come to terms with grief?

JA: As with every aspect of life, Judaism's rituals seek to provide outlets for emotions rather than submerge them. Our tradition understands the immediate response to the crises we experience and seeks to vest them with meaning in the context of our relationship with the divine. Thus when death comes the family's anger, its total withdrawal, is acknowledged. Certain normal religious functions are suspended. In our anger, we can hardly be expected to praise God. After the funeral the family remains at home for 7 days, desisting from its regular habits and allowing friends to come to the house for communal prayer rather than going to the synagogue. After that week, and until 30 days after the death, normal activities are resumed, while some personal habits are still restricted, for which one would have no inclination anyway. For the 10 months following, one does not engage in any activities that might be interpreted as unduly entertaining or engaging in levity. Eleven months after death, family and friends gather to consecrate a memorial at gravesite. This ritual demonstrates the "closing of the grave," a symbol that grief must now be set aside and we must come to terms again with life.

The most modern understanding of the grief syndrome acknowledges stages of emergence from it. Jewish ritual is designed to guide us from the most abject sorrow to renewed composure, allowing for time to bring its healing to the bereaved.

ER: Chaplain Laursen, what extra help can a person find in dealing with death and grief?

EL: Workshops, seminars, and retreats for clergy and laypersons are effective in helping them express their feelings and thoughts about death and grief. People of all ages have participated in these groups. Most of them have felt threatened at first, but after permitting themselves to become involved in the dialogue and in the process of reflection, they have found that some of their fears were lessened. These are subjects that we all prefer to avoid, but by bringing them into the open and confronting them we may be able to deal with death, and life, in a more realistic and wholesome manner. Members of communities in which such experiences take place have developed rich resources for ministering to one another when confronted by death and grief. They can be open with one another to a far greater degree than exists in the usual "denial" of real feelings.

I am convinced that this entire process of opening up to each other makes it possible for persons suffering all kinds of diseases of body, mind, and spirit to live more fully and to limit to some degree the destructive elements that threaten us.

ER: Unlike most of the people who support the patient and his family, the clergy continues to serve the family after the patient's death by helping them through the process of grieving. The ritual of a funeral service and a postfuneral meal for family and friends is as much a supportive gesture toward the bereaved as an opportunity to say farewell to the deceased. Following these brief distractions, the survivors may experience a deeper state of shock than they did at the time of death. The period of mourning begins. There is no way to shorten or lessen the grieving process, although it can be shared and the pain, in part, alleviated through the compassion of others.

PART NINE

Dealing with death

27

When cancer is terminal

Death is a part of life. We all must die sometime—we don't know when. Yet we persist in thinking of death as something that happens to other people. We do not accept our mortality until a crisis forces us to contemplate nonbeing. Even then, we may fight, bargain, and connive to gain more time, but life is elusive as well as precious. It may be snuffed out at a moment's notice or drain away slowly with disease or old age. And although physicians fight to preserve life at almost any cost in time, money, or effort, we also know a day will come when the time is right to let a person die.

In partnership with the physician, cancer patients face many difficult issues. Throughout treatment they share in medical decisions, and if the cancer becomes progressively worse, they will at some point discuss with their physician matters concerning their dying. For example, people often ask that no extraordinary measures be taken to keep them alive when there is no longer any hope of a good quality of life. Other decisions involve a choice of where to die—home, hospital, nursing home, or hospice. Funeral arrangements are also often discussed between patient and physician.

We are all concerned with maintaining dignity in life as well as in dying, and we share certain standards as to what constitutes an acceptable level of dignity. The cancer patient may gradually feel that level recede as he or she experiences diminishing control over personal destiny. A loss of privacy and ability to influence one's present or one's future may become more of a concern than dying. The question may arise whether life is worth living under the circumstances and whether euthanasia is not the best solution. Implementing such a request is neither ethical nor legal, but, under the current official guidelines of medical practice, maximum comfort with a minimum of suffering can be promised. A physician can also promise not to interfere with the natural process of dying by keeping a patient alive with special life-sustaining equipment. A patient has a right to die and to issue a directive to the physician to see that this wish is honored.

There is a growing movement in the United States toward the right to die. A recent example of this movement occurred in October 1981 when the Washington, D.C., City Council gave preliminary approval to a "death with dignity" ordinance that legalizes a request by adults not to be kept alive by life-sustaining procedures when their condition is terminal. As a protection for doctors against malpractice suits, the signatures of at least two doctors are required to carry out this request. The ordinance ensures that the wishes of the dying person are honored by subjecting doctors who do not comply with the request to civil penalties of up to $5000, plus suspension or revocation of their license. As of the autumn of 1981, 10 states have adopted similar laws: Arkansas, California, Idaho, Kansas, Nevada, New Mexico, North Carolina, Oregon, Texas, and Washington.

When the question arises of where to die, some patients choose the hospital, where they can be close to trained personnel and special equipment. They may prefer the hospital because they fear that dying at home will add to the family's physical and emotional burdens and thus, perhaps, to their own. However, most people prefer to spend their remaining days at home, where they will have more peace than in the hospital and be in familiar surroundings. Extra help is available to solve some problems of home care. Social service agencies, paramedical people such as licensed vocational nurses and nurses' aides, and civic and professional groups such as the American Cancer Society—all offer support. The Cancer Society is often able to provide hospital beds, walkers, bedside toilets, and other equipment and, in certain cities, it helps defray the cost of x-ray examinations and treatments and drugs and arranges transportation to and from treatment.

The advantages of going home vary from patient to patient. One of my patients was in the terminal stages of disease when she asked to go home. She could barely walk, had lost her appetite, and required intravenous feeding. Her weight loss exceeded 50 pounds. To carry out her wish, we requested help from the American Cancer Society, which provided a walker and a wheelchair and arranged for nursing care at home. The move was made, and the resulting emotional lift contributed to a few extra rewarding days of life.

But at other times my judgment has been wrong. I have sent a patient home when the family was not prepared to accept the burden or to fulfill the patient's needs, and have later been told how destructive the experience was for the patient as well as the family. The stress of prolonged illness often creates unresolvable problems. Other members of the family need to continue with their daily activities, yet they may feel guilty for doing so. A patient may simultaneously feel guilty for being a burden and resentful that he or she is not receiving sufficient attention and sympathy.

Today more people die in nursing homes and hospitals than at home. Dying in this manner, separated from familiar sights and sounds, can be a doubly lonely ordeal, increasing natural feelings of isolation and abandonment. But if one had to choose between a hospital and a nursing home, I would recommend the former. Nursing homes are frequently run strictly for financial gain and may not have the more elaborate facilities of a regular hospital. Many of these homes will need to be upgraded before they can provide the proper warmth and dignity for anyone, especially for the dying.

An ideal institution for the dying is St. Christopher's Hospice, in London.* Founded by Dr. Cicely Saunders in 1967, St. Christopher's is a research,

---

*The discussion about hospices is taken from an article by Melvin J. Krant, M.D., entitled "Hospice Philosophy in Late-Stage Cancer Care," *J.A.M.A.* **245** (10), March 13, 1981.

treatment, and teaching facility devoted to meeting the needs of the dying and the long-term sick. Its aims are both control of physical pain and understanding of the emotional and spiritual problems of patients and their families. Dr. Saunders wants her patients to live until they die. The atmosphere is informal, the building designed for maximum openness, space, and light. Families are encouraged to visit at any hour of the day; the staff becomes as friendly with them as with the patients. Children are welcome visitors, and there is a day-care center for the staff's children. Dr. Saunders describes St. Christopher's as offering "intensive personal care," and she feels that it is what staff members do beyond their strictly medical duties that counts most.

Dr. Saunders believes that constant pain needs constant control, so drugs are given regularly rather than when the need arises. This reassures patients that they will not suffer and forestalls the fear and anxiety that can intensify pain. The goal is to be free of pain, but alert. Drugs are usually given orally rather than by injection, to increase a patient's feelings of independence and to make it easier for him to go home for weekends or longer. The number of patients who are in their own homes at any given time equals the number of patients in the hospice. On the other hand, the hospice has a wing for elderly people, who may live there for years. For dying patients, St. Christopher's provides the opportunity for them and their families to say a loving good-by, and this is what families will remember: a time of sadness but not of depression, when the person dear to them received affection and physical relief.

Since the founding of St. Christopher's, the term "hospice" has become part of the language in U.S. medicine. Several different forms of hospice units have emerged, helping to ease some of the problems associated with both home and hospital care. In some communities a hospice unit is a segregated ward in the hospital with an associated staff of physicians, bedside nurses, home-coordinating nurses, and social workers managing inpatient care and supporting at-home care through interaction with other community resources. Most units in the United States have developed as out-of-hospital home-care agencies, coordinating inpatient services through a loose affiliation with neighboring hospitals.

In some settings, where the hospice unit has not been created separately, a group of hospital-based personnel that includes a physician, nurse, social worker, and chaplain is available for consultation and support to patients throughout the institution.

A few free-standing hospices have also been constructed. These low-technology inpatient facilities admit only terminal patients and are often associated with a home-care program.

The hospice movement is beginning to fill a void in the medical and psychological care of the terminally ill. However, the hospice team should not replace the concerned physician. Patients and families need continuity of care, and physicians should not relinquish their involvement when a patient is admitted to a hospice service. They should remain as physician-of-record, working with the terminal care staff.

A person can sign a directive to his physician and choose the place where he or she will die. The only thing one cannot dictate is *when* he or she will die. There are no yardsticks to measure that delicate, highly individual time. Often I have seen a patient and thought that this was his or her time, only to find that patient so improved in the next few days that he or she returned home a week later. That is why I no longer feel that I or anyone else has the ability to predict when another person will die. I prefer to withhold judgment, visit patients frequently, and continually reassess their condition.

The medical aspects of the terminal phase of the disease are of deep concern to a patient. When should anticancer therapy be stopped? Will the pain be controlled? My general rule is to administer therapy as long as a patient responds well and has the potential for a reasonably good quality of life. But when all feasible therapies have been administered and a patient shows signs of rapid deterioration, the continuation of therapy can cause more discomfort than the cancer. From that time I recommend surgery, radiotherapy, or chemotherapy only as a means of relieving pain or of improving general comfort. However, if a patient's condition should once again stabilize after the withdrawal of active therapy, and if it should appear that he or she could still gain some good time, I would immediately reinstitute active therapy. The decision to cease anticancer treatment is never irrevocable, and often the desire to live will push a patient to try for another remission, or even a few more days of life.

There is an effective therapy to combat any degree of discomfort or pain. I find the most effective procedure is simply to correlate the medication with the complaint. If a patient is nauseated, I give him antinausea medicine. If the problem is inability to sleep, I prescribe sedatives—barbiturate or nonbarbiturate, depending on tolerance. And if there is pain, I use an appropriate analgesic or narcotic, as often as needed. The drugs can be administered in pill form, as a suppository, or by injection. Some patients even learn to administer their own shots, as a diabetic does, under medical supervision. Addiction is not a concern when a person has advanced cancer. Moreover, most patients report a tendency to use fewer drugs when they know drugs are readily available. The need for narcotics can also be lessened not only by surgery, radiotherapy, or chemotherapy, but by acupuncture, nerve blocks (created electrically, chemically, or surgically), or other methods.

As the final days approach for a patient, I continue to base my decisions on my medical knowledge and my patient's needs and preferences. Our contract is still in effect. I am always ready to be candid. I consider it necessary to reassess each day exactly how much a person really wants to hear. A patient may subtly indicate the preference for a period of reticence between us concerning the gravity of his or her situation. For instance, I remember a woman who was in the terminal phase of her disease. She had been through the trials of all the standard and experimental anticancer therapies, and she knew how poor her prospects were. In the past she and I, with her family, had held many frank discussions concerning her progress. Nevertheless, she said to me, "Am I going to die now?" She followed this with, "I know I have cancer, I know it's really bad, I want you to tell me but please don't tell me."

The sentence was uninterrupted. There was no pause in her speech.

With whom do you level, and how do you level? I replied, "No. Your gynecologist says the tumor has receded. Your weakness is due to your therapy and to not eating." Misleading? Yes, but she did not ask the definitive question. I am certain she knew the real answer, and on a subsequent visit when her spirits were improved, I knew I had been right to reply as I had because it fulfilled her emotional need of the moment and assured her of my continuing support.

At other times I may postpone giving patients a candid appraisal of their medical status. Discomfort and pain from progressive disease or the side effects of a drug can affect a person's ability to accept bad news. A depressed patient may interpret any pessimistic statement as a prognosis of imminent death, so I see no sense in making them feel worse by telling them their x-ray films show progressive disease or their blood counts are more abnormal than yesterday.

Most people know when they are dying and are sensitive to the suffering of those around them. Yet sometimes when they express a desire for peace, they are made to feel guilty by relatives who prefer to keep them alive under any conditions. To resolve in advance the possibility of such a conflict, many patients make a verbal agreement with their physician to sign a document called a Living Will that states their request not to be kept alive by artificial means or heroic measures when there is no reasonable expectation of recovery (see Appendix III).

For some patients there is a preterminal phase that involves a slow descent into a coma. At this time a patient is still alert enough to take comfort in talking with his or her family or the medical staff, and anything or anyone especially dear to the person should be made available. He or she may want to spend time with a particular relative, friend, child, or even a pet.

However, I must repeat that there are no prophets or prognosticators among physicians who are capable of deciding when a person is going to die. We have only clinical judgment as to the time remaining for any patient. Moreover, no one can prejudge the value of extra days or hours. Some time ago a patient of mine was dying, with marked jaundice, of a massive malignancy that was obstructing his liver. Not wanting him to suffer any longer, I left a verbal order with the interns and the resident that when he died no resuscitative efforts should be employed. About half an hour later the patient had a cardiac arrest. Neither the intern nor the resident were in the room, and the nursing staff had changed for the morning shift; the nurse naturally ordered the cardiac resuscitative unit, and the patient was revived. He lived another 48 hours, and in that time several relatives arrived from the Midwest and were able to visit with him. In addition, a brother from whom he had been estranged for 20 years flew to San Francisco, and they were reunited. He also had warm, emotionally satisfying talks with his wife and children about their life together.

Such communication is invaluable. It is natural for a dying person to experience a renewed sensitivity to the meaning of life and to want to convey special messages to those close to him. However, these thoughts are not always expressed, either because of awkwardness at expressing deep feelings or because of a reluctance to speak of death. Whatever the reason, survivors are often left without a final message.

Saying good-by before death can be a comfort to everyone concerned—family, friends, and patient. I have often participated in such a farewell to life by encouraging patients and key family members to make a tape-recording together. The recording may include a family history, or anecdotes, or it may lead to a philosophical conversation on life and death. A physician or nurse can often be instrumental in helping people break their silence by initiating similar conversations.

People who find it difficult to speak of their feelings sometimes write a letter expressing their thoughts and love. Such a letter often contains hopes for the future happiness of their loved one, in effect giving them permission to seek joy and fulfillment in the next phase of their lives.

For example, I recently received a copy of a letter sent by a young woman to her husband several months before she died. She wrote of their life together, her happiness with him, and her sadness that it would end soon. She also told him he would need to return to active living, and that he should marry again when he met the right person.

It doesn't matter how eloquently or awkwardly such thoughts are expressed. This conscious, deliberate communication can relieve the stress of silence between two people and bring them closer together. Remorse and guilt in both people may be assuaged. The person who is dying may gain peace of mind, while the survivor experiences a bond that can be a solace during mourning.

When a patient goes into a final state of coma, I keep him or her comfortable. This may require a moderate amount of hydration—intravenous feeding and keeping the mouth moist—as well as frequent turning and skin care. In certain cases I may continue to administer narcotics or sedatives at regular intervals even after the patient is comatose, if there appears to be restlessness or pain. This reassures the family that any pain or discomfort is being alleviated.

Death is never easy to accept, no matter what the cause. Family members need special attention throughout the ordeal, but especially in those final days. Help may come from within the family, or from friends, but physicians, nurses, clergy, social workers, and hospital volunteers are also available and ready to listen. I always hope that families will find solace in the knowledge that the loved one received good medical care and sensitive emotional support, that he or she lived as long and as well as possible under adverse conditions, and that all possible comfort was provided to ease the process of dying.

28

Grief and recovery

Grief is a normal, necessary psychological process that helps a person adapt to the loss of a loved one. The survivor is depressed and often withdraws from former interests, activities, and even friends. Grief is a very personal experience, and even among members of a family who lose the same person, the subjective experience of the loss will be different for each one. The closer the relationship, the greater the loss.

For an adult the psychological work of grief is connected with remembering and reliving the experiences shared with the person who has died. Grief is not a consciously determined task; rather, it is set in motion automatically and proceeds at the rate that is *bearable* for the individual. Grieving is painful because, as one remembers good times as well as bad, the very process of remembering requires a continuing recognition that the person loved is not there now.

Grief involves intense mental anguish, remorse, and sorrow. The outward behavior of grief is identical to depression. But these are mere words, and can in no way suffice to describe the deep emotional inburst of pain and shock experienced by a person who mourns. He or she has lost love, goals, friendship, security, none of which is immediately replaceable.

The depth of grief is unpredictable, because it reflects so many factors—the availability of support from family, children, and friends; culture, religion, degree of preparation for the event, and many others. And there is no universal approach to the process of grieving, although in our society many people follow specified religious procedures. Each of the major religions observes a degree of ritual, quite similar in format, when dealing with death.

As a physician who deals with these problems frequently, I try to prepare a patient's family and friends as well as possible for an anticipated death. I do this by providing medical information and holding family conferences on the patient's progress. Yet no matter how thoroughly I have prepared them, the family will still experience shock and momentary disbelief when the death occurs. In addition, questions will be asked and decisions required of them. Will there be a postmortem? What funeral arrangements must be made? This is where I can be helpful, because at such a time those close to the patient are not thinking or remembering clearly. If the disease was chronic, funeral arrangements have often been completed, or at least initiated, by the family.

When the funeral is over, the family, as well as the members of the medical team that has been involved with the patient, need time for their sorrow to abate. At this time I usually write the family a letter expressing both sympathy and hope for the future. I also review the patient's medical problem and the therapy given, and provide pertinent autopsy information. This alleviates any questions or misunderstandings among family members about what actually occurred, especially in the final days, when their comprehension may have been clouded by concern for the patient.

In my letter I also discuss the supportive role played by the family during the patient's illness. In almost every case the care and assistance given by the family, in the hospital or at home, has contributed to better medical care for the patient, and I acknowledge the help they gave the doctors and nurses. Finally I mention the normality of grieving, in addition to reminding them that there will be a time when life will be less painful. I may say, "Life will be very difficult following your loss, yet with time, the assistance and support of your children and family, and your own perseverance and courage, you will build a new life that will have both happiness and quality." I also invite them to visit me at any time if they feel I can help them with their problems of readjustment.

During the first few weeks, phone calls, visitors, and cards of sympathy distract the attention of the grief-stricken. Then suddenly the attention diminishes and one is left alone with the problem of the future. Often there is a denial of mourning, an attempt to hold back tears and suppress grief. Crying is believed by some people to be a sign of weakness.

Sometimes grief occurs simultaneously with unrelenting depression, in which the survivor becomes obsessed with the loss. When this happens, the crisis has become chronic and debilitating for the survivor, whose persistent, unremitting loneliness, helplessness, guilt, shame, and anger may lead to a regressed state, in which case professional help may be required to alleviate these problems.

In more normal grief, friends and other family members may try to prevent the bereaved from living in the past. They may try to create diversions to lessen the person's emotional suffering. These efforts are helpful and important. However, grief must be allowed to run its course.

In March of 1975 I invited Janet Segal to the monthly conference with the Patient Service volunteers at Mount Zion Hospital. The topic was grief and recovery. After opening the meeting with some remarks on the mechanisms of grief and adaptation to loss, I asked Janet to describe her own experiences since Mort's death, 1 year earlier (see Chap. 11).

Janet Segal: It's hard to know where to start. During this last year I have had wildly fluctuating moods and attitudes and have been better or less able to handle what my life is now compared to what it was before. Mort and I were married almost 10 years and had a blessed and easy life. Neither of us, by personality, lived in the future, and so our life together didn't end with many regrets about things we hadn't done or were waiting to do. So I would keep thinking about all the good things that had happened, but each time I did this—and it is still true today—I would have to face the fact that Mort is gone and will not be back. Our children, Josh and Rebecca, are now 4 and 6; and the fact that they won't have the influence of this most remarkable man is still, and will probably always be, hard for me to accept.

I feel guilty because I complain. What we had in a relatively short time was probably a whole lot better than many people experience all their lives. It seems ungrateful to complain, but I do. I had thought I would go through a maturing process in my grief, and reach a point where I would face the fact of Mort's death and accept it graciously. It is just in the course of the last week, while talking to a friend, that I realize I'm not ever going to accept it. Never, never, never!

The last year has not been a completely sad year for me. I don't feel that my life ended with Mort's death or that good things won't happen, because they have, and I expected they would. Of course, there were the circumstances at the end of his life. All that he was going through, his suffering, was finished, and that was a relief. But, you know, I may live to be 120 years old and have some wild life beyond anything I could imagine in the future—I think that's perfectly possible—but I will never—no matter what happens in the future—I will never be able to accept graciously that Mort died when he did, and how he did.

In the course of the last year, I have been through different phases of grief. The phases seem to be repetitive and very short. At times I can be overcome and almost nonfunctional with grief, sad thoughts, resentment, and anger. I wonder what I would be like if I didn't have the children to spur me to action and decisions and all the other things.

I might otherwise have apathy or become one of those people who sit in the corner and put the drapes over their head and everyone would have to work to get me to move. The children saved me from that. They've also had a year of grieving and also have a lot of pleasant memories of Mort. Josh has always been able, without any concerted effort, to talk about Mort or refer to him, because Mort was a big person in our lives and is just naturally a part of our conversations, or record, or reference.

Josh will say, "Was that a car like Mort's?" or "Remember when Daddy took us here?" or "That's Mort's book." For me this has been helpful.

ER: The effect of a parental loss on children is deep. A few months ago, when I said good-by to Josh after a visit, he replied accusingly, "Ernie, you're not going to come back, just like my daddy."

JS: One thing I wonder about is my decision that the children should not see Mort after he died. They saw him the morning he died, and he was able to recognize them and talk to them and joke a little. Then they went out of the room and an hour later Mort died.

I did not have them come back and see Mort, and that is out of my childhood. I went to wakes with open caskets and remember thinking, "That's not what Grandma looked like," and for me that image remained. I felt this particularly for Josh and Rebecca. I did not want that image of Mort to be their most vivid memory of him, and I was concerned that it would be. They had known him such a short time and wouldn't have a store of images to draw on.

They have had a lot of questions since then, and I don't know but what maybe they would have felt better if they had seen him. But I made the decision for them. I still think it was right, but there is one step they can't quite put together. The last time they saw Mort, he was alive; and the next time, after I told them he had died, there was the funeral and his body was in a casket.

They have asked me the same questions many times since then. "Was Daddy's whole body in the box? Was he wearing clothes?"

Josh became very angry immediately after Mort's death. He had always been a friendly type, but then he was positively furious. His anger manifested itself with physical displays—throwing things, and so forth.

Rebecca knew Mort better. She reacted in a more "adult" way. She would be overcome with sobbing and want to talk, but was unable to talk because she just could not get the words out. As the months went by she became more able to say the words that Mort was dead and that she would never be able to touch him again.

Josh would on occasion say things like, "I wish I were dead, because if I were dead then I could see Daddy. Then I would be with Mort." I still don't think the children have accepted it either.

I had a lot of preparation before Mort died, because we knew it was going to happen and both of us talked about things and did some reading. What I'm trying to say is, I was better able to handle it because of the preparation.

Grieving is a selfish experience, but I guess, a necessary one. Grief is more intense the closer you are to the person who has died. You may have various parts of that relationship filled by other people, so that instead of one person, or one source, there are many sources. In that case the sum of the parts still doesn't equal the whole. Nevertheless, I've had a lot of support and for that I am very grateful.

The people who have helped me most through the grieving period are those who knew Mort, his complexities and his interests, because they know what he was really like. The support that comes from someone who knew the person—the talk, the conversation, the reminiscing, or the arguing about, or whatever—is most helpful. In the grieving thing it is sort of hard for me to hold myself together. It has been hard some of the time. Right now I don't think I have a lot left to give to someone else who is grieving.

ER: We all grieve after personal tragedies and losses. We progress from shock to recovery and, with time, move toward a new life. Anger and disbelief subside. Throughout the period of mourning, the concern and support of friends help the bereaved until a time comes when grief lessens. Life goes on, and the bereaved person joins in.

To the survivor grief may seem endless and recovery impossible. Nevertheless, a process does begin whereby grief and recovery occur simultaneously, in alternating patterns and moods. Of course, nothing is ever quite the same. The attitudes of the survivor may be permanently altered by the long acquaintance with illness, suffering, and death, and quite likely he or she will emerge from the ordeal a stronger, more mature person.

The means and length of time required for recovery will vary. Those who are alone will have a more difficult time and may need additional and continuing support from clergy, social workers, or the medical team to help them through their period of grief.

Slowly a new pattern of life evolves. At first the bereaved may feel guilty when experiencing brief episodes of enjoyment. To feel happiness may seem inappropriate, even traitorous. Yet it is these interludes of enjoyment that gradually create new hope. When they accumulate, they will coalesce into a vision of the future, and the survivor will be able to acknowledge emotionally what he or she always knew intellectually, that vitality and involvement with others will return.

Little by little the painful memories of suffering and illness become less poignant, and it is easier to revive and enjoy thoughts of earlier, happier times. While cherishing these memories the bereaved may also derive courage from them by identifying with the positive qualities of the person who is gone. At the same time will come recognition with diminishing guilt that one's own needs continue. This is the turning point.

There is no prescribed time that elapses before a grieving person begins to mobilize his or her interests and energy for the present and the future. There is no line of demarcation between grief and recovery. Old memories are kept alive while new ones are being created.

PART TEN

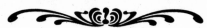

Conclusion

29

Choosing life

Look to this day for it is life,
For yesterday is already a dream,
And tomorrow is only a vision.
But today, well lived, makes every yesterday
A dream of happiness and every tomorrow a vision of hope.
SANSKRIT PROVERB

The purpose of life is to live. The goal of the physician who treats cancer patients is not only to administer medical therapy but to help them live as normally as possible while undergoing treatment.

There is a widespread belief that a diagnosis of cancer is an automatic death sentence. This is not true. Today 43% of all cancer patients are cured; and the majority of those who are not cured are leading active, productive lives with the same odds and life expectancy as people who live with other chronic diseases.

Of course, a cure for cancer is not just around the corner. No one breakthrough will produce all the answers; the answers will come one by one, as they have until now. Nevertheless, in 1982, 14 types of cancer are curable when they are diagnosed at an advanced stage. New forms of cancer will be added to this list because new discoveries are constantly being made and known techniques perfected. New methods of giving radiation therapy, new chemotherapeutic drugs and combinations of drugs, the use of adjuvant chemotherapy, hormonal therapy, and experimental therapies such as immunotherapy and hyperthermia all give hope for the future.

In spite of the promise of these medical advances, living with cancer is an anxious, fearful time. Undergoing therapy and experiencing the side effects of treatment involve compromise. This compromise consists in accepting what has happened and at the same time in being willing to fight for your life. But no matter how well informed you become about current therapies and available treatment alternatives, you still feel a loss of control over your fate because you must trust the judgment of cancer specialists and pray for good luck. One day you are hopeful, the next day full of gloom.

Not all patients are able to live well with cancer because cancer, like heart disease, may not respond to the best of treatment or the strongest will to live. When treatment fails to stop the spread of tumor, or when a recurrence comes after a long remission, the heartbreak and frustration are more than a person can bear. I can only admire the determination and endurance of people under these grievous circumstances. They are facing the toughest time in their lives. Some patients even contemplate suicide, and I wonder what I would do under such circumstances. However, as a physician, I find suicide to be a very uncommon event. At our lowest ebb, there is a small flame, an inner strength. Call it what you will—fear of dying, the will to live, or sheer determination. Whatever it is, there is a toughness in all of us that makes us try again—and opt for life.

Many patients tell me that the uncertainties of living with cancer can make life more meaningful. The smallest pleasures—flowers, the sky, sunshine—are intensified. Much hypocrisy is eliminated. When such patients can reduce some of the bitterness and anger they feel toward cancer and what it has done to their life, they find there is still room for enjoyment.

In my approach to cancer therapy, I have in mind the words of Theodore Roosevelt: "It is hard to fail, but it is worse never to have tried to succeed." Success and victory have many definitions. For me, victory consists of achieving the best quality of life possible under the circumstances for each patient.

Sometimes we are able to survive a current crisis because of the way we coped with a crisis in the past. We acquire resilience; we learn how tough we really are and develop confidence in our ability to endure. By turning to these inner resources and the resources offered by members of the medical team, a cancer patient has the best chance of maintaining a good quality of life while living with cancer. Attention to nutrition and to muscle strength can have marked physical and emotional benefits for a patient. Knowledgeable, sensitive nurses and physicians can assuage fear and offer reassurance as well as good medical care. Medical social workers can help with insurance problems, or arrange for home care or participation in a discussion group. Every patient should be aware of these services.

Thus help is available from people in many professions who understand your needs. These needs can also be met by other cancer patients who have formed support groups. Use them all. We are here to help each other. How you live with cancer is your choice.

All cancer patients must live with their disease. The decision on how to approach the problem is theirs. With the proper support from family, friends, and the medical team, and with their own inner resources of courage and hope, they can continue to live a meaningful life.

> *Choose life—only that and always, and at whatever*
> *risk. To let life leak out, to let it wear away by the*
> *mere passage of time, to withhold giving it and*
> *spreading it, is to choose nothing.*

SISTER HELEN KELLEY

I

A patient's bill of rights

The American Hospital Association presents a Patient's Bill of Rights* with the expectation that observance of these rights will contribute to more effective patient care and greater satisfaction for the patient, his physician, and the hospital organization. Further, the association presents these rights in the expectation that they will be supported by the hospital on behalf of its patients, as an integral part of the healing process. It is recognized that a personal relationship between the physician and the patient is essential for the provision of proper medical care. The traditional physician-patient relationship takes on a new dimension when care is rendered within an organizational structure. Legal precedent has established that the institution itself also has a responsibility to the patient. It is in recognition of these factors that these rights are affirmed.

1. The patient has the right to considerate and respectful care.
2. The patient has the right to obtain from his physician complete current information concerning his diagnosis, treatment, and prognosis in terms the patient can be reasonably expected to understand. When it is not medically advisable to give such information to the patient, the information should be made available to an appropriate person in his behalf. He has the right to know by name the physician responsible for coordinating his care.
3. The patient has the right to receive from his physician information necessary to give informed consent prior to the start of any procedure and/or treatment. Except in emergencies, such information for informed consent should include but not necessarily be limited to the specific procedure and/or treatment, the medically significant risks involved, and the probable duration of incapacitation. Where medically significant alternatives for care or treatment exist, or when the patient requests information concerning medical alternatives, the patient has the right to such information. The patient also has the right to know the name of the person responsible for the procedures and/or treatment.
4. The patient has the right to refuse treatment to the extent permitted by law, and to be informed of the medical consequences of his action.

*Approved by the House of Delegates of the American Hospital Association, February 6, 1973.

5. The patient has the right to every consideration of his privacy concerning his own medical care program. Case discussion, consultation, examination, and treatment are confidential and should be conducted discreetly. Those not directly involved in his care must have the permission of the patient to be present.

6. The patient has the right to expect that all communications and records pertaining to his care should be treated as confidential.

7. The patient has the right to expect that within its capacity a hospital must make reasonable response to the request of a patient for services. The hospital must provide evaluation, service, and/or referral as indicated by the urgency of the case. When medically permissible a patient may be transferred to another facility only after he has received complete information and explanation concerning the needs for and alternatives to such a transfer. The institution to which the patient is to be transferred must first have accepted the patient for transfer.

8. The patient has the right to obtain information as to any relationship of his hospital to other health care and educational institutions insofar as his care is concerned. The patient has the right to obtain information as to the existence of any professional relationships among individuals, by name, who are treating him.

9. The patient has the right to be advised if the hospital proposes to engage in or perform human experimentation affecting his care or treatment. The patient has the right to refuse to participate in such research projects.

10. The patient has the right to expect reasonable continuity of care. He has the right to know in advance what appointment times and physicians are available and where. The patient has the right to expect that the hospital will provide a mechanism whereby he is informed by his physician or a delegate of the physician of the patient's continuing health care requirements following discharge.

11. The patient has the right to examine and receive an explanation of his bill regardless of source of payment.

12. The patient has the right to know what hospital rules and regulations apply to his conduct as a patient.

No catalogue of rights can guarantee for the patient the kind of treatment he has a right to expect. A hospital has many functions to perform, including the prevention and treatment of disease, the education of both health professionals and patients, and the conduct of clinical research. All these activities must be conducted with an overriding concern for the patient, and, above all, the recognition of his dignity as a human being. Success in achieving this recognition assures success in the defense of the rights of the patient.

II

Informed consent form

Date: _____ Name of patient: _____

I, the undersigned, consent for Dr. _____
and/or associates or assistants of his choice to perform the following procedure upon me:

and/or to do any other procedure that (his) (their) judgment may dictate to
be advisable for my well-being.

The nature of the procedure has been explained to me and no warranty
or guarantee has been made as to the results.

With these conditions, I willingly volunteer to aid in the research study
but reserve the right to discontinue at any time and without the necessity of
giving a reason.

Patient's signature _____

Witness _____

III

The living will

DIRECTIVE TO MY PHYSICIAN

This directive is written while I am of sound mind and fully competent.

I insist that I have complete right of self-determination. That includes complete right of refusal of any medical or surgical treatment unless a court order affirms that my decision would bring undue or unexpected hardship on my family or society.

Therefore:

If I become incompetent, in consideration of my legal rights to refuse medical or surgical treatment regardless of the consequences to my health and life, I hereby direct and order my physician, or any physician in charge of my care, to cease and refrain from any medical or surgical treatment which would prolong my life if I am in a condition of:

1. Unconsciousness from which I cannot recover.
2. Unconsciousness over a period of 6 months.
3. Mental incompetency that is irreversible.

However, although mentally incompetent, I must be informed of the situation, and if I wish to be treated, I am to be treated in spite of my original request made while competent.

If there is any reasonable doubt of the diagnosis of my illness and prognosis, then consultation with available specialists is suggested but need not be considered mandatory.

This directive to my physician also applies to any hospital or sanitarium in which I may be at the time of my illness and relieves them of any and all responsibility in the action or lack of action of any physician acting according to my demands.

If any action is taken contrary to these expressed demands, I hereby request my next of kin or legal representative to consider—and if necessary, to take—legal action against those involved.

If any of my next of kin oppose this directive, their opposition is to be considered without legal grounds because I remove any right of my next of kin who oppose me in this directive to speak for me.

I hereby absolve my physician or any physician taking care of me from any legal liability pertaining to the fulfillment of my demands.

Date _____   Signed _____

Witness _____   Accepted _____

IV

Glossary

acute infection an infection of viral or bacterial origin that develops and progresses rapidly, as opposed to a chronic infection, which may have a prolonged course.

adjuvant programs the administration of chemotherapy to patients from whom all known cancer has been surgically removed. This may destroy small amounts of undetected cancer.

alkylating agents a family of chemotherapeutic drugs that combine with DNA (genetic substance) to prevent normal cell division.

amphetamines drugs that stimulate a patient's nervous system.

analgesic a drug used for reducing pain.

androgens male sex hormones.

anemia the condition of having less than the normal amount of hemoglobin or red cells in the blood.

angiogram the process of visualizing an x-ray image of the blood vessel through the introduction of a substance that renders the blood vessels radiopaque (capable of blocking x rays).

anticoagulants drugs that reduce the blood's ability to clot.

antimetabolites a family of chemotherapeutic drugs that interfere with the processes of DNA production, and thus prevent normal cell division.

antioxidant any substance that delays the process of oxidation.

arterial system a branching pattern of vessels by which blood is distributed from the heart to all tissues of the body.

arthritic disease a broad category of diseases that result in pain or decreased flexibility of joints.

asbestosis scarring of the lungs from prolonged inhalation of asbestos dust.

atrophy a reduction in size of an organ or cell that had previously reached a larger size.

atrophied withered or reduced in bulk.

bacteria one-celled primitive plant organisms widely encountered in nature, capable of causing disease in humans.

barbiturates a specific class of drugs capable of inducing relaxation, narcosis, sleep, or unconsciousness.

BCG (Bacillus Calmette-Guérin) a form of the tuberculosis bacterium, used primarily for TB vaccination, which can act as an excellent stimulant to the immune system.

benign not malignant.

biopsy the surgical removal of a small portion of tissue for diagnosis.

blood chemistry panels multiple chemical determinations prepared by an automated method from a single sample of blood.

blood clot a solid composed of blood components held together by interlacing strands of fibrin (the major protein of blood coagulation).

blood count a laboratory study to evaluate the amount of white cells, red cells, and platelets.

blood transfusion the introduction of whole blood (red cells and/or plasma) into the circulation to replace blood lost or to correct anemia.

bone marrow a soft substance found within bone cavities, ordinarily composed of fat and developing red cells, white cells, and platelets.

bone-marrow examination the process of removing bone marrow from the cavity by withdrawing it through a needle for pathological examination.

Burkitt's lymphoma a lymphoma originally described in Africa as readily cured by chemotherapy.

cancer the proliferation of malignant cells that have the capability for invasion of normal tissues.

carcinogen any cancer-producing substance or agent.

carcinoid a potentially malignant tumor arising in the wall of the gastrointestinal tract or bronchial tree, capable of secreting substances causing diarrhea, flushing, or rapid heartbeat.

cardiac of or pertaining to the heart.

cardiac arrest a situation in which the heart ceases to function.

catheter a hollow tube (rubber, plastic, glass, or metal) for introduction into a body cavity (e.g., the bladder) to drain fluid.

cell-cycle specific chemotherapeutic drugs that kill only cells that are in the process of division.

cervix the lower portion of the uterus, which protrudes into the vagina and forms a portion of the birth canal during delivery.

charged particles portions of an atom that are attracted to either the positive or the negative pole of an electric field.

chemotherapy the treatment of disease by chemicals (drugs) introduced into the bloodstream by injection or taken by mouth as tablets.

choriocarcinoma a carcinoma composed of cells arising from the placenta or, rarely, in the testes.

chromosomes material in a cell made of DNA which carries the genes.

chronic defining a disease process that develops over a long period of time and progresses slowly.

cobalt, cobalt treatment radiotherapy using gamma rays generated from the breakdown of radioactive cobalt-60.

cobalt-60 a radioactive isotope of the element cobalt used in radiation treatment.

codeine a narcotic analgesic drug prepared from the stems of the opium poppy, used for control of pain and treatment of cough and diarrhea.

colostomy formation of an artificial anus in the abdominal wall, so the colon can drain feces into a bag (see *ostomy*).

coma a condition of decreased mental function in which the individual is incapable of responding to any stimulus, including painful stimuli.

consultation the formal process of soliciting the opinion of a specialist.

coronary thrombosis blockage of the arteries serving the heart muscle, resulting in death of a portion of the heart.

cyanotic a blue appearance of the skin, lips, or fingernails as the result of low oxygen content of the circulating blood.

cyst a fluid-filled sac of tissue; a cyst may be malignant or benign.

Demerol a potent synthetic narcotic analgesic related to morphine.

diagnosis the process by which a disease is identified.

diagnostic procedures studies designed to yield information about the nature and extent of disease in a patient.

digestive tract the esophagus, stomach, and intestines and colon, including such other organs involved in digestion as the liver and the pancreas.

diuretics drugs that increase the elimination of water and salts (urine) from the body.

DNA abbreviation for deoxyribonucleic acid, the building block of the genes, responsible for the passing of hereditary characteristics from cell to cell.

dolophine a synthetic narcotic (methadone) analgesic related to morphine.

edema the accumulation of fluid within the tissues.

electrocardiogram a method of evaluating heart rhythm and muscle function by the measurement of the heart's electrical impulses.

electrons negatively charged particles making up the outer shell of atoms; electron beam is a form of radiotherapy used for treating the skin.

enzymes proteins that assist the occurrence of specific chemical reactions; the increase of certain enzymes in the blood may be a measure of certain diseases.

Epstein-Barr virus a virus that is known to cause infectious mononucleosis and has been associated with the Burkitt's lymphoma and certain cancers of the head and neck.

estrogens female sex hormones.

euthanasia (1) an easy or calm death (Greek: *eu* = well, *thanatos* = death); (2) the act of causing death painlessly, to end suffering. The second definition is the one generally used in medical contexts.

excision surgical removal of tissue.

exploratory surgery undertaken to investigate a situation that diagnostic tests have failed to clarify.

foci in cancer diagnosis, minute deposits of cancer cells that are undetectable by ordinary methods of examination.

four-drug chemotherapy program, multidrug chemotherapy the use of several chemotherapeutic agents at one time to improve the chance of response.

friable fragile, as in a tumor that easily disintegrates during attempted excision.

gamma rays a unit of radium or radiation dosage.

gene a portion of DNA capable of transmitting a single characteristic from parent to progeny.

genetics a branch of biology that deals with heredity and the study of the differences and disease risk between parents and children.

hemangiopericytoma a rapidly growing, highly malignant cancer arising from the walls of blood vessels.

hematologist a physician (internist) specializing in the study of blood diseases.

hematoma a blood lump in the skin following a local hemorrhage.

herpes an acute viral inflammation of the skin or mucous membranes characterized by the development of groups of vesicles or blisters.

history and physical examination the routine by which information is obtained from patients and their physical characteristics are assessed.

Hodgkin's disease a form of lymphoma that arises in a single lymph node and may spread to local, then distant lymph nodes and finally to other tissues commonly including the spleen, liver, and bone marrow.

hormonal anticancer therapy a form of therapy that takes advantage of the fact that certain cancers will stabilize or shrink if a certain hormone is added or removed.

hormones naturally occurring substances that are released by the endocrine organs and circulate in the blood, stimulating or turning off the growth or activity of specific target cells or organs.

hydration defines the status of the patient with regard to body water; a patient may be dehydrated, well hydrated, or excessively hydrated (edematous).

ice blanket a blanket cooled with ice water or a refrigerant on which a patient lies to reduce body temperature.

immune identifies the state of adequate defense against a particular infection or possibly against a certain cancer.

immunology the study of the body's natural defense mechanism and of the diseases that result from deficient or inappropriate defense responses.

immunotherapy a method of cancer therapy that stimulates the body defenses (the immune system) to attack cancer cells or modify a specific disease status.

infectious mononucleosis a viral infection involving the blood and organs.

inflammation the triggering of local body defenses resulting in the outpouring of defensive cells (leukocytes) from the circulation into the tissues, frequently with associated pain and swelling.

"informed consent" a legal standard defining how much a patient must know about the potential benefits and risks of therapy before being able to agree to undergo it knowledgeably with legal responsibility for the result.

infuse to introduce any liquid foreign substance into a vein or artery.

intern a physician in the first year of training following graduation from medical school.

internist a specialist in internal medicine, dealing with the nonsurgical treatment of diseases.

intestinal tract esophagus, stomach, small bowel, and colon.

intramuscular literally, within the muscle; usually refers to the injection of a drug into the muscle, whence it is absorbed into the circulation.

intravenous (IV) the administration of a drug or of fluid directly into the vein.

intravenous pyelogram the intravenous administration of a radiopaque dye that is concentrated and excreted by the kidneys, making the kidneys and drainage system visible with x rays.

irrigation washing with a stream of water or other fluid.

isotopic scan a class of diagnostic procedures for assessing organs (liver, bone, brain) in which particular radioactive substances are introduced intravenously; the relative concentrations of these substances are detected by their radioactivity, yielding information about cancerous involvement of specific structures.

jaundice the accumulation of bilirubin, a breakdown product of hemoglobin, resulting in yellowish discoloration of the skin and of the white portion of the eyes; this is indicative of liver disease or blockage of the major bile ducts.

keratosis a disease of the skin characterized by an overgrowth of the top layer of the skin.

Laetrile a cancer "cure" promoted by unethical practitioners and having no proved demonstrable value; otherwise known as amygdalin or vitamin B_{17}.

laparotomy any surgical procedure that involves entering the abdominal cavity.

laryngectomy the surgical removal of the larynx, or voice box.

leukemia a malignant proliferation of white blood-forming cells in the bone marrow; cancer of the blood cells. There are two types of acute leukemia: lymphocytic and myelogenous.

linear accelerator a machine used for certain cancers requiring special techniques of radiotherapy.

lob a natural division or segment of an organ.

localized with reference to cancer, this means confined to the site of origin without evidence of spread or metastasis.

lucid alert and aware of one's surroundings.

LVNs licensed vocational nurses; technical functions that they may legally perform are limited.

lymph nodes organized clusters of lymphocytes through which the tissue fluids drain upon returning to the blood circulation; they act as the first line of defense, filtering out and destroying infective organisms or cancer cells and initiating the generalized immune response.

lymphangiogram a diagnostic method by which radiopaque dye is introduced into the lymph channels that drain tissue fluids to the blood circulation; this dye is filtered by the lymph nodes, making them visible on x-ray film, and cancerous involvement of lymph nodes is evaluated by this test.

lymphocytes a family of white blood cells responsible for the production of antibodies and for the direct destruction of invading organisms or cancer cells.

lymphoma a group of malignant diseases of the lymph nodes or lymphatic tissues, which are divided into Hodgkin's disease and Non–Hodgkin's lymphoma (histiocytic, nodular and diffuse lymphomas, and Burkitt's lymphoma).

malignant having the potentiality of being lethal if not successfully treated. All cancers are malignant by definition.

mastectomy the surgical removal of the breast.

megadose a very large dose that exceeds many times the normal dose.

melanoma a cancer of the pigment cells of the skin, usually arising in a preexisting pigmented area (mole).

mesothelioma a primary tumor of the covering of the lungs or heart.

metabolism the process of transformation of foods or compounds into substances needed for body function or energy resources.

metastasized, metastatic the establishment of a second site or multiple sites of cancer remote from the primary or original site.

modality a general class or method of treatment. The basic modalities of cancer therapy include surgery, radiation, medical (chemotherapy or hormonal) therapy, and experimental immunotherapy.

multimodality therapy the use of more than one modality for cure or palliation of cancer.

mutation a change in DNA or a cell that alters the genetic potential of chromosomes and their offspring. It may be a response to a chemical substance and the daughter cells may be cancerous.

myelogram the introduction of radiopaque dye into the sac surrounding the spinal cord, a process that makes it possible to see tumor involvement of the spinal cord or nerve roots on x-ray film.

narcotics a legal term defining euphoric and analgesic substances whose use is closely regulated by the federal government; natural and synthetic relatives or morphine make up the major class of narcotics.

nasopharyngeal cancer a cancer of the nose or throat.

neurologic pertaining to the nervous system.

neutron an atomic particle; if increased in number in an element, will result in an isotope.

nitrates and nitrites compounds of the salt of nitric acid that are used to preserve food.

nodes see *lymph nodes.*

noncell-cycle specific chemotherapeutic drugs capable of destroying cells that are not in active division.

oncologist an internist who has subspecialized in cancer therapy and has expertise in both chemotherapy and the handling of problems arising during the course of the disease.

oophorectomy the surgical removal of an ovary.

opacity, opaque the property of being impervious to light or to x rays (radiopaque); the opposite of radiolucent.

osteosarcoma tumor of the bone.

ostomy a surgically created passage connecting an internal organ with the skin for purposes of excretion (see *colostomy*).

ovarian carcinoma cancer of the ovary.

ovary the female gonad, responsible for the production of ova (eggs) and of female sex hormones.

Pap smear Papanicoulaou smear, a screening diagnostic procedure for the rapid detection of precancerous and cancerous conditions of the cervix.

paramedical refers to skilled nonphysician personnel who participate in providing care.

Parkinson's disease a degenerative disease of the brain resulting in tremor and rigidity of the muscles.

pathologist a physician skilled in the examination of tissues and in the performance and interpretation of laboratory studies.

percodan a narcotic analgesic compound related to morphine.

perivascular about or surrounding blood vessels.

pi mesons subatomic particles of an element.

polyps nodular growths of tissue from the lining of nasal, gastrointestinal, urinary tract, or uterus, which can be benign or malignant.

prognosis an estimate of the outcome of a disease process based on the status of the patient and accumulated information about the disease and its treatment.

progression the advancement or worsening of a cancer with respect to size.

promyelocytic a stage of acute leukemia.

prophylactic treatment designed to prevent a disease or a complication that has not yet become evident.

prostate an organ located at the bladder neck in males. It produces some components of the semen.

prosthetic an artificial structure designed to replace or approximate a normal one.

protons positively charged particles, which with neutrons make up the atomic nucleus.

psychosomatic pertaining to the mind and body, an affliction with emotional disturbance reflected in physical or mental components.

pulmonary embolus a life-threatening condition in which a blood clot becomes dislodged from a vein and travels to a branch of an artery carrying blood to the lungs (pulmonary artery).

radiation, radiation therapy the use of radiation for control or cure of cancer.

radical an extensive operation to remove the site of cancer and adjacent structures and lymph nodes.

radioactive isotope an element that has undergone spontaneous or artificial decomposition and may emit radiation.

radiolucent transmitting x rays easily (e.g., the lungs are normally radiolucent).

radium a highly radioactive metallic element that can be used in radiation therapy for cancer.

radiosensitive describes a cancer that responds readily to small dosages of radiation; the opposite is radioresistant.

regression the diminution of cancerous involvement, usually as the result of therapy; it is manifested by decreased size of the tumor (tumors) or its clinical evidence in fewer locations.

relapse the reappearance of cancer following a period of remission or absence of evident active disease.

remission the temporary disappearance of evident active cancer, occurring either spontaneously or as the result of therapy.

resection the surgical removal of tissue.

resident a physician who is undergoing specialized hospital training after internship.

residual disease, residual tumor cancer left behind following the palliative removal of cancerous tissue.

resuscitation, resuscitative a procedure designed to restore and sustain normal function in an individual who has undergone failure of respiration or of heartbeat.

reverse isolation isolation to prevent visitors or hospital staff from carrying an infection into a patient's room; gowns, gloves, and masks are worn by those who enter.

sarcoma a cancer of the connective tissue. For example, osteogenic sarcoma (bone), rhabdomyosarcoma (muscle), ewingsarcoma, (long bones).

scans see *isotopic scan.*

sciatic nerve a large nerve originating within the buttock and coursing down the back of the thigh.

sedatives drugs used to induce drowsiness or sleep.

seizure an abnormal discharge by brain cells resulting in involuntary movement, unusual behavior, or periods of unconsciousness.

selenium an element resembling sulfur.

semicomatose in a partial coma or state of unconsciousness.

sepsis bacterial growth within the bloodstream.

spleen an organ adjacent to the stomach, composed mainly of lymphocytes.

staging an organized process of ascertaining the extent of spread of a cancer.

STP a nonapproved drug that stimulates the nervous system.

subcutaneous cyst a cyst located beneath the skin, usually benign (see *cyst*).

suppository a drug administered by insertion into the anus, where it is gradually absorbed into the bloodstream; vaginal suppositories are used to treat local conditions and are not absorbed.

symptom a manifestation or complaint of disease as described by the patient, as opposed to one found by the doctor's examination; the latter is referred to as a "sign."

systemic disease disease that involves virtually all parts of the body.

terminal a condition of decline toward death, from which not even a brief reversal can be anticipated.

testicular mass a firm swelling involving a testis, or testicle, the male gonad.

therapeutic procedure a procedure intended to offer palliation or cure of a condition or a disease.

thoracic of or pertaining to the thorax, the chest—the rib cage and all organs within it.

toxicity the property of producing unpleasant or dangerous side effects.

tumor a mass or swelling. In itself the word "tumor" carries no connotation of either benignity or malignancy.

ulcer an erosion of normal tissue resulting from corrosive chemicals (i.e., acids), infection, impaired circulation, or cancerous involvement.

vasectomy the surgical interruption of the spermatic cords, the tubes that carry sperm cells from the testicles to the penis; the operation results in sterilization.

vital structure an organ whose unimpaired functioning is essential for life.

Wilms' tumor a kidney cancer most commonly seen in children.

xeromammogram x-ray examination of the breasts by a new method that improves the detail representation of soft tissues and facilitates the diagnosis of minute areas of cancer.

V

National cancer organizations

REGIONAL TOLL-FREE NUMBERS
FOR CANCER INFORMATION SERVICE

Alaska	1-800-638-6070	Massachusetts	1-800-952-7420
California		Minnesota	1-800-582-5262
(from area codes 213,		Montana	1-800-525-0231
714, and 805)	1-800-252-9066	New Hampshire	1-800-225-7034
Colorado	1-800-332-1850	New Jersey	800-523-3586
Connecticut	1-800-922-0824	New Mexico	1-800-525-0231
Delaware	1-800-523-3586	New York City	(212) 794-7982
District of Columbia		New York State	1-800-462-7255
(includes suburban Maryland		North Carolina	1-800-672-0943
and northern Virginia)	(202) 636-5700	North Dakota	1-800-328-5188
Florida	1-800-432-5953	Ohio	800-282-6522
Georgia	1-800-327-7332	Pennsylvania	1-800-822-3963
Hawaii		South Dakota	1-800-328-5188
Oahu	524-1234	Texas	1-800-392-2040
Neighbor islands, ask		Vermont	1-800-225-7034
operator for	Enterprise 6702	Washington	1-800-552-7212
Illinois	800-972-0586	Wisconsin	1-800-362-8038
Kentucky	800-432-9321	Wyoming	1-800-525-0231
Maine	1-800-225-7034	All other areas	800-638-6694
Maryland	800-492-1444		

Organizations and programs offering services to the cancer patient and the family

Organization	General description
National organizations and affiliates American Cancer Society* 777 Third Ave. New York, N.Y. 10017	Voluntary organization offering programs of cancer research, education, and patient service and rehabilitation.
CanSurmount	Composed of patient, family member, trained volunteer (also a cancer patient), health professional. Volunteers visit hospitals and homes.
I Can Cope	Addresses the educational and psychological needs of people with cancer.
International Association of Laryngectomees	Voluntary umbrella organization of 225 local clubs (varying names) that promote and support total rehabilitation program. Volunteers visit hospitals.
Reach to Recovery (Breast Cancer)	Provides rehabilitation support for women who have had mastectomies. Volunteers visit hospitals.
Cancer Information Service†	Telephone information and referral service, supplemented by printed materials.
The Concern for Dying 250 W. 57th St. New York, N.Y. 10019	Nonprofit educational organization distributes the living will, a document that records patient wishes concerning treatment.
Leukemia Society of America 211 E. 43rd St. New York, N.Y. 10017	Offers financial assistance and consultation services for referrals to other means of local support to cancer patients with leukemia and allied disorders.
Make Today Count P.O. Box 303 Burlington, Iowa 52601	More than 200 chapters comprising patients and family members, with the general goal of living each day as fully and completely as possible.
The National Hospice Organization 301 Tower, Suite 506 301 Maple Ave. W. Vienna, Va. 22181	Membership organization consisting of groups providing or preparing to provide hospice care; institutions concerned with care of the terminally ill and their families.

*For information on the following programs, contact the American Cancer Society.
†See list of telephone numbers and areas served.

Psychological and emotional support; education	Medical, physical logistical support	Financial and employment assistance
Programs to support psychological and physical rehabilitation of patients. Patient education and information.	Equipment loans for care of homebound, blood programs, surgical dressings, medication. Transportation to and from treatment, e.g., volunteer drivers or taxi fare reimbursement.	Financial counseling Assistance with employment problems.
Patient and family education and information.	. . .	. . .
Educational program to provide information and psychological support.	. . .	. . .
Support and education programs for persons who have had laryngectomees.	. . .	Program to inform employees about reemployability of laryngectomees.
Information on rehabilitative exercises. Psychological support.	Demonstrate rehabilitative exercises. Provide temporary prosthesis.	. . .
Information on local and regional resources and programs.	Information on local and regional resources and programs.	Information on local and regional resources and programs.
Provides copies of living will and referral to local sources of same.	. . .	. . .
. . .	. . .	Financial assistance to outpatients for drugs, laboratory costs associated with blood transfusions, transportation, and radiation therapy.
Peer emotional support.	. . .	. . .
Literature, information, and referral to local and regional resources.	Literature, information, and referral to local and regional resources.	. . .

continued.

Organizations and programs offering services to the cancer patient and the family

Organization	General description
United Cancer Council, Inc. 1803 N. Meridian St. Indianapolis, Ind. 46202	Federation of voluntary cancer agencies that seek the control of cancer through a three-point program of service, education, and research. Agencies are funded by the United Way of Giving.
United Ostomy Association 1111 Wilshire Blvd. Los Angeles, Ca. 90017	Nonprofit organization with more than 500 chapters in United States and Canada. General goal is to provide ostomy patients with mutual aid, moral support, and education. Members visit hospitals.
Regional organizations and programs Cancer Call PAC (People Against Cancer) American Cancer Society 37 S. Wabash Ave. Chicago, Ill. 60603	Emotional support telephone service; volunteers are recovered cancer patients and family members.
Cancer Care, Inc., of the National Cancer Foundation* One Park Ave. New York, N.Y. 10016	Voluntary social service agency providing professional counseling and planning to patients with advanced cancer and their families.
TOUCH, Coordinator, Cancer Control Program University of Alabama in Birmingham 104 Old Hillman Bldg. Birmingham, Ala. 35294	General goal is to provide assistance to cancer patients and their families in forming realistic, positive attitudes toward cancer and its treatment.
Psychosocial Counseling Service UCLA-Jonsson Comprehensive Cancer Center 1100 Glendon Ave. Suite 844 Los Angeles, Ca. 90024	Telephone counseling service directed to psychosocial needs of patients and care givers.

*Direct services in tristate metropolitan areas of New York, New Jersey, and Connecticut.

Psychological and emotional support; education	Medical, physical logistical support	Financial and employment assistance
Health promotion and educacation programs and therapy groups.	Screening, nursing, homemaking, medication, prostheses.	. . .
Publish ostomy information. Peer support.	Encourage development of better equipment and supplies. Promote better management techniques.	Insurance programs for members include hospital income plan and major medical plan.
Trained volunteers provide emotional support, information, and appropriate referrals.	. . .	. . .
Programs of professional consultation and education. Public education.	Nursing care, homemaker, home-health aids, housekeepers.	Financial assistance offered.
Peer emotional support. Continuing education on treatment methods.	. . .	. . .
Trained mental health professionals directly counsel cancer patients, family members, and friends. Provide referrals to other sources of assistance.	. . .	. . .

VI

Bibliography

Ahmed, P., editor: Living and dying with cancer, Amsterdam, 1980, Elsevier/North-Holland.

Alsop, S.: Stay of execution, Philadelphia, 1973, Lippincott.

American Cancer Society: Cancer facts and figures, New York, 1980.

American Cancer Society: Unproven methods of cancer management, New York, 1971.

Ashenburg, N.J.: Employability and insurability of the cancer patient, paper presented to New York State Cancer Program ASSO, Inc., annual meeting, Nov. 8, 1975, Rochester, N.Y.

Barofsky, I.: Job discrimination of cancer patients: what we know and what we need to know, paper presented to the Virginia Division of the American Cancer Society, March 12, 1981.

Barofsky, I., Gielen, A. C., and Clovelle, P.: Returning to work: a measure of the efficacy of medical treatment, paper prepared for the Health Services Research and Development Center of Johns Hopkins Medical Institutions and Division of Health Education, the Johns Hopkins School of Hygiene and Public Health, Baltimore, Md.

Breast cancer digest, National Institutes of Health, 1979, Department of HEW Publ. No. 80-1691.

Brody, J. E.: You can fight cancer and win, New York, 1977, Quadrangle/The New York Times Book Co.

Brody, J. E.: (Diet Book, 1981)

Cabrins, J.: The cancer problem, Sci. Am. **233**:64-77, 1975.

DeVita, V. T., and Kershner, L. M.: Cancer, the curable disease, Am. Pharm., April 1980.

DeVita, V. Jr., Hellman, S., and Rosenberg, S. A.: Cancer principles and practice of oncology, Philadelphia, 1981, Lippincott.

Epstein, S. S.: The politics of cancer, San Francisco, 1970, Sierra Club Books.

Everson, T. C., and Cole, W. H.: Spontaneous regression of cancer, Philadelphia, 1966, Saunders.

Feifel, H., editor: The meaning of death, New York, 1959, McGraw-Hill.

Feldman, F.: Work and cancer health histories (series): White collar workers (1976); Blue collar workers (1978); Young workers (1981); Studies of the experience of recovered patients, California Division, American Cancer Society.

Guidelines for the cancer-related checkup, Ca—A Cancer Journal for Clinicians, July/August 1980.

Hammond, E., Cuyler, et al.: Smoking and cancer in the U.S., Prev. Med. **9**:169-173, 1980.

Hammond, E., Cuyler, and the American Cancer Society: Cancer prevention study, New York, 1979, American Cancer Society.

Hoover, R.: Saccharin—bitter aftertaste? N. Engl. J. Med. **302**:573-575, 1980.

Israel, L.: Conquering cancer, New York, 1978, Random House.

Kushner, R.: Why me? New York, 1977, New American Library, Signet Press.

Leib, S., and Remeker, M.: Understanding cancer, Palo Alto, Ca., 1979, Bull Publishing Co.

Levitt, P., Guralnick, E., Kagan, R., and Gilbert, H.: The cancer reference book, New York and London, 1979, Paddington Press, Ltd.

MacMahon, B., et al.: Coffee and cancer of the pancreas, N. Engl. J. Med., March 1981.

McWaters, D., Thompson, M., and Remaker, M.: Preventing cancer, Palo Alto, Ca., 1981, Bull Publishing Co.

Moira, M., and Potts, E.: Choices—realistic alternatives in cancer treatment, New York, 1980, Avon Books.

Mullen, B. D.: The ostomy book: living comfortably with colostomies, ileostomies, and urostomies, Palo Alto, Ca., Bull Publishing Co.

National Cancer Institute: The breast cancer digest, Washington, D.C., April 1979.

National Cancer Institute: Coping with cancer, Washington, D.C., 1980.

Northern California Cancer

NCCP Diet Book

Office on Smoking and Health, U.S. Public Health Service: Smoking and health: a report of the Surgeon General, Washington, D.C., 1971.

Opinion Research Corporation: Policies and practices of insurance carriers affecting applicants for group insurance, prepared under contract J938-0214 for the U.S. Department of Labor, Princeton, N.J.

Raffmen, R.: Using marijuana in the reduction of nausea associated with chemotherapy, Seattle, Wa., Murray Publishing Co.

Reif, A.: The causes of cancer, Am. Sci. **69**:437–447, 1981.

Richards, V.: Cancer: the wayward cell, Berkeley, Ca., 1978, University of California Press.

Rosenbaum, E., and Rosenbaum, I.: A comprehensive guide for cancer patients and their families, Palo Alto, Ca., 1980, Bull Publishing Co.

Rosenbaum, E., and Rosenbaum, I.: Decision for life, Palo Alto, Ca., 1980, Bull Publishing Co.

Rosenbaum, E., and Rosenbaum, I.: Nutrition for the cancer patient, Palo Alto, Ca., 1980, Bull Publishing Co.

Rosenbaum, E., and Rosenbaum, I.: Sexuality and cancer, Palo Alto, Ca., 1980, Bull Publishing Co.

Rosenbaum, E., and Rosenbaum, I.: Rehabilitation exercises for cancer patients, Palo Alto, Ca., 1980, Bull Publishing Co.

Ryan, C., and Ryan, K. M.: A private battle, New York, 1979, Simon & Schuster.

Shimkin, M. B.: Contrary to nature, Washington, D.C., 1979, U.S. Department of Health, Education and Welfare.

Shimkin, M. B.: Science and cancer, Washington, D.C., 1980, U.S. Department of Health and Human Services.

Spletter, M.: A woman's choice: new options in breast cancer, Boston, 1982, Beacon Press.

Stoddard, S.: The hospice movement, New York, 1978, Stein and Day.

U.S. Food and Drug Administration, FDA Office of Public Affairs, Rockville, Md. 20857 (HHS Publ. No. 80-4022).

U.S. Department of Health and Human Services, Public Health Service, National Institutes of Health (three publications): Taking time; Chemotherapy and you; Radiation therapy and you.

Wynder, E. L.: Dietary habits and cancer epidemiology, Cancer **43**:1955–1961, 1979.

Zilbergeld, B., and Ullman, J.: Male sexuality, Boston, 1978, Little, Brown.